AF689473

Multiple Risk Factors in Cardiovascular Disease

Multiple Risk Factors in Cardiovascular Disease

Edited by
Akira Yamamoto
Vice Director of the Research Institute
National Cardiovascular Center
Osaka, Japan

Churchill Livingstone
Tokyo Osaka Edinburgh London
Madrid Melbourne Milan New York

CHURCHILL LIVINGSTONE
Medical Division of Longman Group UK Ltd

© Churchill Livingstone Japan K.K. 1994
All rights reserved, including that of translation into other languages. No part of this publication may be reproduced, stored in a retrieval system, or transmitted in any form or by any means, electronic or mechanical, including photocopying, recording, or otherwise, without either the prior written permission of the Publisher (Churchill Livingstone Japan) or by a license permitting restricted copying.

First edition 1994
ISBN 4-89370-088-X C 3047

Published by CHURCHILL LIVINGSTONE JAPAN K.K.
Head Office: K.I.T. Bldg., 2-8-16 Yutenji, Meguro-ku, Tokyo 153, Japan
Osaka Office: 7F, Manabe-Doshomachi Bldg., 1-4-6 Doshomachi, Chuo-ku, Osaka 541, Japan

Distributed in Japan by Churchill Livingstone Japan K. K., K.I.T. Bldg., 2-8-16 Yutenji, Meguro-ku, Tokyo 113; in the United States of America by Churchill Livingstone Fulfillment Center, 5S 250 Frontenac Road, Naperville, IL 60563-1711; and in the United Kingdom and the rest of the world by Churchill Livingstone, Robert Stevenson House, 1-3 Baxter's Place, Leith Walk, Edinburgh EH1 3AF, UK, and associated companies, branches, and representatives throughout the world

The publication of this book is supported by the educational grants from Sankyo Co., Kissei Pharmaceutical Co., Banyu Pharmaceutical Co., Pfizer Pharmaceutical Inc., Marion Merrell Dow K.K., Daiichi Pharmaceutical Co., and Ohtsuka Pharmaceutical Co.

Printed in Japan

PREFACE

The First International Symposium on Multiple Risk Factors in Cardiovascular Disease was held in Washington, DC, in 1990. We felt greatly honored that Osaka had been selected for the second meeting in 1992.

Atherosclerotic diseases, which occupy the major part of cardiovascular diseases, are based on the combination of many risk factors, such as hyperlipidemia, glucose intolerance, hypertension, and smoking. It is important in the practical point of view in prevention and treatment of atherosclerosis to understand the nature and weight of such risk factors in individual cases and make a proper manage in nutrition, diathesis, and underlying diseases. The symposium achieved in providing newest informations of the recent research development and the strategy for the intervention of the risk factors. The organizing committee is particularly indebted to all the participants of the meeting for their contribution in delivering informations of high quality.

At first we could not decide a plan to publish the proceeding of the symposium. After the meeting, opinion arose to leave a commemorative material and we decided to publish a monograph composed of representative papers from each session of the meeting. We asked the authors to include the most up-to-date knowledge in each field in addition to the contents that were presented in the meeting at Osaka. We hope this will help everyone to get an idea of the scope of the Multiple Risk Factors Symposium and access to the future meetings.

March 31, 1994.

Akira Yamamoto
Chairman of the Local Organizing
Committee of the Second International
Symposium on Multiple Risk Factors
in Cardiovascular Disease

The Second International Symposium on Multiple Risk Factors in Cardiovascular Disease

Chairmen:
A. M. Gotto, Jr. (*Houston, TX, USA*)
R. Paoletti (*Milan, Italy*)
Y. Goto (*Isehara, Japan*)
T. Omae (*Suita, Japan*)

Chairman of the Local Organizing Committee:
A. Yamamoto (*Suita, Japan*)

Advisory Committee:
C. Kawai (*Kyoto, Japan*)
H. Manabe (*Osaka, Japan*)
C. Naito (*Tokyo, Japan*)
T. Shimao (*Tokyo, Japan*)
S. Tarui (*Osaka, Japan*)
K. Tanaka (*Fukuoka, Japan*)

Local Scientific Program Committee:
Chairman: A. Yamamoto (*Suita, Japan*)
Y. Akanuma (*Tokyo, Japan*)
K. Arakawa (*Fukuoka, Japan*)
M. Asano (*Tokyo, Japan*)
T. Kita (*Kyoto, Japan*)
M. Kuramochi (*Numazu, Japan*)
Y. Matsuzawa (*Osaka, Japan*)
T. Matsuda (*Kanazawa, Japan*)
H. Nakamura (*Tokorozawa, Japan*)
Y. Saito (*Chiba, Japan*)
A. Sumiyoshi (*Miyazaki, Japan*)
H. Toshima (*Kurume, Japan*)
H. Yamaguchi (*Tokyo, Japan*)
T. Yasugi (*Tokyo, Japan*)
M. Yokoyama (*Kobe, Japan*)

International Advisory Board:
G. Assmann (*Münster, Germany*)
V. W. Brown (*Washington, D.C., USA*)
A. V. Chobanian (*Boston, MA, USA*)
J. Davignon (*Montreal, Canada*)
J. L. De Gennes (*Paris, France*)
De Witt S. Goodman (*New York, NY, USA*)†
C. Lenfant (*Bethesda, MD, USA*)
B. Lewis (*London, UK*)
A. N. Orekov (*Moscow, Russia*)
G. M. Reaven (*Stanford, CA, USA*)
Y. Stein (*Jerusalem, Israel*)
A. Zanchetti, (*Milan, Italy*)
K. T. Lee (*Pusan, Korea*)†
M.-P. She (*Beijing, China*)
J. Chen (*Taipei, Taiwan*)

† deceased

In Appreciation:
The organizing committee is grateful to all the contributors who so generously support the organization.

Sankyo Co.
Kissei Pharmaceutical Co.
Banyu Pharmaceutical Co.
Pfizer Pharmaceutical Inc.
Marion Merrell Dow K.K.
Daiichi Pharmaceutical Co.
Ohtsuka Pharmaceutical Co.

Parke-Davis Warner Lambert
Eisai Co.
Sandoz Pharmaceuticals
Zeneca
Bayer AG
Kanegafuchi Chemical Industry Co.
To-so Manufacturing Co.
Daiichi Pure Chemicals Co.
Daikin
Terumo Corporation
Cosmo Bio
Suntory, Ltd.
Ono Pharmaceutical Co.
Sumitomo Pharmaceutical Co.
Osaka Pharmaceutical Manufacturers Association
The Pharmaceutical Manufacturers Association of Tokyo
The Life Insurance Association of Japan
Keidanren
National Rice Association of Japan
International Olive Oil Council
The Commemorative Association for the Japan World Exposition

CONTENTS

SECTION 1.
EPIDEMIOLOGY

Multiple Risk Factors in Cardiovascular Disease, ed. by A. Yamamoto, Churchill Livingstone Japan, Tokyo, pp. 3–6 (1994)

EPIDEMIOLOGY OF CARDIOVASCULAR RISK FACTORS IN ITALY

Salvatore PANICO,*1 Rocco GALASSO,*1 Eduardo FARINARO,*2 Antonio ASTI,*1 Paola RESCIGNO,*1 Camilla AMBROSCA,*1 and Egidio CELENTANO*1

*1 *Institute of Internal Medicine and Metabolic Disease, and*
*2 *Hygiene and Preventive Medicine — Community Medicine,*
Faculty of Medicine, University "Federico II" Naples

Key words: cardiovascular disease, risk factors, epidemiology, Italy, trend

Some specific cultural and geographic characteristics of the Italian population are always of interest as far as the epidemiology of cardiovascular disease (CVD) is concerned.

Most of the interest in the country from a cardiovascular epidemiology point of view is due to its participation in the Seven Countries Study (Keys 1980). Since then, Italy has always been included in the area of "Mediterranean advantage" for CVD, and specifically for coronary heart disease (CHD) risk.

The interest in the Italian population from an epidemiological viewpoint is also due to the fact that in going from Northern to Southern Italy two concurrent trends are apparent:

1. The passage from a Continental way of eating, much closer to Central European habits, to a more Mediterranean style. This gives a unique opportunity to observe a relatively homogeneous population — from an ethnic and cultural point of view — with a varied intake of food and other nutrients.
2. The different frequency of CVD, that is higher in the North than in the South.

CVD is the most frequent cause of death in Italy: 38% of deaths in men and 49% in women are due to this disease, with CHD and stroke as the major contributors. CVD also represents the main cause of morbidity and premature disability in the country. Moreover, the increase in life expectancy over the last 15 years has changed the demographic structure of the population, especially the female component, reinforcing the priority of CVD prevention and compression of morbidity at community level.

However, Italy has one of the lowest rates of all the economically developed countries, generally attributable to the healthy dietary habits — low consumption of animal fat and high consumption of vegetables and fruit — especially for those Italians living in the Mediterranean part of the country (Keys 1980; Farchi et *al* 1989; Trevisan *et al* 1990a, b).

MAJOR RISK FACTORS IN THE ITALIAN POPULATION

The epidemiological studies carried out in Italy in the last few decades have confirmed that the classical major risk factors also play

*1 via S. Pansini 5, 80131 Naples, Italy.

an etiological role in the Italian population (Menotti *et al* 1983, 1985; Spagnolo *et al* 1989). The strict relationship between the risk and these factors, detectable in population studies all over the world, has also confirmed by these studies.

In addition, a recent analysis performed within the framework of the RIFLE Project (the Italian Pooling Project, collecting data from 52 cohorts, most of which were randomly selected from the adult population in different parts of the country) has indicated the importance of major established risk factors (serum cholesterol, blood pressure, and smoking) in determining cardiovascular events (Menotti *et al* 1993).

Data on the distribution of cardiovascular risk factors are available in three successive "generations" of epidemiological studies carried out in Italy over three time-periods (1978–79, 1983–1984, 1985–1986). Most of these investigations were conducted on random samples of the Italian population aged 20–59 years, with a uniform geographical representation, in both sexes. Highly standardized procedures were adopted for biological measurements, and a questionnaire on dietary habits was administered in some of them. They have been recently reviewed in order to investigate any changes in risk factors over the last 15 years in Italy (Menotti *et al* 1992; Panico 1993). The most interesting papers are the ones examining the relationship between dietary habits and cardiovascular risk.

Italians who habitually consume high quantities of food rich in animal fats have higher plasma cholesterol, triglycerides, glucose and raised systolic and diastolic blood pressure compared with those consuming less animal fat (Trevisan *et al* 1990a). In addition, there is a linear trend in the association between the intake of atherogenic food items, indicated by means of a dietary atherogenic index score, and both the plasma cholesterol and blood pressure in the two sexes. The analysis was made by examining tertiles of the distribution of the index and the mean level of plasma cholesterol and systolic blood pressure in the three tertiles were calculated after adjusting for age, body mass index, and the amount of fat in the diet.

The use of monounsaturated fats (due to the consumption of olive oil) has been shown to contribute to the lower levels of plasma cholesterol and blood pressure (Trevisan *et al* 1990b). The INTERSALT Study has also included in its world-wide analyses data coming from 4 Italian centers, in different parts of the country and involving about 800 individuals aged 20–59 years of both sexes (Farinaro *et al 1991*). According to the specific analyses of the Italian centers it was confirmed that salt intake, alcohol consumption and obesity also influence blood pressure in the Italian population. The specific contributions of the level of sodium excretion (as a group indicator of salt intake), and alcohol consumption to the systolic blood pressure were available separately and free from the specific effects of potassium excretion, body mass index, and age. No sex difference was found, therefore the findings are applicable to both men and women. The data on the relationship between alcohol consumption and blood pressure, coming from another population-based investigation, could also be used as a cross check, confirming a progressive increase in blood pressure and a progressive increase in alcohol intake starting from about the level of moderate consumption — 40 g/day for women, 60 g/day for men (Trevisan *et al* 1987).

Information relating dietary habits to the incidence of CVD and mortality in Italian population groups is available from the Italian component of the Seven Countries Study (Farchi *et al* 1989). In this study none of the analyses carried out was able to identify the specific influence of single nutrients, since the individuals were classified according to an overall pattern of nutrients. According to this original analysis, the individuals at high risk of CHD were found in the group characterized by the highest alcohol and lowest carbohydrate intake. It should be recalled that the data pool from all the countries participating in the study had confirmed that dietary fats were determinants of CHD.

Data from an original Italian nutritional investigation are also available. In a group of families living in Southern Italy — where the Mediterranean diet is the norm — an experiment was carried out to study the influence of dietary changes on plasma cholesterol and blood pressure (Ferro-Luzzi *et al* 1987). Changing the diet for six weeks, by increasing the intake of animal fat and reducing the polyunsaturated/saturated (P/S) fat ratio, the plasma cholesterol and blood pressure increased significantly, but returned to their original levels after resuming the normal diet. The opposite was observed in a specular experiment in Finnish families: decreasing the animal fat consumption and increasing the P/S ratio lead to reduction in plasma cholesterol and blood pressure (Enholm *et al* 1982).

TRENDS IN CARDIOVASCULAR RISK FACTORS IN ITALY

The mortality rates for CHD in the three regions (North, Center, and South), passing from the Continental to the Mediterranean part, decrease steadily for both sexes. This change is apparent for stroke in men but not in women. The differences in the three regions, however, had become less marked at the end of 90s.

As in many other developed countries, the mortality trends over the last 15–20 years in Italy showed a decline in CVD.

This decline is quite clear (about 50%) with some small differences in the three different geographical regions of the country (North, Center, and South).

Most of the decline in CVD mortality rates reported involves males and stroke. Less evident, but still detectable (especially in men), is the decline in myocardial infarction, which seems to be more rapid in Northern Italy.

The reasons for this decline in Italy and the differences among the three regions are not easy to explain, not only because of the known intrinsic problems involving the comparison of vital statistics with analytical data, but also because over the last 15–20 years, unlike other economically developed countries, the socio-economic growth has been quite rapid. Perhaps some environmental and lifestyle factors are involved and need to be disentangled. However, as pointed out earlier, a recent attempt has been made to explain the CVD mortality trends in Italy. Again this relies on the data from the three generations of studies mentioned above.

When comparing the late 70s with the late 80s, systolic blood pressure declined significantly by 6.5% in women and 3.3% in men, the diastolic blood pressure declined significantly by 3.6% in women and 2.5% in men, and the body mass index fell significantly by 0.6% in women and 0.4% in men, whereas no significant changes were detected in the serum cholesterol in both sexes. A significant increase in the percentage of smokers and the number of cigarette smoked has been found in women while there has been a significant decrease in men.

The interpretation of these data is not simple. The attributable risk may be greater for factors changing favorably (e.g. blood pressure) than for factors changing inconsistently between sexes and among regions (e.g. smoking and plasma cholesterol).

The favorable change in blood pressure may well be due to both a decrease in the prevalence (higher in women than in men) and an increase the number of treated hypertensives (again higher in women than in men).

Looking at several pieces of data coming from the three different regions of the country, the decrease in smoking in men is higher in the North, where a favorable change in serum cholesterol is also reported, counterbalanced by an unfavorable change in the South. This may be due to what has been called the "loss of the Mediterranean advantage," due to very recent changes in dietary habits in most Southern areas of the country. Actually, in the North the decline for all

CVD, stroke and CHD has been more marked.

Nevertheless, other lifestyle changes and/or biological variables may well be responsible for the change in CVD mortality trends.

As in many other economically developed countries, the explanation of the decline deserved for women is complex, and confused by the fact that it started earlier than in men. Insufficient information is available for speculation.

SUMMARY

CVD is the major cause of death, morbidity and disability in Italy. Classical major risk factors (diet, plasma cholesterol, blood pressure, cigarette smoking) have been found to play the major etiological role in the Italian population just as they have in other developed countries.

As far as dietary factors are concerned, fats have been found to be associated with the major risk factors (plasma cholesterol and blood pressure) and the incidence and mortality from CVD. Mono-unsaturated fats derived from the heavy consumption of olive oil appear to have a favorable effect on cardiovascular risk.

Trends in CVD mortality are in line with those observed in other developed countries with a decline essentially attributable to a reduction in stroke. These changes in mortality rates may be mainly attributable to changes in major risk factors in all the regions of the countries investigated.

REFERENCES

Enholm C, Huttunen JK, Pietinen P 1982 Effect of diet on serum lipoprotein in a population with a high risk of coronary heart disease. N Engl J Med 307: 850–854

Farchi G, Mariotti S, Menotti A, Seccareccia F, Torsello S, Fidanza F 1989 Diet and 20-y mortality in two rural population groups of middle-aged men in Italy. Am J Clin Nutr 50: 1095–1099

Farinaro E, Trevisan M, Jossa F *et al* 1991 INTERSALT in Italy: Findings and community health implications. J Hum Hypertens 5: 15–19

Ferro-Luzzi A, Strazzullo P, Scaccini C *et al* 1987 Changing the Mediterranean diet: Effect on blood lipids. Am J Clin Nutr 40: 1027–1032

Keys A 1980 Seven countries study: A multivariate analysis of death and coronary heart disease in 10 Years. Harvard University Press, Cambridge, MA, USA

Menotti A 1993 The RIFLE Project: Preliminary results. Paper presented at the 3rd International Conference on Preventive Cardiology, June, Oslo

Menotti A, Farchi G, Seccareccia F, Capocaccia R, Conti S 1983 La predizione a breve termine degli eventi coronarici nel Progetto Romano di Prevenzione della Cardiopatia Coronarica. Clin Ter Cardiov 2: 193–199

Menotti A, Conti S, Dima F *et al* 1985 Incidence of coronary heart disease in two generations of men exposed to different levels of risk factors. Acta Cardiol 40: 307–312

Menotti A, Scanga M, Responsible Investigators of the RF2, OB43, MICOL Research Group 1992 Recent trends in selected coronary risk factors in Italy. Int J Epidemiol 21: 883–892

Panico S 1993 Cardiovascular risk factors in Italian women in the last 15 years. Paper presented at the 3rd International Conference on Preventive Cardiology, June, Oslo

Spagnolo A, Menotti A, Giampaoli S *et al* 1989 High density lipoprotein cholesterol distribution and its predictive power in some Italian population studies. Eur J Epidemiol 5: 328–335

Trevisan M, Krogh V, Farinaro E, Panico S, Mancini M 1987 Alcohol consumption, drinking pattern and blood pressure: Analysis of data from the Italian National Research Council Study. Int J Epidemiol 16: 520–527

Trevisan M, Krogh V, Freudenheim J *et al* 1990a Diet and coronary heart disease risk factor in population with varied intake. Prev Med 19: 231–236

Trevisan M, Krogh V, Freudenheim J *et al* 1990b Consumption of olive oil, butter and vegetable oils and coronary heart disease risk factors. JAMA 263: 688–693

Multiple Risk Factors in Cardiovascular Disease, ed. by A. Yamamoto, Churchill Livingstone Japan, Tokyo, pp. 7–10 (1994)

CARDIOVASCULAR RISK FACTORS IN ELDERLY MEN: THE HONOLULU HEART PROGRAM

Katsuhiko YANO, J. David CURB, Charles J. MACLEAN, Ellen B. MARCUS, Abraham KAGAN, and Po-Huang CHYOU

*Honolulu Heart Program, Kuakini Medical Center**

Key words: Asian-Americans, coronary heart disease, cerebrovascular disease, prospective study, risk factor

The importance of major risk factors for cardiovascular disease such as hypertension, elevated serum cholesterol and cigarette smoking has been well established in the young and middle-aged. The predictive value of these risk factors is less clear and controversial in the elderly.

Kannel and Gordon (1980) reported on the basis of the 20-year follow-up data from the Framingham Study that the impact of serum cholesterol and cigarette smoking diminished with advancing age and ceased to be significant after age 65. However, more recent reports from the Framingham Study (Harris *et al* 1988) and other studies (Barret-Connor *et al* 1984; Benfante & Reed 1990; Benfante *et al* 1991) have shown that hypertension, elevated serum cholesterol and cigarette smoking continue to be significant risk factors for coronary heart disease (CHD) among the elderly.

This report presents data describing the effects of cardiovascular risk factors on the incidence of CHD and stroke as well as on total mortality in elderly Japanese men living in Hawaii compared with middle-aged men who were free of CHD and stroke at entry and were followed for an average of 15 years.

STUDY POPULATION AND OUTCOMES

The Honolulu Heart Program (HHP) is a prospective epidemiological study of CHD and stroke among men of Japanese ancestry who were born between 1900 and 1919 and were living on Oahu Island in 1965. Approximately 8,000 eligible men, aged 45–68, participated in the initial examination during 1965–1968. Repeat examinations were carried out two and six years later with response rates of 95% and 90%, respectively. Also, the entire cohort has been followed from the beginning of the study to identify new cases of CHD and stroke as well as all deaths by continuous monitoring of hospital discharges, death certificates, medical examiner's cases and obituary notices in local newspapers. Approximately 1.5% of the cohort were lost to follow-up during the study period.

In this present report, 6,107 men who completed the third examination (1971–

* 347 North Kuakini Street, Honolulu, HI 96817, USA.
This study was supported by the National Heart, Lung, and Blood Institute Contract No. NO1-HC-02901.

1974) and were free of CHD and stroke formed the study population. They were divided into two groups: 3,369 men aged 50–59 (mean age 56) and 2,738 men aged 60–74 (mean age 65). The former was called the middle-aged group and the latter the elderly group.

During the subsequent follow-up period to the end of 1988 (average 15 years), we identified the following numbers of new events: 268 definite CHD (non-fatal myocardial infarction and CHD death), 83 thromboembolic (TE) stroke, 39 hemorrhagic (HEM) stroke, and 509 deaths from all causes in the middle-aged group; and 277 definite CHD, 152 TE stroke, 42 HEM stroke, and 882 deaths in the elderly group.

ASSOCIATION OF RISK FACTORS WITH OUTCOMES

The associations of known cardiovascular risk factors with the four outcomes were evaluated using the Cox regression model (Cox 1972). The risk factors were measured at the third examination and included resting heart rate (per minute), systolic and diastolic blood pressures (mmHg), hypertension with blood pressure ≥ 160/95 or on antihypertensive medication (0,1), serum cholesterol (mg/dl), body mass index (kg/m^2), history of diabetes(0,1), current cigarette smoking (0,1), and current alcohol intake (0,1).

First, the association of each risk factor with each outcome was evaluated using bivariate Cox regression, with age as the covariate, in the two age groups separately. Then, the significance of the difference in regression coefficients between the two age groups was tested using a two-sided t test. In this analysis, almost all risk factors were significantly associated with each outcome, and there was no significant difference in the regression coefficients between the two age groups, except for blood pressure or hypertension which showed significantly weaker associations with HEM stroke in the elderly group than in the middle-aged group although the associations remained significant in both age groups.

In the next step of the analysis, the independent contributions of these risk factors to the prediction of each outcome were evaluated using multivariate Cox regression where age and all risk factors were simultaneously included in the model. Systolic and diastolic blood pressures were excluded because of their high correlations with each other, as well as with hypertension.

TABLE I. Summary of Multivariate Cox Regression Analyses on Four Outcomes in the Two Age Groups

Risk factor	Men aged 50–59				Men aged 60–74			
	Definite CHD	TE stroke	HEM stroke	Total mortality	Definite CHD	TE stroke	HEM stroke	Total mortality
Age (years)	NS	*	NS	*	**	***	NS	***
Hypertension (0,1)	***	***	**	***	***	**	NS	***
Heart rate (per min)	NS	NS	NS	NS	NS	NS	NS	***
Serum cholesterol (mg/dl)	***	NS	(**)	(*)	***	**	(*)	NS
Body mas index (kg/m^2)	***	NS	NS	NS	NS	*	(*)	(*)
Diabetes (0,1)	***	***	NS	*	***	**	NS	**
Cigarette smoking (0,1)	**	***	*	***	***	***	**	***
Alcohol intake (0,1)	(**)	NS	NS	NS	(*)	NS	NS	NS

CHD, coronary heart disease; TE, thromboembolic; HEM, hemorrhagic.
Level of significance for the association with outcome: NS $p > 0.05$; * $p \le 0.05$; ** $p \le 0.01$; *** $p \le 0.001$.
( ) indicates negative regression coefficients (inverse relationship).

As shown in Table I, which summarizes the results of the multivariate Cox regression, hypertension was strongly associated with all outcomes in both age groups, except that the association with HEM stroke in elderly men was of borderline significance (p = 0.07). Likewise, cigarette smoking was strongly associated with all outcomes in both age groups, although the association with HEM stroke in middle-aged men was only weakly significant. Diabetes was strongly associated with all outcomes except for HEM stroke in both age groups. Serum cholesterol was a strong risk factor for CHD, but was inversely related to HEM stroke in both age groups. Alcohol intake was inversely related to CHD in both age groups, but no significant association was shown with all other outcomes. Body mass index showed irregular relationships to each outcome in the two age groups. Resting heart rate was significantly associated only with total mortality in elderly men.

Thus, hypertension and cigarette smoking were the most potent and universal risk factors in both age groups, and the general patterns of the relationship between individual risk factors and the four outcomes appeared to be similar in the two age groups.

EFFECTS OF MULTIPLE RISK FACTORS UPON OUTCOMES

The effects of coexisting multiple risk factors upon the four outcomes were assessed in the two age groups separately by estimating the age-adjusted relative risks and 95% confidence intervals for men with one, two, three, and four or more risk factors, using the risk for men with no risk factors as a reference group. The significance of trends in the relative risks were tested using a Cox regression model with age and the number of risk factors as independent variables in the two age groups separately. Differences in the trend of the relative risks of each outcome between the two age groups were examined statistically using a large-sample Z test for equal slopes (Kleinbaum & Kupper 1978).

As shown in Table II, the relative risks increased progressively with an increase in the number of coexisting risk factors for all outcomes in both age groups and these trends were highly significant except for HEM stroke in the older group. The increasing trend of relative risks was significantly greater in middle-aged men compared with elderly men only for HEM stroke.

TABLE II. Age-adjusted Relative Risks[a] and 95% Confidence Intervals (in parentheses) of Study Outcomes by Number of Coexisting Risk Factors in the Two Age Groups

Number of risk factors	Man aged 50–59				Men aged 60–74			
	Definite CHD	TE stroke	HEM stroke	Total mortality	Definite CHD	TE stroke	HEM stroke	Total mortality
1	1.3 (0.8–2.1)	6.9 (0.5–90.4)	0.8 (0.2–4.2)	1.6 (1.0–2.5)	1.8 (1.0–3.0)	1.2 (0.6–2.5)	2.1 (0.5–9.2)	1.3 (1.0–1.8)
2	2.2 (1.4–3.6)	17.0 (2.3–124.4)	0.6 (0.2–1.9)	2.1 (1.3–3.3)	3.1 (1.8–5.2)	2.7 (1.4–5.1)	1.8 (0.4–8.3)	1.7 (1.3–2.2)
3	3.3 (2.0–5.5)	22.0 (3.0–164.5)	3.0 (0.7–13.1)	2.9 (1.8–4.6)	5.1 (3.0–8.7)	3.1 (1.6–6.1)	3.7 (0.8–16.6)	2.1 (1.6–2.8)
4 or more	5.8 (3.4–10.1)	42.0 (5.5–321.3)	9.6 (2.2–42.6)	3.6 (2.2–6.0)	5.4 (2.8–10.1)	6.0 (2.8–12.9)	6.2 (1.3–30.9)	2.4 (1.7–3.4)
Significance test for trend[b]	$p < 0.0001$	$p < 0.0001$	$p < 0.0001$	$p < 0.0001$	$p < 0.0001$	$p < 0.0001$	NS	$p < 0.0001$

[a] Relative risks were estimated using men with no risk factors as reference group.
[b] Significance tests for trend were done in the two age groups separately using bivariate Cox regression with age and the number of risk factors as independent variables.

SUMMARY

Based on the 15-year follow-up data in the Honolulu Heart Program, the effects of cardiovascular risk factors upon CHD and stroke incidence and total mortality among 3,369 middle-aged men (aged 50–59) and 2,738 elderly men (aged 60–74) were compared.

In general, these effects were quite similar in the two age groups. The only exception was that hypertension and blood pressure were less strongly associated with HEM stroke in the elderly group than in the middle-aged group although the associations were highly significant after adjustment for age in both age groups.

From the multivariate analyses, hypertension and cigarette smoking were the most potent and universal independent risk factors in both age groups. High serum cholesterol was a strong risk factor for CHD, whereas it was protective against HEM stroke in both age groups.

The relative risks of all outcomes increased progressively with an increase in the number of coexisting risk factors. There was no difference in the slope of these trends between the two age groups except for HEM stroke which was significantly greater for middle-aged than for elderly men. These results appear to support the notion that preventive measures relating to cardiovascular risk factors should be taken by elderly men as well as by their middle-aged counterparts.

REFERENCES

Barrett-Connor E, Suarez L, Khaw K, Criqui MH, Wingard DL 1984 Ischemic heart disease risk factors after age 65. J Chronic Dis 37: 903–908

Benfante R, Reed D 1990 Is elevated serum cholesterol level a risk factor for coronary heart disease in the elderly? JAMA 263: 393–396

Benfante R, Reed DM, Frank J 1991 Does cigarette smoking have an independent effect on coronary heart disease in the elderly? Am J Public Health 81: 897–899

Cox DR 1972 Regression models and life tables. J R Stat Soc, Ser B 34: 187–200

Harris T, Cook EF, Kannel B 1988 Proportional hazards analysis of risk factors for coronary heart disease in individuals aged 65 or older. The Framingham Study. J Am Geriatr Soc 36: 1023–1028

Kannel WB, Gordon T 1980 Cardiovascular risk factor in the aged: The Framingham Study. *In*: Haynes JA, Stallones L (Eds), Second conference on the epidemiology of aging. U.S. Department of Health and Human Services, National Institute of Health, NIH Publication No. 80-909, pp 65–89

Keinbaum DG, Kupper LL 1978 Applied Regression Analysis and Other Multivariable Methods. Duxbury Press, North Scituate, Massachusetts, pp 99–102

Multiple Risk Factors in Cardiovascular Disease, ed. by A. Yamamoto, Churchill Livingstone Japan, Tokyo, pp. 11–14 (1994)

ASSOCIATION OF A WESTERNIZED LIFESTYLE AND ISCHEMIC HEART DISEASE IN THE JAPANESE

Genshi EGUSA, Hitoshi HARA, and Michio YAMAKIDO

*Second Department of Internal Medicine, Hiroshima University School of Medicine**

Key words: westernized lifestyle, Japanese-American, hyperlipidemia, hyperinsulinemia, ischemic heart disease

After World War II, the lifestyle of the Japanese became markedly westernized. The suggestion that the changes in lifestyle imposed by "westernization" are associated with the development of ischemic heart disease (IHD) has been confirmed by the results of epidemiological surveys conducted in Asians in England (Tunstall *et al* 1975).

Thus, it is important for the Japanese to identify the characteristics of a westernized lifestyle that are associated with the development of IHD. With this objective, we carried out a medical survey of Japanese-Americans living in the United States (Hawaii and Los Angeles) and Japanese living in Hiroshima over the period 1978 to 1988.

WESTERNIZED LIFESTYLE IN THE JAPANESE: DIET AND PHYSICAL ACTIVITY

The dietary survey revealed that the total energy intake of male and female Japanese-Americans did not differ significantly from that of their Japanese counterparts. However, in the Japanese-Americans, the intake of animal fat and simple carbohydrates (especially fructose) was markedly greater than in the Japanese while the intake of complex carbohydrate was lower. While the total energy intake of both the Japanese and Japanese-Americans was very similar to that found in the NIHON-SAN Study conducted in the 1970s (Kagan *et al* 1974), the difference between the two groups in terms of the intake of animal fat and simple carbohydrates found in the former study was more marked, suggesting that the eating habits of the Japanese had become more westernized during the intervening 20 years.

The proportion of the Japanese-Americans who engaged in strenuous physical activity was lower in comparison with native Japanese, while the proportion who engaged in light or moderate physical activity was higher.

Thus, the characteristics of the westernized lifestyle in the Japanese were an increased intake of animal fat and simple carbohydrates without an accompanying increase in total energy intake, or reduction in physical activity.

WESTERNIZED LIFESTYLE AND RISK FACTORS FOR IHD

Serum Lipids, Hypertension and Smoking

We examined several factors associated with both a westernized lifestyle and the risk of IHD in both groups. Both the serum choles-

* 1-2-3 Kasumi, Minami-ku, Hiroshima 734, Japan.

terol (CH) and triglyceride (TG) levels in the Japanese-Americans were 30 to 50 mg/dl higher than in the native Japanese, for both sexes and in all age groups (Fig. 1). These levels in the Japanese-Americans were also higher than those in Caucasians in the United States reported in a recent ARIC study (Brown *et al* 1993). The elevated intake of animal fat and simple carbohydrates in the Japanese-Americans, even though it is less than that in Caucasian-Americans, might have an effect on their serum CH and TG levels.

Thus, the capacity to metabolize nutrients exhibited by the Japanese, who have consumed a traditional Japanese diet for generations, might not be able to deal with a highly westernized diet without producing changes in serum CH and TG levels. The serum CH in other Asian groups living in foreign countries is reported to be lower than that of Caucasians in the same country.

The two groups did not differ as far as the prevalence of hypertension was concerned (WHO criteria) and the percentage of current smokers in the Japanese-American group (39%) was lower than that in the Japanese living in Hiroshima (53%).

Obesity

It has been reported that the waist-hip ratio of people resident in England but of South Asian descent is higher than that of Caucasians and is true for in both sexes (Mckeigue *et al* 1991). We found that the waist-hip ratio of Japanese-Americans was significantly higher than that of native Japanese both male and female, even after adjustment for body mass index. Thus, a westernized lifestyle clearly influences the distribution of body fat not only among Japanese but also other Asians.

Diabetes

We found a significantly higher prevalence of diabetes in Japanese-Americans. The age-sex adjusted prevalence of diabetes was 6.2% in Hiroshima, 18.9% in Hawaii, and 13.7% in Los Angeles. Furthermore, the Japanese-Americans had significantly higher serum insulin concentrations than the native Japanese, both before and after glucose loading, following adjustment for age, body mass index and blood glucose. Thus, westernized eating habits, reduced physical activity and upper body obesity may have influenced insulin resistance and contributed to the

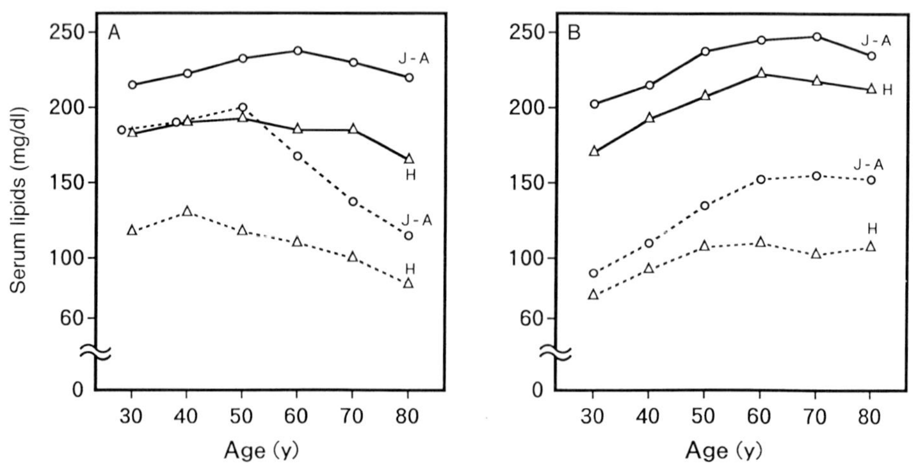

Fig. 1. Mean serum cholesterol (——) and triglycerides (----) in Japanese-Americans (J-A) and Japanese living in Hiroshima (H). A, male; B, female.

development of diabetes in the Japanese-Americans. A markedly higher prevalence of diabetes, as well as higher blood pressure, higher plasma TG and lower high-density lipoprotein choresterol (HDL-CH) concentrations associated with insulin resistance have also been reported in South Asian residents in England in comparison with native Caucasians.

ASSOCIATION OF A WESTERNIZED LIFESTYLE AND IHD

Several epidemiological studies have indicated that the change of lifestyle as a result of emigration is associated with increased IHD-related mortality and morbidity in people of South Asian descent (Tunstall *et al* 1975). We found that the prevalence of abnormal Q waves in resting electrocardiograms (ECGs) in Japanese-Americans was three to four times higher than in Japanese living in Hiroshima . Furthermore, a survey of the causes of death in Hawaii revealed that the changes in death rates due to cancer and cerebrovascular disease over the past twenty years among Japanese-Americans have been very similar to that in Caucasians, whereas the death rate due to IHD among Japanese-Americans has increased markedly and is approaching that in Caucasians. Thus, a westernized lifestyle may influence many risk factors for atherosclerosis and accelerate the development of IHD in Japanese-Americans, as well as in other residents of Asian descent.

Hypercholesterolemia is an important coronary risk factor in most industrialized countries. The plasma CH of immigrants from the Indian subcontinent residing in Britain is lower than that of indigenous Caucasians, but the IHD mortality rate is disproportionately greater in the former. The effects of other established risk factors for IHD, including smoking, hypertension and hemostatic activity, do not account for the higher IHD mortality rate in this population. On the other hand, the mean fasting and post-load serum insulin and TG levels in South Asian people are higher than those in European men, while the HDL-CH level is lower. Thus, metabolic disturbances associated with insulin resistance might underlie the higher rates of IHD in these populations (Mckeigue *et al* 1993). Compared with the native Japanese in our study, the Japanese-Americans exhibited apparently higher fasting and post-load plasma insulin and TG levels. Moreover, the fasting plasma insulin level in the Japanese-Americans, but not in the native Japanese, was positively correlated with plasma TG and blood pressure and negatively correlated with HDL-CH. Thus, the Japanese-Americans have important coronary risk factors, insulin resistance syndrome in addition to hypercholesterolemia, compared with the native Japanese. The avoidance of excessively westernized dietary habits, the control of obesity, and the greater physical activity in the native Japanese are beneficial in maintaining low rate of diabetes and IHD in this group.

SUMMARY

The westernized dietary habits of the Japanese are characterized by an increased consumption of animal fat and simple carbohydrates and a decreased intake of complex carbohydrates without any increase in calorie intake. Decreased physical activity is also apparently associated with a westernized lifestyle. These changes amplify many risk factors for atherosclerosis and are strongly associated with the development of IHD.

The incidence of both cerebral bleeding and pulmonary tuberculosis, which were formerly the primary causes of death in Japan, has decreased markedly in the past thirty years. On the other hand, our results indicate that IHD will become an important cause of death in Japanese with a westernized lifestyle. It is important for the management of our health that excessive westernization of the Japanese lifestyle is avoided.

REFERENCES

Brown SA, Hutchinson R, Morrisett J *et al* 1993 Plasma lipid, lipoprotein cholesterol, and apoprotein distributions in selected US communities: The atherosclerosis risk in communities (ARIC) study. Arterioscler Thromb 13: 1139–1158

Kagan A, Harris BR, Winkelstein W *et al* 1974 Epidemiologic studies of coronary heart disease and stroke in Japanese men living in Japan, Hawaii and California: Demographic, physical, dietary and biochemical characteristics. J Chronic Dis 27: 345–364

Mckeigue PM, Shah B, Marmot MG 1991 Relation of central obesity and insulin resistance with high diabetes prevalence and cardiovascular risk in South Asians. Lancet 337: 382–386

Mckeigue PM, Ferrie JE, Pierpoint T 1993 Association of early-onset coronary heart disease in South Asia men with glucose intolerance and hyperinsulinemia. Circulation 87: 152–161

Tunstall PH, Clayton D, Morris JN *et al* 1975 Coronary heart-attacks in east London. Lancet ii: 833–838

Multiple Risk Factors in Cardiovascular Disease, ed. by A. Yamamoto, Churchill Livingstone Japan, Tokyo, pp. 15–18 (1994)

INTERRELATIONSHIPS OF CIGARETTE SMOKING, BLOOD PRESSURE, AND SERUM LIPIDS IN SINGAPORE

Kenneth Hughes

*Department of Community, Occupational and Family Medicine National University of Singapore**

Key words: interrelationships, cigarette smoking, blood pressure, lipids

Cigarette smoking, blood pressure, and serum lipids are established major risk factors for coronary heart disease, though the mechanisms of their actions are not yet fully understood. Knowledge of their interrelationship will help elucidate these mechanisms and also be of importance in the prevention of coronary heart disease. However, there have been inconsistencies in their relationships reported in different studies, partially due to differences in the control of confounding factors.

Singapore is an island state which in June 1984 had a population of 2.53 million consisting of Chinese, Malays, Indians, and others. Singaporeans now have a high standard of living with the two commonest causes of death being cardiovascular disease and cancer.

A cross-sectional population-based survey of cardiovascular risk factors was carried out in Singapore from 1982 to 1985 and the methodology used has been described (Hughes *et al* 1990). The risk factors were measured by standardized techniques and details have been reported of the analyses of the relationships between the different cardiovascular risk factors (Hughes *et al* 1993). This present paper reviews the relationships between cigarette smoking and blood pressure, cigarette smoking and serum lipids, and blood pressure and serum lipids, and compares them with other studies.

This study in Singapore was carried out on a random sample of the general population and involved 2,143 Chinese, Malays, and Indians aged 18–69 years . For cigarette smoking, only males are analyzed because of the small proportion of females in Singapore who smoke. As far as serum lipids are concerned, only subjects who had fasted for at least 10 hours (94%) were used for triglyceride measurement but both fasting and non-fasting subjects were used to determine low density lipoprotein (LDL) cholesterol and high density lipoprotein (HDL) cholesterol.

There was control of the possible confounding due to age, ethnic group, body mass index, alcohol consumption, and physical activity. For blood pressure and serum lipids partial correlation coefficients were calculated using the REG procedure of the SAS statistical package. For the relationships between cigarette smoking and blood pressure and cigarette smoking and serum lipids use of this form of analysis was not appropriate because of the high proportion of non-

* Singapore 0511.

smokers. Hence mean values of blood pressure and lipids were calculated (with adjustment by analysis of covariance using the GLM procedure of the SAS package) in non-smokers, light smokers (1–10 cigs/day), moderate smokers (11–20 cigs/day), and heavy smokers (> 20 cigs/day).

CIGARETTE SMOKING AND BLOOD PRESSURE

Figure 1 shows the relationship between the factors for males in Singapore. There is an inverse relationship between current cigarette smoking behavior and mean systolic blood pressure which, though not marked, has a dose-response effect suggesting that it is causal. Compared with non-smokers, there are falls of 1.3 mmHg ($p = 0.319$) in light smokers, 3.8 mmHg ($p = 0.001$) in moderate smokers, and 4.6 mmHg ($p = 0.012$) in heavy smokers. Overall, the mean systolic blood pressure of smokers (120.6) is lower than that of non-smokers (123.5) by 2.9 mmHg ($p = 0.002$).

There is no clear relationship with diastolic pressure though all-smokers have a slightly lower level (74.6 mmHg) than non-smokers (75.8 mmHg) by 1.2 mmHg ($p = 0.057$).

Lower blood pressures in cigarette smokers compared with non-smokers have been found in the Tecumseh Study (Higgins & Kjelsberg 1967), the Normative Aging Study (Seltzer 1974), and the Albany Study without the difference being statistically significant (Gordon & Doyle 1986). No clear relationship was found in the Evans County Study (Greene *et al* 1977), Framingham Study although smokers did have slightly lower levels (Gordon *et al* 1975), and the British Regional Heart Study although the lowest levels were present in the heaviest smokers (Shaper *et al* 1981).

Other studies have examined the effect of cessation of cigarette smoking on blood pressure. One found an increase, especially in systolic pressure (Williams *et al* 1979), while two found no change (Greene *et al* 1977; Gordon *et al* 1975). A randomized controlled trial also found no change (Rabkin 1984) while the Multiple Risk Factor Intervention Trial (MRFIT) found an increase in those becoming hypertensive, although weight gain was considered to have contributed to this (Gerace *et al* 1991).

While cigarette smoking produces an immediate and transient elevation of blood pressure the question is whether there is any cumulative effect. The epidemiological evi-

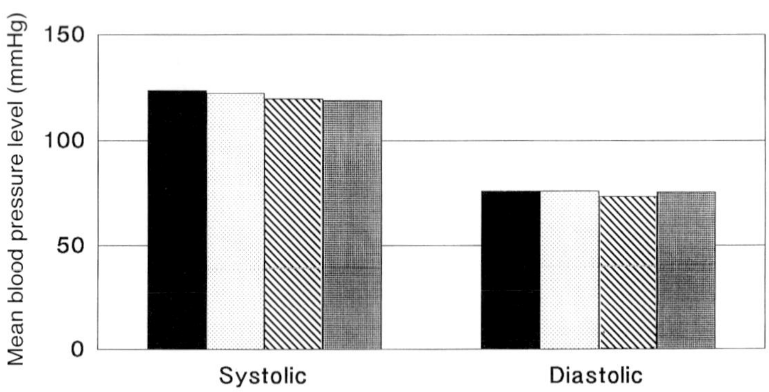

Fig. 1. Mean blood pressures (adjusted by analysis of covariance for ethnic group, age, body mass index, alcohol consumption, and physical activity) by current cigarette smoking behavior, males aged 18–69 years.
■, none; □, light (1–10 cigs/day); ▧, moderate (11–20 cigs/day); ▦, heavy (>20 cigs/day).

dence indicates that cigarette smoking does not lead to higher blood pressure but whether it has no effect at all or produces a modest lowering is not clear.

CIGARETTE SMOKING AND SERUM LIPIDS

Figure 2 shows the data for males in Singapore. Although there is no evidence of a relationship between smoking and LDL-cholesterol, there is an inverse relationship

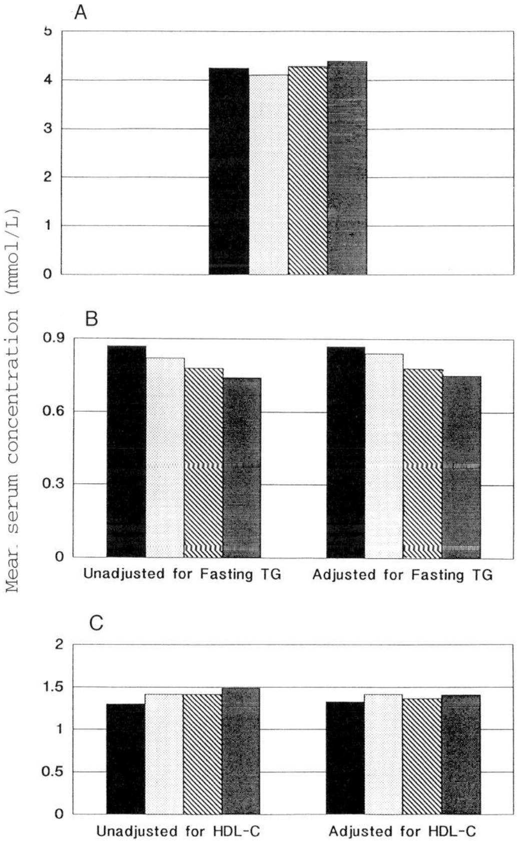

Fig. 2. Mean serum lipid levels (adjusted by analysis of covariance for ethnic group, age, body mass index, alcohol consumption, and physical activity) by current cigarette smoking behavior, males aged 18–69 years.
A, LDL-cholesterol; B, HDL-cholesterol; C, fasting triglyceride. ■, none; □, light (1–10 cigs/day); ▧, moderate (11–20 cigs/day); ▦, heavy (>20 cigs/day). TG, triglyceride.

with HDL-cholesterol. Compared with non-smokers light smokers exhibit a fall of 0.05 mmol/L ($p = 0.064$), moderate smokers 0.09 mmol/L ($p < 0.001$) and heavy smokers 0.13 mmol/L ($p < 0.001$). All smokers have a lower mean level than non-smokers, the difference being 0.08 mmol/L ($p < 0.001$).

In this population, as in others, HDL-cholesterol and fasting triglyceride are themselves inversely related with a partial correlation coefficient for males of –0.34 ($p < 0.001$). However, the relationship between smoking and HDL-cholesterol is still present after adjusting for fasting triglyceride, with corresponding falls of 0.03 mmol/L ($p = 0.314$), 0.09 mmol/L ($p < 0.001$), and 0.12 mmol/L ($p = 0.004$). All smokers have a lower mean level than non-smokers with the difference being 0.07 mmol/L ($p < 0.001$). The dose-response effect suggests a causal relationship.

There is a direct relationship between smoking and fasting triglyceride, (although there is not a uniform dose-response effect), with light, moderate and heavy smokers exhibiting rises of 0.12 mmol/L ($p = 0.066$), 0.12 mmol/L ($p = 0.052$), and 0.19 mmol/L ($p = 0.067$) compared with non-smokers. All-smokers have higher values than non-smokers, the difference being 0.13 mmol/L ($p = 0.008$). However, this relationship is abolished on adjustment for HDL-cholesterol.

A meta-analysis of studies investigating the relationship between cigarette smoking and serum lipids concluded that cigarette smoking is associated with higher serum concentrations of LDL-cholesterol and triglyceride, and lower serum concentrations of HDL-cholesterol (Craig *et al* 1989). However, the different studies had variable degrees of control for confounding. Also, for LDL-cholesterol, a difference between non-smokers and smokers was only present for heavy smokers and not for light or moderate smokers while, for total cholesterol, the dose-response effect was not particularly strong. This suggests, despite the authors' conclusion, that there is no causal relationship between smoking and LDL-cholesterol which is what has been found in Singapore.

This meta-analysis (Craig *et al* 1989) also found, as in Singapore, a direct dose-dependent relationship between cigarette smoking and triglyceride and a dose-dependent inverse relationship between smoking and HDL-cholesterol. However, in Singapore, it has been shown that after adjusting for the other factor the relationship remains for HDL-cholesterol but not for fasting triglyceride suggesting that the causal relationship is with HDL-cholesterol and the one with triglyceride is due to confounding from HDL-cholesterol. No other study seems to have made this adjustment.

As in Singapore, the Lipid Research Clinics Program found a dose-dependent inverse association between cigarette smoking and HDL-cholesterol which was independent of age, obesity, alcohol intake, and regular exercise (Criqui *et al* 1980).

Further evidence for these relationships between cigarette smoking and lipids (i.e. a causal one only with HDL-cholesterol) is provided from trials of men giving up smoking. Two found an increase in HDL-cholesterol but no change in LDL-cholesterol or triglyceride (Stubbe *et al* 1982; Rabkin 1984), while MRFIT found an increase in HDL-cholesterol but no difference in LDL-cholesterol (Gerace *et al* 1991).

How cigarette smoking lowers HDL-cholesterol is not clear, although recent research suggests that it may act by increasing lipase activity and/or through insulin resistance and hyperinsulinemia. However, whatever the mechanism, it may well be part of the explanation for the adverse effect of cigarette smoking on coronary heart disease.

BLOOD PRESSURE AND SERUM LIPIDS

This relationship in Singapore has been examined by calculating partial correlation coefficients (r), adjusting for age, ethnic group, body mass index, alcohol consumption, and physical activity. For blood pressure and LDL-cholesterol, the coefficients are low and statistically insignificant for both sexes: males (systolic, $r = -0.03$, $p = 0.353$ and diastolic, $r = -0.02$, $p = 0.490$) and females (systolic, $r = 0.06$, $p = 0.053$ and diastolic, $r = 0.04$, $p = 0.172$). This also applies to HDL-cholesterol: males (systolic, $r = -0.02$, $p = 0.527$ and diastolic, $r = -0.03$, $p = 0.382$) and females (systolic, $r = 0.03$, $p = 0.278$ and diastolic, $r = 0.02$, $p = 0.599$).

However, for fasting triglyceride, the coefficients are higher (although still not particularly high) and statistically significant for males (systolic, $r = 0.06$, $p = 0.066$ and diastolic, $r = 0.12$, $p < 0.001$) and females (systolic, $r = 0.11$, $p < 0.001$ and diastolic, $r = 0.13$, $p < 0.001$).

The Tecumseh Study (Ostrander 1976) and Chicago Community Surveys (Stamler *et al* 1975) found no correlation between blood pressure and total cholesterol after adjusting for relative weight. While some studies have found such a correlation, generally there has been inadequate control of confounding or the correlation coefficients have been very low (less than 0.1). However, the Tromso Study (Bonaa & Thelle 1991) was an exception.

The Tromso Study also found that blood pressure was related to triglyceride although the relationship was weak in lean subjects and, as far as HDL-cholesterol was concerned, only in subgroups with high alcohol consumption (Bonaa & Thelle 1991). In a British general population study HDL-cholesterol and the HDL-cholesterol/total cholesterol ratio were not related to blood pressure after control of confounding (Williams *et al* 1979). Comparing hypertensives with controls, another study found the former to have higher triglyceride but there was no difference in LDL-cholesterol and HDL-cholesterol (Catalano *et al* 1991).

Hence the biological relationships between blood pressure and serum lipids have not yet been fully clarified. However, on balance, the epidemiological evidence indicates that there are no important relationships after adjusting for relative weight, except for a modest one relating to fasting triglyceride.

CONCLUSION

This survey of the general population in Singapore has found relationships between cigarette smoking and systolic blood pressure (inverse), cigarette smoking and serum HDL-cholesterol (inverse), and blood pressure and serum fasting triglyceride (direct), with no evidence of other relationships among these major cardiovascular risk factors.

SUMMARY

Cardiovascular risk factors were measured by standardized techniques in a cross-sectional random sample of the entire population of Singapore. For the analysis of 2,143 subjects aged 18–69 years, possible confounding from ethnic group, age, body mass index, alcohol consumption, and physical activity was controlled. Cigarette smoking in males was inversely related to systolic blood pressure and compared with non-smokers, there were reductions of 1.3 mmHg (1.1%) in light smokers, 3.8 mmHg (3.1%) in moderate smokers, and 4.6 mmHg (3.7%) in heavy smokers. There was no clear relationship with diastolic blood pressure. Cigarette smoking in males was inversely related to high density lipoprotein cholesterol, even after further adjustment for fasting triglyceride, and compared with non-smokers there were reductions of 0.03 mmol/L (3.4%) in light smokers, 0.09 mmol/L (10.3%) in moderate smokers and 0.12 mmol/L (13.8%) in heavy smokers. Cigarette smoking in males was directly related to fasting triglyceride but this disappeared on adjusting for high density lipoprotein cholesterol. Cigarette smoking was not related to low density lipoprotein cholesterol. There were no relationships between blood pressure and serum lipids except for modest direct ones with fasting triglyceride, the partial correlation coefficients being as shown: — males: systolic, $r = 0.06$, $p = 0.066$ and diastolic, $r = 0.12$, $p < 0.001$ and females: systolic, $r = 0.11$, $p < 0.001$ and diastolic, $r = 0.13$, $p < 0.001$. These results were compared with those from other surveys.

REFERENCES

Bonaa KH, Thelle DS 1991 Association between blood pressure and serum lipids in a population. The Tromso Study. Circulation 83: 1305–1314

Catalano M, Aronica A, Carzaniga G, Seregni R, Libretti A 1991 Serum lipids and apolipoproteins in patients with essential hypertension. Atherosclerosis 87: 17–22

Craig WY, Palomaki GE, Haddow JE 1989 Cigarette smoking and serum lipid and lipoprotein concentrations: an analysis of published data. Br Med J 298: 784–788

Criqui MH, Wallace RB, Heiss G, Mishkel M, Schonfeld G, Jones GTL 1980 Cigarette smoking and plasma high-density lipoprotein cholesterol: The Lipid Research Clinics Program Prevalence Study. Circulation 62 (Suppl IV): 70–76

Gerace TA, Hollis J, Ockene JK, Svendsen K 1991 Smoking cessation and change in diastolic blood pressure, body weight, and plasma lipids. MRFIT Research Group. Prev Med 20: 602–620

Gordon T, Doyle JT 1986 Alcohol consumption and its relationship to smoking, weight, blood pressure, and blood lipids: The Albany Study. Arch Intern Med 146: 262–265

Gordon T, Kannel WB, Dawber TR, McGee D 1975 Changes associated with quitting cigarette smoking: The Framingham Study. Am Heart J 90: 322–328

Greene SB, Aavedal MJ, Tyroler HA, Davis CE, Hames CG 1977 Smoking habits and blood pressure change: A seven year follow-up. J Chronic Dis 30: 401–413

Higgins MW, Kjelsberg M 1967 Characteristics of smokers and non-smokers in Tecumseh, Michigan. II. The distribution of selected physical measurements and physiologic variables and the prevalence of certain diseases in smokers and nonsmokers. Am J Epidemiol 86: 60–77

Hughes K, Yeo PPB, Lun KC *et al* 1990 Cardiovascular diseases in Chinese, Malays, and Indians in Singapore. II. Differences in

risk factor levels. J Epidemiol Community Health 44: 29–35
Hughes K, Leong WP, Sothy SP, Lun KC, Yeo PBB 1993 Relationships between cigarette smoking, blood pressure and serum lipids in the Singapore general population. Int J Epidemiol 22: 637–643
Ostrander LD 1976 Coronary risk factors in a community. Findings in Tecumseh, Michigan. Circulation 53: 152–156
Rabkin SW 1984 Effects of cigarette smoking cessation on risk factors for coronary atherosclerosis: A control clinical trial. Atherosclerosis 53: 173–184
Seltzer CC 1974 Effect of smoking on blood pressure. Am Heart J 87: 558–564
Shaper AG, Pocock SJ, Walker M, Cohen NM, Wale CJ, Thomson AG 1981 British Regional Heart Study: Cardiovascular risk factors in middle-aged men in 24 towns. Br Med J 283: 179–186
Stamler J, Stamler R, Rhomberg P *et al* 1975 Multivariate analysis of the relationship of six variables to blood pressure: Findings from Chicago Community Surveys, 1965–1971. J Chronic Dis 28: 499–525
Stubbe I, Eskilsson J, Nilsson-Ehle P 1982 High-density lipoprotein concentrations increase after stopping smoking. Br Med J 284: 1511–1513
Williams P, Robinson D, Bailey A 1979 High-density lipoprotein and coronary risk factors in normal men. Lancet i: 72–75

Multiple Risk Factors in Cardiovascular Disease, ed. by A. Yamamoto, Churchill Livingstone Japan, Tokyo, pp. 21–24 (1994)

THE SEVEN COUNTRIES STUDY: A HISTORIC ADVENTURE IN SCIENCE

Henry Blackburn*[1] and Hironori Toshima*[2]

*[1] *Division of Epidemiology, School of Public Health, University of Minnesota, and* *[2] *Third Department of Medicine, School of Medicine, Kurume University*

Key words: cardiovascular disease epidemiology, Seven Countries Study, risk factors

Keys and collaborators hypothesized early on that differences in population rates of cardiovascular disease (CVD), and of individual risk within populations, were related to lifestyle and physical risk factors, including the composition of the diet. To examine this hypothesis, the Seven Countries Study (SCS) cross-sectional surveys were conducted starting in 1958, among samples of men aged 40 59, in fourteen areas of seven countries with known differences in the composition of the diet and in the purported rates of heart disease: Yugoslavia, Italy, and Greece, representing Mediterranean diets and lifestyle, the Netherlands and Finland, for northern Europe, Japan and the USA. Baseline survey participants were entered into cohorts and both the diseased and disease-free men were followed for up to 30 years in most areas. The study was unique for its time, with adequately-sized "chunk" samples of all men in the area, with standardized risk factor and disease measurements, training of teams and quality control of field procedures, and central coding and analysis of data. The SCS became the prototypical population comparison study, made across a wide range of diet and disease experience, analyzed in cross-section and in long-term follow-up.

BACKGROUND

The SCS developed out of an abundant set of observations made by a number of clinicians and investigators, emerging independently and in embryonic form in each of the seven countries. There was, in the late 1950's, a readiness to accept new ideas, along with a preparedness for effective research among disciplines and across cultures. Keys and colleagues at Minnesota were prepared, using quantitative thinking and computational skills, to link ideas, bridge disciplines, and apply methods appropriate to the scientific question. Researchers in several parts of the world were examining similar issues; Karvonen in the Finnish group, Fidanza and Puddu in the Italian group, Buzina and Djordjevic in the two Yugoslavian groups, Aravanis and Dontas in the Greek group, Kimura and Toshima in the Japanese group, and Dalderup and colleagues in the Dutch group. Each had already begun explorations of CVD and risk phenomena as they existed

*[1] 1300 South 2nd St, Suite 300, Minneapolis, MN 55454, USA.
*[2] Asahi, Kurume 830, Japan.

outside the clinical setting, in the general population, testing hypotheses about the causal role of diet, physical activity and lifestyle. Back in Minnesota, Keys, Grande, and Anderson were also making crucial metabolic experiments on the precise effects on serum cholesterol of diet changes. Essential to the whole development were the observations of Paul Dudley White of Boston and Noboru Kimura in Kyushu, who put into stark and simple terms the contrasts in CVD frequency and arterial pathology seen around the world.

BEGINNINGS

Meetings between these remarkable people were stimulated by Ancel Keys, the ideas for collaborative research rapidly took hold, and active work soon began. Pilot studies with the Finns in 1956 and the Italians and Greeks in 1957, demonstrated the feasibility of the SCS in the field. A central coordinating grant to Keys from NIH allowed the definitive cohort surveys to begin in Yugoslavia in 1958, while the U.S. Railroad Study preceded them in 1957 under a separate grant to Henry Taylor.

Fortunately for the SCS, National Heart Foundations and other groups in those days were ready to support the early phases of these activities. The U.S. Railroad Study, in which Taylor and Blackburn developed and tested much of the methodology for the larger project, profited from the support of the new National Heart Institute (NHI). Keys played the central role, putting all the ideas together in a clear proposal to the NHI for collaborative research among the seven countries. He possessed the international contacts, the vision and the experience to move forward this major enterprise. The special experience and knowledge of each of the SCS principal investigators in their professional fields, as well as the geography and culture of their lands, along with their clinical contacts and political clout, enabled the whole SCS operation to be put in motion.

COORDINATION

As remarkable as these beginnings was the later emergence of leadership in the SCS, from various places, always where and when it was needed. Ancel Keys' leadership was essential to organize the study, prepare the initial collaborative proposal and, over the years, to bring out the three major monographs: the 1967 Acta Med Scand Supplement (Keys *et al* 1967), the 1970 Circulation Supplement (Keys *et al* 1970), and the 1980 Oxford Press monograph (Keys *et al* 1980). Each of these efforts was a tour de force which brought the diverse findings together in a way that no other investigator or editorial board could have done as cogently and effectively. However, other leadership appeared when the SCS came under its greatest threat; the central grant expired in the late 1960's, and soon after Dr. Keys retired and his base of operations was constrained. This was paralleled by our necessarily intense preoccupation in Minnesota with new activities to assure the survival and growth of the Laboratory of Physiological Hygiene, then and still, a largely self-supporting academic institution. Thus, in the late 1960's, much of the SCS energy, data collection and coordinating responsibility was transferred to the capable hands of Alessandro Menotti and the Rome center.

NEW DIRECTIONS

Since then, an important new axis of leadership has developed between the Netherlands, Rome and Finland, with a rich collegial sharing of ideas, initiatives and new data collection for new research. The SCS owes much to the enterprise of Kromhout, Menotti and Nissinen for this development. Daan Kromhout has taken the initiative in extending the dietary analyses and in sponsoring a major historical monograph on the SCS. Hironori Toshima organized a remarkable 35th anniversary meeting, along with publication of the scientific proceedings.

In addition to the long list of SCS "firsts," the study continues to redefine its mission and hypotheses. For example, there is every evidence of continued success in long-term follow-up of survival in the cohorts. Dr. Keys continues to study survival and longevity related to characteristics at entry. In addition, researches by several investigators seek to explain further the large differences in population CVD rates, and the individual differences in risk with respect to differences, and to changes over time, in diet and other risk factors.

STRENGTHS AND LIMITATIONS

Of course, there are problems. The SCS has a relatively small number of units to compare, with few degrees of freedom for the ecological correlations. Early on making these correlations at all was criticized. Some have criticized the selection of the geographic areas, the varied occupational composition of the populations compared, and the obvious technical limitations of measurement and classification across areas by national teams, often under difficult field survey conditions. It is true that improvements have since been made in the configuration of populations for such internal and international comparisons, for example, by random selection of greater numbers of units.

But the SCS was not only "state-of-the-art" for its time, it was bold and foresighted in its concepts and thrust. As we realize increasingly today, the ecological associations of habitual diet, other risk factors, and population rates of disease, alone and in themselves a rather weak base for causal inference, are, nevertheless, in the presence of strong congruent evidence from the laboratory and clinic, among the more valuable indicators of the true forces underlying mass diseases. When the evidence is consistent, population correlations of behavior, risk factors and disease may indicate the major determinants of different population rates of disease.

CONTRIBUTIONS

The SCS, perhaps more than any other scientific study, has directed attention to the causes of population rates of disease in contrast to the causes of individual risk. It has documented large population differences in disease rates and in the average risk factor levels related to those different rates. It has demonstrated the degree to which the composition of the diet, particularly saturated fatty acids, and mean population serum cholesterol levels, and their changes over time, effectively predict present and future population rates of coronary heart disease (CHD).

The regressions derived from the ecological correlations of risk and CVD in the SCS as a whole have provided the "rule," while departure from this has disclosed important "exceptions," such as the excess of CHD in east Finland, the high rate of hemorrhagic stoke and low coronary rates in southern Japan, and the paradox of Crete, with a high fat diet, mid-range serum cholesterol levels, and low CHD rates. These findings, in turn, have provided the impetus to research on mass CVD determinants other than dietary saturated fatty acids, including omega-3 and monounsaturated fatty acids, fibers and, more recently, anti-oxidants.

Finally, the SCS, a pioneering epidemiological exploration, has laid a major foundation stone on which has been built new preventive research and interventions, extending to the laboratory and to the clinic and then back again to whole populations. It has been an adventure in ideas and methods and collegiality, and in the organization of effective scientific collaboration. In the end, this adventure has come to influence profoundly our thinking, practice and policy in cardiovascular medicine, and thereby, to influence public health.

SUMMARY

The SCS has become a classic in science for its pioneering effort in CVD epidemiology. It provides a powerful lesson to science: that mass risk phenomena determine the population rates and the preventive strategies of CVD. The idea of the SCS arose in various forms in the minds of individuals capable of integrating laboratory, clinical and population evidence.

The SCS was the first to make systematic comparisons of CVD rates and characteristics of risk in contrasting cultures. It was the first to combine cross-sectional surveys with long-term follow-up among cohorts. It was the first to compute population (ecologic) correlations between lifestyle and risk factors and between risk factors and disease, and their changes over time. It was the first to apply multivariate regression coefficients derived in one population to findings in men of the same age in another, thereby demonstrating that the major CVD risk factors are universal but that the force of a risk factor differs among contrasting populations. The SCS has had a major influence on the thinking methods and research into the causes and prevention of CVD, and on public health.

Here we briefly review the history, results, and effect on public health of the SCS.

REFERENCES

Keys A, Blackburn HW, Van Buchem *et al* 1967. Epidemiological studies related to coronary heart disease: Characteristics of men aged 40–59 in seven countries. Acta Med Scand, 460 (Suppl 180): 1–392

Keys A, Blackburn H, Menotti A *et al 1970*. Coronary heart disease in seven countries. Circulation (Suppl 1): 1–211

Keys A, Aravanis C, Blackburn H *et al 1980*. Seven countries. A multivariate analysis of death and coronary heart disease. Harvard University Press, Cambridge Mass and London, pp 1–381

Multiple Risk Factors in Cardiovascular Disease, ed. by A. Yamamoto, Churchill Livingstone Japan, Tokyo, pp. 25–35 (1994)

THE SPECIAL EFFECTS OF SEVERAL RISK FACTORS ON PROGRESSION OF ATHEROSCLEROSIS IN YOUNG PEOPLE IN THE USA

Robert W. WISSLER* and the PDAY Research Group

* *Department of Pathology and the PDAY Coordinating Center, The University of Chicago*

Key words: atherosclerotic plaques, risk factors, progression, young people, arterial wall

The multicenter study of the Pathobiological Determinants of Atherosclerosis in Youth (PDAY) is now in its 9th year of active support by the National Heart, Lung, and Blood Institute. This period of activity is now divided into five phases. During phase one, which was a two-year period devoted to a feasibility study, all the original sixteen centers which were approved and funded in 1985 took part in a carefully rehearsed collection of over 100 cases, obtained at the originally approved eleven collection centers. These were all located at forensic pathology laboratories, throughout the U.S., and all the cases were confined to the specified age range of 15 to 35 years. At the end of the feasibility period, we reported our success at collecting cases following a highly structured protocol and manual of procedures. We also reported the accomplishment of the carefully planned preservation, distribution, and risk factor analysis of the samples and of the data collected, as well as the successful initiation of a number of the proposed pathobiological analyses at most of the centers which had been approved for special study. Two of the collection centers were dropped, and the study was approved and funded for phase two.

Starting in 1987, this was a three-year period of intensive collection, sample preservation, processing, distribution, risk factor analysis and histochemical production of high resolution fat stains as well as connective tissue stains from the ten 'core' samples which had been established as a result of the feasibility study. The computerized analysis as well as the grading of arterial lesions by pathologists, both of which methods appeared to offer valuable and complementary data on the lesion extent and severity, were approved for inclusion and the statistical center at San Antonio was judged to be highly effective for receiving and processing the numerous items of data coming from all of the centers. The study proceeded for three years of active collection, processing, and core data retrieval. The special pathobiological studies which are carried out at eleven centers got underway. Some of the most valuable and unique features of this study are given in Table I.

At the end of phase two (the three years of intensive collection, preservation, process-

* Chicago, IL 60637 USA.

Much of the research reported, as well as the preparation of the presentations, were supported by grants No. HL 10-33740 and No. HL 10-45715 from the National Heart, Lung and Blood Institute.

TABLE I. Valuable And Unique Features in the Design and Function of the PDAY Study

1. Multicenter structure makes results more applicable to USA. Age and race distribution leads to significant results in virtually all 'cells' of these categories.
2. Exclusive use of sudden unexpected death cases with no evidence of chronic disease or therapeutic intervention improves study population, as compared with community hospitals and medical centers.
3. Methods of assessing the risk factors of hyperlipidemia, diabetes, smoking, hyperglycemia, as well as immune complexes and DNA polymorphisms in candidate genes for atherosclerosis allow these variables to be quantitated in a large number of cases.
4. The detailed protocol, manual of procedures, and training sessions have provided standard samples of arteries, blood, and other tissues as well as high-quality preservation, processing, and distribution of the PDAY research materials.
5. Relatively short postmortem intervals (average 17 hours) and, in most cases, intervals between death and refrigeration (average 2 hours) help to insure reliable samples.
6. Sampling strategy utilized for each case allows comparison between:
   a) areas of high prevalence vs low prevalence of aortic lesions
   b) thoracic aortic lesions with the abdominal aorta disease.
   c) microscopic features of the LAD coronary artery samples with those of aortic samples.
   d) right coronary artery gross topographic features with the gross morphometric results of aortic intimal lesions
   e) left circumflex chemical analyses with aortic chemical analyses.
   f) immunohistochemical analyses with other gross and microscopic and/or chemical determinations.
7. Computer-assisted gross and microscopic morphometric methods utilized for image processing at Ohio State University in concert with Louisiana State University facilitate rapid, accurate quantitative information on samples and accurate maps of lesion topography.
8. Abundant samples for studies of cell populations, lipoproteins, epitopes of oxidized LDL, etc.
9. Monthly Steering Committee conference calls involving the convener of the Protocol and Manual of procedures committee, have helped insure the smooth functioning of the program.
10. The data review board and the input of the NHLBI scientific staff, especially Momtaz Wassef, Gardner MacMillan, Basil Rifkind, and our center's own scientific advisory committee, have been very valuable.
11. Quality control has been strengthened through monitoring by the University of Texas statistical center; the LSU processing, distribution, morphology, lipid chemistry, and risk factor center; the University of Chicago collection, processing, distribution, macrophotography, histotechnique, and administrative center.
12. Annual scientific days where results are reported and problems are discussed in a mutually interactive and helpful way have made important contributions to success.

LSU, Louisiana State University; LDL, low density lipoprotein; PDAY, Pathobiological Determinants of Atherosclerosis in Youth; LAD, left anterior descending.

ing, distribution, and study), over 2,000 cases had been collected, of which 1,832 were judged suitable in terms of completeness of samples and data, as well as quality, so that they could be utilized for the more definitive 'core' studies and for many of the special pathobiological studies. Once again, the progress of the study was reviewed by a Heart Council-appointed special research review team and, once again, approval was given to go into phase three, the sixth and seventh years of very intensive research using as a basis the 1,832 core cases.

Because there was a relative lack of female cases, although the other variables were well balanced in terms of age, except for the top five years (i.e., 30–34 inclusive), and race (with blacks almost equal to whites in the overall distribution of cases) it was decided, in concert with the staff at the National Heart, Lung, and Blood Institute (NHLBI), to apply for additional funds in order to permit collection at three of the most successful collection centers (Maryland, Vanderbilt, and Chicago) to help provide additional female and older male cases and to preserve, process, and carry out the core analyses of risk factors, extent of lesions, histological slide preparation, etc.

The plans for phase four were approved and funded in 1988. The collection, processing, preservation, and the incorporation of risk factors, histotechnique and computerized data permitted the initiation of phases four and five, with the addition of these much needed additional cases. The funding was for an additional five years and is scheduled to end in late March 1996, but phase four and case collection will end in August 1994. In the meantime, more than 75 full-length manuscripts have been published and numerous abstracts and presentations are on record, often illuminating the exciting preliminary results of additional detailed and time consuming studies which are underway and which were outlined in the plans for the originally funded program (Wissler *et al* 1990, Wissler 1991).

This report is selectively devoted to the results of special studies being carried out at the University of Chicago, which is the only one of the fourteen centers which has had an active role in six of the major activities necessary for PDAY to function successfully. These activities include overall administration, collection of cases, archiving and distribution of all of the frozen specimens, processing and production of all the histo-

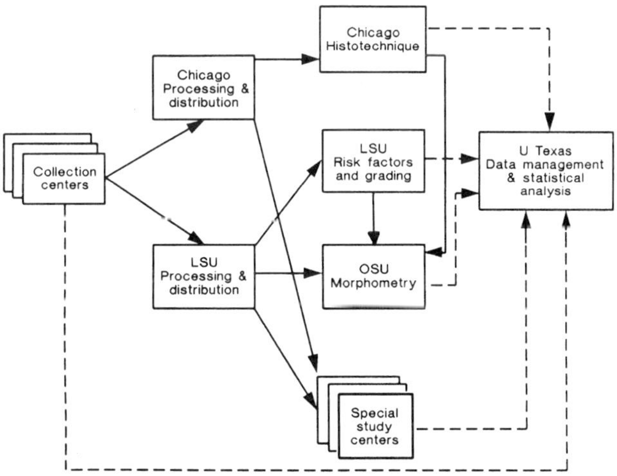

Fig. 1. PDAY materials and data flow.
This diagram indicates how the collection centers interact with the various core centers in preserving and transmitting samples for processing, for risk factor measurements, for statistical evaluation of date, for gross and microscopic morphometry, and for use in the various special studies that are being carried out at a number of centers. This system, which was demonstrated to be workable during a "phase 1 feasibility trial" involving samples, data, and information generation and utilization on more than 200 cases, has now been used successfully in more than 1,500 cases. (Reprinted publisher's permission from R.W. Wissler, 1991; Ann. N.Y. Acad. Sci. 623:26)

technique for the core studies — special studies involving many immunohistochemical and micromorphometric studies in order to learn more about how risk factors, anatomical arterial locations as well as the extent and location of lipid in the lesions influence the components of the developing plaques. The distribution of the various connective tissue elements, the lipid-containing smooth muscle cells and macrophages are included in these studies. Finally, the University of Chicago center conducts all the evaluations of macrophotographs taken at the time the lesions are classified grossly at autopsy.

A diagram of the ways that information and samples are developed and distributed is given in Fig. 1 and constitutes one of the many unique and successful aspects of this study.

PDAY RESEARCH GUIDELINES AND PROCEDURES

Case Samples

The major materials for this study are the six carefully standardized and anatomically positioned 'core' samples of the thoracic and abdominal aorta, as well as the proximal left circumflex and left anterior descending coronary arteries, the latter fixed by pressure perfusion. Half of the aorta and the right coronary arteries were prepared in a standardized way for gross pathological evaluation as well as computer-assisted mapping of the extent and severity of the lesions. The accurately positioned samples of additional tissues such as myocardium, liver, kidneys, spleen, and adipose tissue were obtained for both chemical and microscopic analysis. The specified blood samples were also obtained on most cases. More than 50 standardized samples were obtained from other parts of the arterial system under many different prescribed conditions of preservation including Carnoy's and glutaraldehyde fixation, OCT frozen-specimen preservation, fresh frozen samples for lipid, connective tissue, and vasoactive amine analysis (Fig. 2).

The sampling strategy is also a very valuable attribute of the research program, since it was developed after a careful and painstaking study of arterial lesion distribution by Stary and Cornhill (Cornhill *et al* 1990) prior to the development of the main protocol and manual of procedures, which have been utilized throughout the entire study. This is one of the many other unique features of the study (Table I).

Risk Factor Analysis

As is indicated in Table I under Item 3, the methods of assessing the risk factors of hyperlipemia, diabetes, smoking, hyperglycemia, as well as the methods developed for measuring immune complexes and DNA polymorphisms in candidate genes, have helped make it possible to relate many of the gross and microscopic findings in large numbers of cases to these risk factors. It should be emphasized that the factors listed in Table II have been carefully developed and validated over a period of several years by the group of investigators at Louisiana State University in their monumental community pathology studies. Strong and his group have recently published some of the methodology used for the PDAY study (Strong 1992; Strong *et al* 1992).

The ability to assess risk factors by these methods, even though they provide only a snapshot of the likely state of risk factors at the time of death, is proving to be valuable in correlating the extent and severity of lesions at the time of autopsy with the risk factor measurements (PDAY Research Group 1990, 1993).

Other Remarkable Methodologies and Features

The ingenious methods that Hixson has developed for finding and relating various DNA polymorphisms or genotypes to the extent and severity of lesions constitutes another extremely valuable and unique feature of this study (Hixson & Vernier 1990; Hixson *et al* 1992) in tracking the development of atherosclerosis in young people. The additional remarkable aspects of the core studies

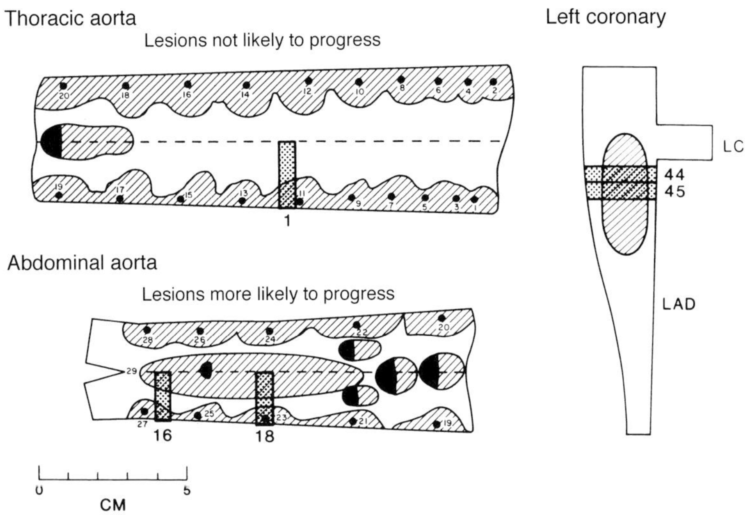

Fig. 2. Diagrammatic form of the strengths and advantages of the core sampling strategy that PDAY is employing on all of its cases.
As can be seen, these samples make it possible to study and to evaluate quantitatively the thoracic aorta core sample area (no. 1) as compared to the standard abdominal aorta areas (nos. 16 and 18). It also makes it possible to evaluate similarly the left anterior descending coronary artery (LAD) standard samples (nos. 44 and 45) and to compare lesion-prone (▨) and lesion-resistant (□) areas in each of these standard samples (□). (Reprinted publisher's permission from R.W. Wissler, 1991; Ann. N.Y. Acad. Sci. 623:26)

TABLE II. Risk Factors Measured at Post-mortem Examination

Risk Factors	Initiating Centers	Marker
Blood Lipids	LSU	Total cholesterol, HDL cholesterol and apolipoprotein concentrations including Lp(a) in postmortem serum
Smoking	LSU	Thiocyanate concentrations in postmortem serum.
Blood Pressure	LSU	Wall thickness of renal arteries and arterioles, and heart weight BW.
Diabetes Mellitus	LSU	Glycosylated hemoglobin concentrations in postmortem red blood cells.
Obesity	All collection centers*	Panniculous adipose thickness: BW/BL and torso indexes
Genetic Factors	SWF	DNA polymer in liver

* OSU, Chicago, Nebraska, Illinois, Georgia, Maryland, West Virginia, Vanderbilt, Albany. LSU, see Table I SWF, Southwest Foundation; OSU, Ohio State University; LP(a), lipoprotein a; HDL, high density lipoprotein; BW, body weight; BW/BL, body weight/body length.

are the skill and experience of the statistical center, which has probably developed the ability to deal with data from autopsy evaluations of atherosclerotic lesions and how they are related to various clinical factors to a more advanced state than any other center in the world. This ability to dispassionately evaluate the findings coming from many laboratories has served both to help validate the data as well as to call attention to a number of hasty generalizations, and to serve as an important quality control feature for all of the studies which are being carried out with PDAY specimens and data.

It is clear at this point in the development of the PDAY study that there are literally hundreds if not thousands of PDAY samples and important pieces of information which can be used for studies by other qualified investigators and which should provide a valuable national resource for future research work in this important field of endeavor.

PATHOBIOLOGICAL RESULTS AT THE UNIVERSITY OF CHICAGO

The special studies conducted at the University of Chicago are proving to be a rich source of information. Many of the results are unexpected and surprising, in view of many of the theories being put forward from *in vitro* studies of the cells and cytokinetic substances which seem to affect endothelium as well as cellular and other important components of the developing atherosclerotic plaque. The six areas of investigation, listed in Table III, and their implications in terms of the relative importance of the findings, represent only a small part of the

TABLE III. University of Chicago Pathobiological and Microscopic Findings with Their Implications: Studies of Small Groups of PDAY Cases to Develop Specific Evidence of Selected Relationships

Pathobiological Findings	Importance
1. The influence of smoking on the localization of antibodies to epitopes of oxidized LDL in developing atherosclerotic lesions (Oyer 1993).	1. One of the major mechanisms by which smoking increases the rate of atherogenesis is by means of oxidized LDL (C. Oyer, B. Berger, R.W. Wissler, and the PDAY Group. Atherosclerosis, in press, 1994).
2. The macrophage population appears to be proportional to the areas where lesions do not progress (Wissler *et al* 1991a, b).	2. The macrophage is acting primarily as a protective cell against the progression of lesions in this age group (Komatsu *et al* 1989).
3. Extracellular lipid is one of the best indicators of the progression of atherosclerotic plaque at the microscopic level (Wissler *et al* 1991b; Kusumi *et al* 1991a).	3. When the cells can no longer metabolize the incoming low density lipoprotein, then the lipid is deposited extracellularly, favoring plaque progression (Wissler *et al* 1991a).
4. Lp(a) localization in young people's lesions is more superficial and definitively localized than it is in advanced atherosclerotic plaques (Kusumi *et al* 1991a, b).	4. This suggests that Lp(a) is exerting its influence in or near the endothelial surface in young people's developing plaques.
5. Apo B and apo E localization in intimal lesions is very diffuse and has little relationship to ORO lipid content or distribution in the intima of lesion prone or lesion resistant areas (Wissler *et al* 1991a, b).	5. The apo B and apo E distribution may be indicating a separate role in the pathogenesis of the developing plaque than the lipid elements.
6. Concentric and inflamed involvement of the intima and inner media of the coronary arteries is rarely found in young people (Wissler *et al* 1991a).	6. But when it is present it frequently is correlated with inculcating immune complexes.

PDAY and LDL, see Table I; Apo, apolipoprotein; ORO, oil red O stain.

numerous special studies which are being pursued in the eleven special study centers. Some of the additional ones have been emphasized in a recent presentation which will soon be published (Wissler 1994).

Concentric Lesions and Circulating Immune Complexes

The findings from the PDAY studies are helping to reinforce the evidence that the rather infrequent and unusual coronary artery concentric lesions, especially when they are accompanied by substantial numbers of mononuclear inflammatory cells, represent a pathogenetic deviation from the usual way that atherosclerosis develops (Wissler *et al* 1985). Although it is a rather slow and tedious process, our studies so far of the occurrence of these relatively rare lesions in the coronary arteries of young people would seem to support the concept that 'atheroarteritis,' as we have designated it, is a special form of atherosclerosis which must be regarded as having a pathogenesis that is quite different from the usual development of classical eccentric initial coronary disease in hyperlipidemic individuals. This concept has been reinforced in a number of ways which have been summarized recently (Wissler 1993). The common denominator of this pattern appears to be chronic and sustained endothelial injury, whether or not it derives from circulating immune complexes (Wissler *et al* 1985, Wissler 1993).

New Classifications of Intermediate Lesions (the Fatty Plaques)

Another remarkable development that has come out of the PDAY study has been the ability to clearly identify and characterize microscopically the small discrete raised plaques that are the next stage in the development of the disease, after the poorly defined and barely elevated fatty streaks. We call these 'intermediate' lesions fatty plaques. These lesions have turned out to be the most common ones we observe in the age groups covered by this study (15–34 years). The close-up macrophotographic transparencies which are obtained from aortic core areas on the majority of cases in the PDAY study have made it possible to correlate the macroscopic findings in early lesions with their microscopic appearances in literally hundreds of cases.

Although it is beyond the scope of this paper to consider the classification of the fatty plaques in detail, this has recently been presented with gross and microscopic illustrations at national and international meetings. Furthermore, it is a product of the PDAY study, which would not have been possible if it were not for this unique opportunity to compare gross and microscopic features of the lesions with complete certainty about where the sample was taken and what it looked like at the time of autopsy, without any embellishment produced by gross staining or any alteration by fixation (Wissler *et al* 1992, 1993). This indeed is a first, and an achievement which we believe will yield a substantial improvement in correlating lesion components with risk factors when we have completed the comparison of the different microscopic forms of the 'fatty plaques' with the results of the risk factor analysis in several hundred cases, a goal we are actively pursuing (Wissler *et al* 1994 in press).

GROSS FINDINGS

The studies being reported from the 'pathologist quantitative evaluation' of the extent and severity of lesions (Strong *et al* 1992; PDAY Research Group 1990), as well as the computer-assisted quantitation and mapping of the topographic features and the extent and severity of aortic and coronary lesions (Cornhill *et al* 1990; Cornhill & Herderick 1993) are introducing many new concepts of pathogenesis which have never been previously appreciated. Some of these are presented in Table IV. Here it is apparent that these two types of evaluations of the fixed and lipid-stained gross specimens of aorta and coronary arteries, as well as the micromorphometry of aortic samples of the

TABLE IV. Major Gross Findings* and Their Implications (A Three Year Study of 1,532 PDAY Cases)

Gross Findings	Importance
1. All cases show fatty streaks of the aorta.	1. The fatty streak is a ubiquitous lesion among young people in the USA.
2. Coronary fatty streaks increase in incidence from 50% to 75% between 15 and 35 years of age.	2. Coronary disease develops in young people, but at a much slower rate than aortic disease.
3. Raised lesions in the right coronary artery increase with age in all sex and age groups and with topography similar to that of fatty streaks.	3. Fatty plaques develop from fatty streaks.
4. Fibrous plaques and calcified lesions are unusual in all arterial segments up to the age of 35.	4. The disease rarely reaches an advanced stage before the age of 35.
5. The abdominal aorta shows the most severe involvement in all race, sex, and age groups.	5. The abdominal aorta is particularly vulnerable to progression of atherosclerosis.
6. Smoking is a very strong risk factor for raised lesions in the abdominal aorta especially, and its effects can be seen as early as 15 years of age.	6. Smoking needs to be prevented at an early age if damage to the artery is to be avoided.
7. The more elevated end of the blood pressure spectrum as measured in the small renal arteries increases the risk for raised lesions in all arterial segments.	7. Hypertension carries an increased risk of accelerated atherosclerosis in all parts of the arterial system.
8. Highly significant interactions of sex and race with hypertension.	8. The well known association of this disease with both race and gender can be noted in the development of atherosclerosis in the very' young.
9. Correlation of abdominal fat-pad thickness with extent of right coronary artery atherosclerosis but not with aortic atherosclerosis.	9. Obesity may carry a special risk for coronary disease.
10. Highly significant correlation of elevated glycosylated hemoglobin values with the extent of the atheromatous process.	10. Impaired glucose tolerance may exert its atherogenic effect long before there is any evidence of overt diabetes.

* All of these findings have been extended to plaque morphometry and topography (mapping) of the extent and patterns of plaque locations at the morphometry center at Ohio State University using computer-assisted macro- and micromorphometric methods.

cross-sections of the proximal left anterior descending artery (LAD) fixed by pressure perfusion are calling attention to two very important aspects of the pathogenesis of atherosclerosis which have been poorly appreciated previously.

- Some of the risk factors affect some parts of the arterial tree much more than others and not necessarily the 'lesion-prone' part of the lower abdominal aorta.
- Many of the risk factors can be observed to have a real effect on lesion extent and severity much earlier than might be appreciated if one did not have a systematic quantitative study of the standardized samples of arteries and their developing atheromatosis from a large number of individuals such as that provided by PDAY.

This was first reported in the paper published on smoking and hyperlipidemia in

JAMA in 1990 (PDAY Research Group 1990). Similar findings are now being obtained in relation to hyperglycemia, hypertension, abdominal obesity, and the end is not yet in sight.

We can look forward to a number of new observations regarding the effects of lipoprotein(a) (Lp(a)) at the gross and microscopic level, as Kuzumi's studies are continued and extended. We can also anticipate many more innovative observations as well as the quantitative effects of the many additional genetic abnormalities found to have an effect at the artery wall and lesion level.

The study has not reached its peak in terms of revelations about new relationships of age, race and sex to lesion development. In fact, the extended period of collection of female cases afforded by the peer review system of NHLBI is sure to increase substantially our knowledge regarding the sex-linked differences in atherosclerotic lesions developing during these important second, third, and fourth decades of life, an age period in which our knowledge has been limited in the past.

SUMMARY

In this brief communication I have tried to reflect some of the most noteworthy features and accomplishments of this unique research program, widely known as PDAY, during its relatively brief productive period. We have overcome many obstacles and pursued our search for those factors responsible for the progression or protection against progression of this pervasive disease process. There can be little doubt from the results produced thus far that progression does in fact begin in the late teens or early 20's for many individuals, while in others atherosclerosis hardly progresses at all, even in the most disease-prone parts of the arterial tree. The knowledge we have gained, which helps explain this huge difference, is proving to be of enormous value to the developing specialty of Preventive Cardiology.

We are proud of what we have accomplished so far, and we trust that the large store of highly valuable and usable, anatomically well defined, fixed and frozen arterial and other tissue samples can be preserved and utilized. When combined with the large amounts of quantitative anatomical, anthropometric, and risk factor data plus the large collection of microscopic slides, photographs, and computer images, this constitutes an incomparable record of atherogenesis in young people in the late twentieth century. We hope and trust that these unique research materials will be utilized by numerous enterprising investigators for many years to come to the ultimate benefit of people everywhere.

Acknowledgments
The author and the PDAY Research Group are grateful for the assistance of Alexander Arguelles, Gertrud Friedman, Mary C. Gorney, Laura Hiltscher and Blanche Berger for their skillful help in preparing this presentation and this manuscript.

REFERENCES

Cornhill JF, Herderick EE 1993 Arterial disease in young people. *In*: DH Blankenhorn (Ed) American Journal of Cardiology Continuing Education Series. Atherogenesis and regression. Part I. Development of atherosclerosis. Cahners Healthcare Communications, New York

Cornhill JF, Herderick EE, Stary HC 1990 Topography of human aortic sudanophilic lesions in blood flow in large arteries: applications to atherogenesis and clinical medicine. Monogr Atheroscler 15: 13

Hixson JE, Vernier DT 1990 Restriction isotyping of human apolipoprotein E by gene amplification and cleavage with HhaI. J Lipid Res 31: 545

Hixson JE, McGill HC, Strong JP, McMahan CA, and the Pathobiological Determinants of Atherosclerosis in Youth (PDAY) Research Group 1992 Apolipoprotein B insertion/deletion polymorphisms affect atherosclerosis in young black but not young white males. Arterioscler Thromb 12: 1023

Komatsu A, Wissler RW, Vesselinovitch D 1989 Cell populations in atheromatous lesions in young people. Arterosclerosis 9: 709a.

Kusumi Y, Wissler RW 1991a Aortic Lp(a) deposition in young people. FASEB J 5: A1254

Kusumi Y, Wissler RW 1991b The localization of Lp(a) in the aortas of young people. 9th International Symposium on Atherosclerosis. Abstract p 75

Oyer C 1993 The greater extent of epitopes of oxidized low density lipoproteins in the early atherosclerotic lesions of smokers as compared to nonsmokers. Honors manuscript. University of Chicago Bachelor's Honor Thesis

Pathobiological Determinants in Youth (PDAY) Research Group 1990 Relationship of atherosclerosis in young men to serum lipoprotein cholesterol concentrations and smoking: a preliminary report from the PDAY Research Group. JAMA 264: 3018–3024

Pathobiological Determinants in Youth (PDAY) Research Group 1993 Natural history of aortic and coronary atherosclerotic lesions in youth: findings from the PDAY study. Arterioscler Thromb 13: 1291–1298

Strong JP 1992 Atherosclerotic lesions: natural history, risk factors, and topography. Arch Pathol Lab Med 116: 1268

Strong JP, Oalmann MC, Malcom GT, Newman WP III, McMahan CA, and the Pathobiological Determinants of Atherosclerosis in Youth (PDAY) Research Group 1992 Pathobiological Determinants of Atherosclerosis in Youth (PDAY): rationale, methodology, and selected risk factor findings. Cardiovascular Risk Factors 2: 22

Wissler RW 1991 USA multicenter study of the pathobiology of atherosclerosis in youth. Ann NY Acad Sci 623: 26

Wissler RW 1993 Human transplant atheroarteritis and its relationship to other forms of risk factor engendered injury of the artery wall: summarizing presentation. 7th International Münster Symposium, 'Modern Aspects of the Pathogenesis of Atherosclerosis.' Rheinisch-Westfälische Akademie der Wissenschaften, Münster September 27–28 1993

Wissler RW 1994 New insights into the pathogenesis of atherosclerosis as revealed by PDAY. Atherosclerosis 108 (Suppl.) S3–S20

Wissler RW, Vesselinovitch D, Davis HR, Lambert PH, Bekermeier M 1985 A new way to look at atherosclerotic involvement of the artery wall and the functional effects. Ann NY Acad Sci 454: 9

Wissler RW, Vesselinovitch D, Komatsu A 1990 The contribution of studies of atherosclerotic lesions in young people to future research. Ann NY Acad Sci 598: 418

Wissler RW, Komatsu A, Ko C, Kusumi Y, Vesselinovitch D 1991a The cell populations and other components of the atheromatous lesions in young people. *In*: Hauss WH, Wissler RW, Bauch H-J (Eds) New aspects of metabolism and behaviour of mesenchymal cells during the pathogenesis of atherosclerosis. Westdeutscher Verlag, Opladen, p 49

Wissler RW, Komatsu A, Kusumi Y, Curi E, Hiltscher L, Vessel D 1991b Qualitative and quantitative distribution of stainable lipid in the intimal atheromatous lesions of 100 young people, aged 15-34 years. 9th International Symposium on Atherosclerosis. Abstract p 41

Wissler RW, Komatsu A, Curi E, Hiltscher L 1992 Classification of the intermediate atherosclerotic lesions in young people. Abstract XI International Symposium on Drugs Affecting Lipid Metabolism

Wissler RW, Hiltscher L, Gage A, Bekermeier M 1993 A useful classification of the intermediate atherosclerotic lesions in the aortas of young people (gross and microscopic lesions). Poster presented at the 26th Hugh Lofland Conference on Arterial Wall Metabolism, Bowman-Gray School of Medicine, Winston-Salem, North Carolina, 6-8 May 1993

Wissler RW, Hiltscher L, Oinuma T, and the PDAY Research Group 1994 Pathogenesis of atherosclerosis — the lesions of atherosclerosis in the young: from fatty streaks to intermediate lesions. *In*: Fuster V, Ross R, Topol E (Eds) Atherosclerosis and coronary artery disease. Raven Press, New York (in press)

Pathobiological Determinants of Atherosclerosis in Youth (PDAY) Research Group

Directors: Program Director: RW Wissler PhD MD, University of Chicago Associate Directors: AL Robertson Jr MD PhD, University of Illinois; JP Strong MD, Louisiana State University

Steering Committee: JF Cornhill DPhil, Ohio State University; HC McGill Jr MD and CA McMahan PhD, University of Texas Health Science Center at San Antonio; AL Robertson Jr MD PhD, University of Illinois; JP Strong MD, Louisiana State University; RW Wissler PhD MD, University of Chicago

University of Alabama: Department of Medicine: Principal Investigator: S Gay MD, Coinvestigators: RE Gay MD and C-Q Huang MD.(HL-33733); Department of Biochemistry: Principal Investigator: EJ Miller PhD, Coinvestigators: DK Furuto PhD; MS Vail; AJ Narkates (HL-33728)

Albany Medical College: Principal Investigator: A Daoud MD; Coinvestigators: AS Frank PhD; MA Hyer, EC McGovern (HL-33765)

Baylor College of Medicine: Principal Investigator: LC Smith PhD; Coinvestigator: FM Strickland PhD (HL-33750)

University of Chicago; Principal Investigator: RW Wissler PhD MD; Coinvestigators: D Vesselinovitch DVM MS; A Komatsu MD PhD,: Y Kusumi MD; RT Bridenstine MS, RJ Stein MD; RH Kirschner MD; M Bekermeier ASCP; B Berger ASCP; L Hiltscher ASCP (HL-33740)

The University of Illinois: Principal Investigator: AL Robertson Jr MD PhD;_Coinvestigators: RJ Stein MD; EE Emeson MD; L Ghosh MD; HM Yamashiroya PhD; RJ Buschmann PhD; ER Donoghue Jr MD; TL An MD; E Choi MD; N Jones MD; MI Jumbelic MD; MS Kalelkar MD; U Konakci MD; Barry Lifschultz MD; M-L Shen PhD; R Yang MS; VR Gumidyala MD; R Harper BS; F Norris HTL ASCP (HL-33758)

Louisiana State University: Principal Investigator: JP Strong MD; Coinvestigators: GT Malcom PhD; WP Newman III MD; MC Oalmann DrPH; PS Roheim MD; AK Bhattacharyya PhD; MA Guzman PhD; AA Hatem MD; CA Hornick PhD; CD Restrepo MD; RE Tracy MD PhD (HL-33746); CC Breaux MS; SE Hubbard; CS Zsembik; DG Gibbs (HL-33746)

University of Maryland: Principal Investigator: WJ Mergner MD PhD; Coinvestigators: JH Resau PhD; RD Vigorito MS PA; Q-C Yu MD; J Smialek (HL-33752)

Medical College of Georgia: Coprincipal Investigators: AB Chandler MD; RN Rao MD; Coinvestigators: DG Falls MD; BO Spurlock BA; Associate Investigators: KB Sharma MD; JS Sexton MD; Research Assistants: KK Smith HTASCP, GW Forbes (HL-33772)

University of Nebraska: Principal Investigator: BM McManus MD PhD; Coinvestigators: JW Jones MD; TJ Kendall MS; JA Remmenga BS; WC Rogler BS(HL-33778)

Ohio State University: Principal Investigator: JF Cornhill DPhil; Coinvestigators: WR Adrion MD; PM Fardel MD; B Gara MS; E Herderick; J Meimer MS; LR Tate MD (HL-33760)

Southwest Foundation for Biomedical Research: Principal Investigator: JE Hixson PhD; PK Powers (HL-39913)

The University of Texas Health Science Center at San Antonio: Principal Investigator: CA McMahan PhD, Coinvestigators: GM Barnwell PhD; HC McGill Jr MD; YN Marinez MA; TJ Prihoda PhD; HS Wigodsky MD PhD (HL-33749)

Vanderbilt University: Principal Investigator: R Virmani MD; Coinvestigators: JB Atkinson MD PhD; CW Harlan MD (HL-33770)

West Virginia University: Principal Investigator: SN Jagannathan PhD; Coinvestigators: B Caterson PhD; JL Frost MD; K Murali; K Rao MD; S Jagannathan; P Johnson; NF Rodman MD (HL-33748)

Multiple Risk Factors in Cardiovascular Disease, ed. by A. Yamamoto, Churchill Livingstone Japan, Tokyo, pp. 37–40 (1994)

ATHEROSCLEROSIS IN YOUNG JAPANESE

Isamu SAKURAI

*Department of Pathology, Nihon University School of Medicine**

Key words: atherosclerosis, young, coronary artery, aorta, intima

Although it is widely believed that arterial atherosclerosis is a geriatric diseases because ischemic injuries of the target organs such as myocardial or cerebral infarction occurs usually in people past middle-age, atherosclerosis in young people is now being studied by groups as multi-institutional cooperative studies or by individual investigators in Japan (Tanaka *et al* 1988), U.S.A. (PDAY research group 1990, 1993), and other nations. The reasons for this is that it takes a long period of time before ischemic injury caused by atherosclerosis develops in various organs. In other words its subclinical latent period could last for many years, and its initial changes may take place during childhood. Such a long-standing subclinical period makes it difficult to gather information about its pathogenesis and natural history. In addition, it is important in any type of disease to study the initial changes in order to elucidate its etiology and pathogenesis, and to prevent its progression.

A quantitative and qualitative study of various arteries obtained at autopsy in a group of Japanese aged from new-born to 39 years of age was carried out and showed that surface involvement and atherosclerotic index increased with age; the severest effects were seen in the aorta, and then, with decreasing severity, in the coronary and cerebral arteries. In addition, age, serum cholesterol, and blood pressure were significantly and positively correlated with the severity and the area of aorta and coronary arteries affected, while atherosclerosis of cerebral arteries showed a significant correlation only with blood pressure (Tanaka *et al* 1988).

These results indicate that severity and extent of atherosclerosis and the associated risk factors may differ between arteries.

AORTAS VERSUS CORONARY ARTERIES

The occurrence, severity, and extent of lipid deposits, as well as the intimal thickening were shown to be markedly different in aortas compared with coronary arteries in a comparative pathomorphological study of 418 aortas and 326 coronary arteries obtained from autopsies on hospital patients who had died aged from new-born to 40 years of age (Sakurai *et al* 1990).

A macroscopic study of the vessel specimens stained with Sudan IV, occurrence of

* 30-1 Ohyaguchi-kami-machi, Itabashi-ku, Tokyo 173, Japan.

fatty streaks, fibrous plaque and complicated lesions in both vessels of each age group are summarized as shown in Fig. 1. As far as aortic intimas are concerned, 92% of children aged from 1 to 10 had fatty streaks, while in the case of coronary intimas only 5% exhibited fatty streaks. None of the children in this age group had either fibrous plaques or complicated lesions in both vessels. In the group between 11 and 20 years of age, 98% of the aortas showed fatty streaks on the intimas, while only 15% of the coronary arteries had fatty streaks. In the groups over 21 years of age fatty streaks were evident in 100% of the aortas, while this was the case in only 28% of the coronary arteries in the group, 21 to 30 years of age, and in 43% in the group, 31 to 40 years of age.

However, for fibrous plaques, which are believed to be more advanced lesions, the difference in frequency between the aortas and coronary arteries was not so marked. fibrous plaques were found first in the age group 11 to 20 in both aortas and coronary arteries with a 15% frequency for the aortas, and 10% for the coronary arteries. fibrous plaques were found in 54% of the aortas and in 16% in the coronary arteries in the age group 31–40.

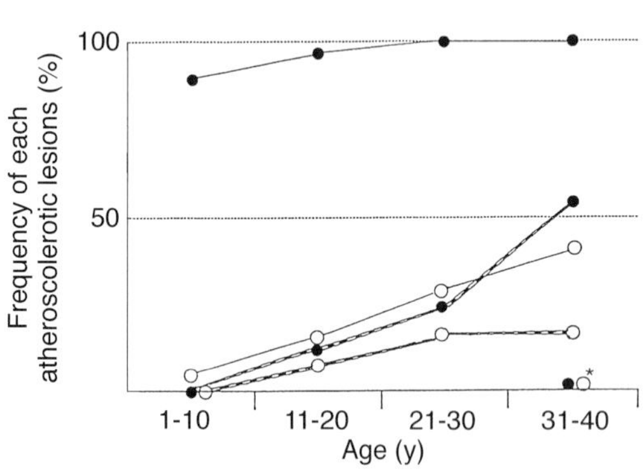

Fig. 1. Frequency of each atherosclerotic lesion in young Japanese — aorta vs coronary. 418 aortas and 326 coronaries. ●—●, fatty streak, aorta; ○—○, fatty streak, coronary; ●═●, fibrous plaque, aorta; ○═○, fibrous plaque, coronary; ●○*, complicated, aorta and coronary.

Complicated lesions were found in both vessels with same frequency, approximately 1%.

In addition, the youngest age at which each lesion was first recognized was at 1 month for a fatty streak in the aortas, but 5 yeas old in the coronary arteries, and 15 years for a fibrous plaque in the aortas and 11 years in the coronary arteries, and 36 years for a complicated lesion in the aortas and 35 years in the coronary arteries.

Furthermore, histologic cross sections from the arteries clearly revealed evidence of a much thicker intima of the coronary arteries than of the aortas, although the incidence of lipid deposits on the intima was significantly lower in the coronary arteries (Sakurai *et al* 1990).

These results indicate that fatty streaks in young people may progress to more advanced lesions, may remain unchanged for long period of time, or may regress. Thus, it seems reasonable to believe that certain pathogenic factors may differ from artery to artery, and that eccentric changes in the coronary intimas in the early period of atherosclerosis may be important for investigating local factors within the arterial walls, which may progress to lumen obstruction by intimal eccentric changes of the affected arterial segment.

CELL POPULATION AND LOCATION OF ECCENTRICALLY THICKENED INTIMAS OF THE CORONARY ARTERIES

Most of the research into the pathogenesis of atherosclerosis may be divided into two major categories: analysis of the constituents of peripheral blood, e.g. serum lipids, platelets and coagulation-fibrinolysis factors, and analysis of the biological actions of various cells and the matrix in arterial walls, e.g. endothelium, macrophages, smooth muscle cells, collagen, and/or glycosaminoglycan. Advanced atherosclerosis, however, is usually characterized by eccentric lumen obstruction at certain local predisposing sites of the arteries. These facts indicate the importance of studying local factors in the arterial wall, which could prove useful in investigating the pathogenesis of atherosclerosis as a disease entity, the most vascular disease resulting in ischemic injury to the heart, brain, and other organs. Therefore, we intend to concentrate on local intimal lesions, characterized morphologically by eccentric changes (Nakamura & Sakurai 1992).

Using immunohistochemical techniques to study the eccentric intimal changes in the arteries to monitor the cell population and location during various stages of intimal thickening, compared with diffuse intimal thickening of the arteries (Nakamura & Sakurai 1992), it became clear that coronary artery intimas frequently tended to have diffuse intimal fibrocellular thickening, in which most of the cells were thought to be smooth muscle cells and fewer macrophages than aortic intimas. Smooth muscle cells tended to be located in the deep layer and macrophages in the subendothelial superficial layer, particularly in diffuse intimal thickening of coronary arteries. Cell location pattern became varied in eccentrically thickened parts of intima of both aortas and coronary arteries. Summaries of the intimal cell populations and their location in intimal eccentrically thickened parts are shown in Fig. 2. With the thickening of intimas and progression of the intimal changes, smooth muscle cells tended to migrate upwards to the superficial layer of intimas, while macrophages moved downwards and both types of cells intermingled. Macrophages could be found in the center of the eccentric elevation, and smooth muscle cells surrounded them in inversed U or doughnut-like shape. Then, eccentric changes can progress to lesions with myxoid changes and to typical atheromatous plaques.

Lipid deposition in the arterial wall is usually seen not only in cells but also in the matrix. The mechanism of lipid binding to connective tissue fibers might be another important factor in the progression of atherosclerosis. Further studies of matrix components and their interaction with cells are need to elucidate the mechanism of lipid accumulation in the intercellular matrix.

Phase	Scheme	SMC	Mø	Histology
1	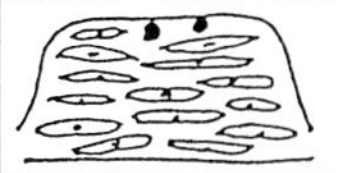	diffuse	none or trace	
2	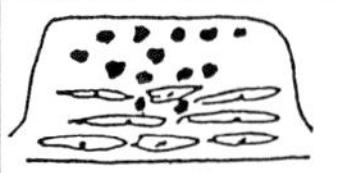	deep	superficial ~ central	
3	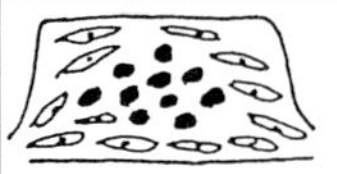	doughnut ~ inverted U	central	
4	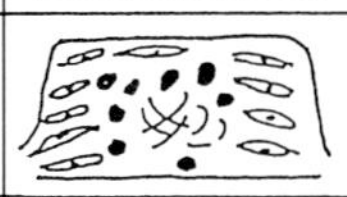			myxoid
5	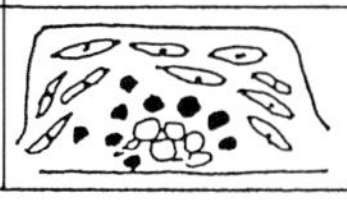			atheroma

Fig. 2. Eccentric intimal thickening of coronary arteries in young subjects — cell distribution and phase.
○SMC, smooth muscle cells; ● Mø, macrophages.

SUMMARY

To study of the pathogenesis of atherosclerosis, it is very important that one should remember that each artery exhibits its own biological activity and characteristics.

In recent years the dietary habits of young Japanese have rapidly changed due to influences from Western countries and this has resulted in an increased intake of more animal protein and fat. This leads us to expect an increasing incidence of ischemic heart disease and cerebral infarction. It is strongly suggested that prevention of atherosclerosis needs to start early in childhood.

REFERENCES

Nakamura H, Sakurai I 1992 Intimal cell population and location in arteries of Japanese children and youth. Angiology 43: 229–243

PDAY Research Group 1990 Relationship of atherosclerosis in young men to serum lipoprotein cholesterol concentrations; a preliminary report from PDAY Research Group. JAMA 264: 3018–3024

PDAY Research Group 1993 Natural history of aortic and coronary atherosclerotic lesions in youth. Arterioscler Thromb 13: 1291–1298

Sakurai I, Miyakawa K, Komatsu A, Sawada T 1990 Atherosclerosis in Japanese youth with reference to differences between each artery. Ann NY Acad Sci 598: 410–417

Tanaka K, Masuda J, Imamura T *et al* 1988 A nation-wide study of atherosclerosis in infants, children and young adults in Japan. Atherosclerosis 72: 143–156

SECTION 2.

CORONARY HEART DISEASE PREVENTION

Multiple Risk Factors in Cardiovascular Disease, ed. by A. Yamamoto, Churchill Livingstone Japan, Tokyo, pp. 43–46 (1994)

STATUS OF THE EUROPEAN GUIDELLNES FOR LIPID MANAGEMENT

Rodolfo Paoletti and Andrea Poli

*Institute of Pharmacological Sciences, University of Milan**

Key words: cholesterol, triglycerides, CHD (coronary heart disease), prevention, lipid control

At the beginning of 1993, the European Atherosclerosis Society (EAS) and the U. S. National Institutes of Health (NIH) released two documents on cardiovascular disease prevention, a topic of great interest to western societies, where these pathological conditions remain the principal public health problem, notwithstanding a decreasing trend (Prevention of Coronary Heart Disease 1992; National Cholesterol Education Program 1994).

One main message emerges from both reports: lipid control plays a key role in the prevention of myocardial infarction and related diseases, but the physician's attention, previously concentrated on risk factors, should now move to the patient.

The EAS document, particularly, suggests the idea of an "individual global risk" as the guideline for the clinical control of the patient at risk of coronary heart disease (CHD). The meaning of this parameter is intuitive: it helps to quantify the possibility that an individual will experience a coronary event, taking into account all the elements which represent risk factors for this condition.

The attitude to the role of lipid profile alteration in the process of atherogenesis is essentially unchanged: both the EAS and NIH reports emphasize its causal role, and confirm that the control of blood cholesterol levels, when they are increased, represents one of the most effective instruments for reducing or reversing the clinical course of atherosclerotic disease.

Specifically, the EAS document suggests that the medical approach toward dislipidemia must be particularly aggressive when the high density lipoprotein (HDL) cholesterol level is below 35 mg/dl in men and 42 mg/dl in women, or when the relationship between total cholesterol and HDL cholesterol is greater than 5. Patients with an low density lipoprotein (LDL)/HDL cholesterol ratio greater than 5, or with familial dislipidemia, must be considered at further increased risk. In familial dislipidemias, in fact, the symptoms of CHD often develop before patients reach the age of forty.

The EAS document underlines the fact that the LDL fraction of total cholesterol is responsible for the atherogenetic process; for this reason, the LDL cholesterol level assumes a role of "indicator" of danger as far as the lipidic profile is concerned; different target values for this parameter must be set

* via Balzaretti 9, 20133 Milan, Italy.

in subjects with different levels of individual overall risk (Tables I and II).

The achievement of an LDL cholesterol level of 155–175 mg/dl will, for example, be satisfactory in subjects with an average overall risk (for example, a patient with a blood cholesterol at the beginning of treatment below 300 mg/dl, without nonlipid risk factors, and a total cholesterol/HDL cholesterol ratio between 4.5 and 5, indicating a good HDL cholesterol level); but the same result would not be considered sufficient in an individual who, because of the presence of a non-lipid risk factor (hypertension, smoking, diabetic disease etc.), or because of a low HDL cholesterol, must be considered at higher risk. In this condition, according to the EAS document, it is appropriate to shift the LDL cholesterol to 135–155 mg/dl.

TABLE I. Target Levels for Total and LDL Cholesterol

Global risk: mildly increased	
e.g.: cholesterol 200–300 mg/dl (5.2–7.8 mmol/liter) no non-lipid risk factors total cholesterol/HDLc ratio 4.5–5.0	
reduce chol. to	195–230 mg/dl (5–6 mmol/liter)
reduce LDLc to	155–175 mg/dl (4–4.5 mmol/liter)
Global risk: increased	
e.g.: cholesterol 200–300 mg/dl (5.2–7.8 mmol/liter) plus one non-lipid risk factor	
or plus HDLc < 39 mg/dl (< 1 mmol/liter)	
reduce chol. to	195 mg/dl (5 mmol/liter)
reduce LDLc to	135–155 mg/dl (3.5–4 mmol/liter)
Global risk: high	
e.g.: presence of CHD or of PVD	
or presence of familial hypercholesterolemia,	
or cholesterol > 300 mg/dl (> 7.8 mmol/liter)	
or cholesterol 200–300 mg/dl (5.2–7.8 mmol/liter) plus two, or one severe, non lipid risk factor	
reduce chol. to	175–195 mg/dl (4.5–5 mmol/liter)
reduce LDLc to	115–135 mg/dl (3–3.5 mmol/liter)

CHD, coronary heart disease; PVD, peripheral vascular disease; LDL, low density lipoproteins; HDL, high density lipoproteins.

TABLE II. Target Levels for LDLc

Patients with established CHD
Some authorities advise for these patients an LDLc target of 95–115 mg/dl (2.5–3.0 mmol/liter)

In individuals with a high coronary risk (for example, patients with established CHD, or with an obstructive vascular pathology involving the carotid or lower limbs, or patients with a plasma cholesterol greater than 300 mg/dl, with familial dislipidemia, or in whom hypercholesterolemia and a pair of non-lipid risk factors coexist) the therapeutic aim will be to reduce the level of LDL cholesterol even further to 115–135 mg/dl.

An "addendum" to the document reminds us that some authors have set a more ambitious target value for individuals already affected by CHD, namely an LDL cholesterol level between 95 and 115 mg/dl.

The overall approach suggested by the U.S. NIH document is substantially similar.

Once again, the indicator which determines the degree and vigor of the intervention is the LDL cholesterol level; a more forceful, and even innovative, message is that the concentration of serum cholesterol linked to this lipoprotein fraction must be reduced back to 100 mg/dl or lower in subjects already affected by CHD (infarction or angina). The NIH report is categoric on this point, underscoring the fact that cholesterol reduction in these patients, as an instrument of secondary prevention, is characterized by a very favorable cost-benefit relationship.

In patients with lower global risk (this concept is similar to the guiding principle of the EAS document), it is sufficient to reduce the LDL cholesterol level to around 130 mg/dl (for example, in individuals with no evidence of clinical CHD but with multiple con-

TABLE III. The U.S. NIH Guidelines for Patients with and without CHD

	LDL cholesterol	
	Level or drug consideration	Goal of therapy
Without CHD and with fewer than 2 risk factors	≥ 190 mg/dl*	< 160 mg/dl
Without CHD and with 2 or more risk factors	≥ 160 mg/dl	< 130 mg/dl
With CHD	≥ 130 mg/dl†	≤ 100 mg/dl

* In men <35 years of age and premenopausal women with LDL cholesterol levels of 190 to 219 mg/dl, drug therapy should be delayed except in high-risk patients such as those with diabetes.

† In CHD patients with LDL cholesterol levels of 100 to 129 mg/dl, the physician should exercise clinical judgment in deciding whether to initiate drug treatment.

comitant risk factors), or even to 160 mg/dl (for example, in individuals without concomitant risk factors) (Table III).

Significantly the American document also proposes the creation of an "ad hoc" category for individuals with a particularly low coronary heart risk (for example, young male subjects or pre-menopausal women). For subjects of this group, the document identifies an LDL cholesterol of around 190 mg/dl as a reasonable and sufficient therapeutic aim. If the level rises above 220 mg/dl then steps must be taken to reduce it. These point are of relevant practical importance since a large fraction of the population is involved.

Also particularly interesting in the NIH report is the emphasis on the role of HDL cholesterol: a high level of this parameter (>60 mg/dl) is an indicator of reduced coronary risk, representing a "negative risk factor", that can balance the presence of another classic coronary risk factor. A 30 year-old subject, for example, should be considered at a low risk, even if he is a smoker, if he has an HDL cholesterol level higher than 60 mg/dl.

A controversial topic as far as the prevention of CHD by means of cholesterol control is concerned, is the elderly. The physician who has to decide whether or not he should treat a dislipidemia in a patient at this stage of life is often worried by understandable doubts and uncertainties.

The NIH document underlines that the benefits deriving from the treatment of hypercholesterolemia appear after a relatively short period (in the order of two years); in absence of concomitant conditions which might limit the expected life-span of the patient, it seems therefore wise to start therapeutic treatment, should the level of serum lipids require it, even in the elderly.

Moving to treatment, both documents emphasize that in control of dislipidemias the dietary approach should precede the pharmacological one.

However, one should consider that the therapeutic target to be reached in patients affected by CHD (an LDL cholesterol level around 100 mg/dl) is very often beyond what can be obtained by hypocholesterolemic dietary treatments, even if they are well conducted. In these specific conditions, it would therefore not seem wise to prolong excessively a restricted lipid diet before starting a targeted pharmacological treatment. For example, in a patient who has already suffered a heart attack, with a starting total cholesterol level around 240 mg/dl, the maximum lowering of plasma cholesterol which can usually be achieved by correctly conducted dieting (about 10–15% in the majority of cases), will not allow the therapeutic aim to be achieved: consequently, in most of these patients, treatment with a hypolipidemic drug will be necessary.

The role of hypertriglyceridemia in the genesis of CHD is analyzed in different ways by the two documents. The EAS document considers hypertriglyceridemia, especially if linked to low HDL cholesterol levels, an important risk factor. This parameter can be controlled by changes in diet and lifestyle; when CHD risk is particularly high, the administration of a specific drug can be considered.

The NIH document, on the other hand, points out that the results of controlled clinical trials investigating the involvement of hypertriglyceridemia in the atherogenesis process cannot be considered conclusive, and that further studies need to be carried out to confirm the validity of the results currently available.

The main message emerging from both reports is that by controlling dislipidemia, within the frame of the overall patient risk, it is possible to effectively prevent CHD.

If the physician and the cardiologist will follow the diagnostic and therapeutic approaches suggested by both the EAS and NIH, the incidence of this disease in the western world will most likely continue decreasing, a trend that has already been apparent for several years.

REFERENCES

National Cholesterol Education Program 1994 Detection, evaluation, and treatment of high blood cholesterol in adults (adult treatment panel II). Circulation 89: 1329–1445

Prevention of Coronary Heart Disease 1992 Scientific background and new clinical guidelines. Recommendation of the European Atherosclerosis Society prepared by the international task force for the prevention of CHD. Nutr Metab Cardiovasc Dis 3: 113–156

Multiple Risk Factors in Cardiovascular Disease, ed. by A. Yamamoto, Churchill Livingstone Japan, Tokyo, pp. 47–52 (1994)

DIETARY CONTROL IN THE PUBLIC AND CORONARY ARTERY DISEASE PREVENTION

John C. LaRosa

*Chancellor of Tulane University Medical Center**

Key words: diet, coronary artery disease, dietary fat, dietary cholesterol, dietary fiber

Questions about diet often come to physicians. This discussion will update some of the dietary issues that have generated interest regarding blood cholesterol and its relationships to both diet and coronary artery disease (CAD).

I SATURATED FAT

The long-held belief that the amount of saturated fat in the diet is directly related both to increased cholesterol and the risk of coronary disease in the population is still intact. Nevertheless, it has become clear that fatty acids are not all equivalent as far as raising blood cholesterol is concerned.

For example, considerable attention has been paid recently to stearic acid, an 18-carbon saturated fatty acid, that does not raise low-density lipoprotein cholesterol (LDL-C) when given in experimental-formula diets (Bonanome & Grundy 1988). It has been hypothesized that this is due to the fact that stearic acid is rapidly converted after absorption to a monounsaturated fat and so does not, like many other saturated fats, increase LDL-C. Nevertheless, excessive quantities of most dietary, saturated fats, whether from animals or vegetable sources such as coconut, palm, or palm kernel oils, are likely to be associated with an undesirable increase in LDL-C and an increased risk in coronary disease. Maintaining total saturated fat below 10% of total calories is still recommended (Summary of NCEP Expert Panel 1993).

II MONOUNSATURATED FAT

For sometime it has been observed that, despite the fact that populations in the Mediterranean Basin take substantial quantities of their calories as fat (about 30% of calories versus about 35% in the United States), the risk of coronary disease among such populations is, nevertheless, quite low. Recent studies with oleic acid, which is the major fatty acid component of olive oil, have provided some possible insights as to the reasons for this difference. Oleic is a monounsaturated fat; that is, it has only one carbon-carbon double bond in its chain. Oleic acid has also been observed in experimental studies to lower LDL-C proportionately more than high-density lipoprotein cholesterol (HDL-C). This is in contradistinc-

* 1430 Tulane Avenue, Box SL-76, Room 1550, New Orleans, LA 70112-2669, USA.

tion to polyunsaturated fats, with more than one carbon-carbon double bond (found in vegetable oils such as corn and safflower oils), which lower both LDL-C and HDL-C. One hypothesis holds that because olive oil, and therefore oleic acid, makes up as much as 50% of the fat intake in Mediterranean diets, LDL-C is lower while HDL-C is maintained in these populations. As a result, the risk of coronary disease is lower.

In fact, not all studies support these differences in lipoprotein effects between mono- and polyunsaturated fats. An alternate explanation may be that oleic acid, when incorporated into LDL particles, makes them more resistant to oxidation. Since it is oxidized LDL that is thought to deposit in the walls of arteries, any antioxidant effect of monounsaturates would render LDL less prone to uptake by arterial wall macrophages and therefore less atherogenic. Finally, the so-called Mediterranean diet may be healthy for other reasons, including the simple fact that it contains less saturated fat.

III TRANS FATTY ACIDS

Not all monounsaturated fats have the same benefits as oleic acid. When polyunsaturated fats are hydrogenated in order to make them more solid at room temperature, one result is the production of elaidic acid. Elaidic acid, a "*trans*" fatty acid, is identical in composition to oleic acid, a "*cis*" fatty acid, in terms of number of carbon, hydrogen, and oxygen atoms. However, a molecule of elaidic acid is shaped differently because the hydrogen atoms are arranged differently around the carbon-carbon double bond. Elaidic acid, the trans fatty acid, has the same dietary effects as a saturated fat, raising rather than lowering LDL-C (Mensink & Katan 1990). Moreover, trans fatty acids have been shown to raise levels of lipoprotein (a), a complex lipoprotein strongly associated with increased coronary risk (Mensink *et al* 1992).

IV FISH OILS

Studies in populations that regularly consume fish as part of their diet indicate that the rates of coronary disease are lower and this is directly related to the amount of fish in the diet (Kromhout *et al* 1985). Clinical trials, in which some patients with established coronary disease were given advice to eat fish as part of their diet, indicated that those who received such advice subsequently had lower rates of recurrent coronary events (Burr 1989). Thus, fish in the diet appears to protect against the development and progression of coronary disease. This may simply indicate that diets that are relatively higher in terms of fish intake are lower in animal fat.

On the other hand, there is evidence that the so-called omega 3 fatty acids, the polyunsaturated fatty acids that are found in high concentrations in fish, have physiological effects that might be expected to reduce the risk of atherosclerosis. These include inhibition of platelet stickiness, increasing HDL-C, and lowering triglycerides (Harris 1989).

On the other hand, many studies on the ingestion of fish oils (as opposed to fish in the diet) indicate that LDL-C may actually rise as a result of fish oil ingestion. Since fish oils interfere with platelet stickiness, there is, moreover, some reason to be concerned that they might be associated with increased risks from hemorrhage. In fact, in populations in which fish oil ingestion is high, there does appear to be an increased morbidity and mortality from disorders such as hemorrhage stroke (Goto 1985).

V DIETARY CHOLESTEROL

The phenomenon of dietary cholesterol, itself, is often overlooked in discussions of diet and coronary disease. It has been known for some time that dietary cholesterol is a relatively minor determinant of the circulating level of cholesterol in the blood. Saturated fat is the major determinant in western diets. Most foods that contain saturated fat are of animal origin and also contain cholesterol. There are, however, some plant foods like coconut oil, palm oil, and palm kernel oil that contain large amounts of saturated fat but no cholesterol. Because of their saturated fat content, these foods are likely to raise LDL-C even though dietary cholesterol may be absent.

On the other hand, there are a few foods, predominantly eggs, that contain large amounts of cholesterol with relatively insignificant amounts of saturated fat. Therefore, concentrating on reducing the amount of eggs in the diet without also lowering animal fat levels is not likely to result in any significant decline in cholesterol.

Dietary cholesterol has also been correlated with the appearance in the blood of a form of LDL that is small and more dense than normal LDL and more easily oxidized (Williams *et al* 1986). This LDL is thought to be more likely to lead to an increased risk of atherogenesis than 'normal' LDL. It has been recently demonstrated that some individuals are very sensitive to cholesterol in the diet, while others do not appear to react to increased blood cholesterol (Lehtimaki *et al* 1992). This observation has little practical value since there are no clinical means available to detect those individuals who will be sensitive to dietary cholesterol. Current recommendations are to limit cholesterol intake to less than 300 mg a day or no more than four egg yolks per week in all forms of food, including baked products (Summary of NCEP Expert Panel 1993).

VI FIBER

Oat bran, psyllium, guar gum, and pectin, all soluble fiber, found in laxatives, fruits, and vegetables, lower LDL-C. Studies indicate that oat bran, as well as other soluble fibers, lower LDL-C about 5% following long-term use (Van Horn *et al* 1986). In addition, dietary fiber has been shown to lower blood sugar and insulin requirements in diabetes (Riccardi & Rivellese 1991).

Insoluble fibers such as wheat bran have no effect on cholesterol (Kestin *et al* 1990), although they may increase stool size and regularize bowel habits and relieve constipation. For a few patients with borderline cholesterol, the addition of fiber to the diet, either in foods or with regular amounts of psyllium in the form of bulk laxatives, may promote a small degree of cholesterol lowering and can be used as an adjunct to a cholesterol-lowering diet or even to cholesterol-lowering drugs. The American Heart Association (AHA) and the National Cholesterol Education Program (NCEP) put no numerical recommendations on dietary fiber but have indicated that western diets are too low in fiber and that fiber contained in vegetables and fruits could be comfortably doubled.

VII ALCOHOL

Alcohol is an addicting drug that, in susceptible individuals, can lead to chronic, debilitating, and often fatal degenerative diseases. Its use presents potential dangers not only for the user but also for others in his or her environment. It is the source of a considerable proportion of all accidental deaths.

In moderation, however, alcohol is enjoyed by many as a dietary supplement. There is little doubt, moreover, that in moderate quantities, it is associated with lower mortality rates from coronary disease. In fact, the overall mortality rates when plotted against alcohol intake show a U-shaped distribution; that is, individuals with an alcohol intake equivalent to one drink a day have lower mortality rates than either teetotalers or heavier drinkers. There appears to be an inverse relationship between alcohol intake and death from coronary disease.

This may be potentially explained by several effects. Alcohol consistently raises HDL-C, lowers platelet stickiness and fibrinogen levels, all with favorable effects on coronary risk. In fact, the entire 'French Paradox', i.e., the observation that in France, dietary saturated fat is poorly correlated with CAD risk, is explainable by the large per capita intake of alcohol (in the form of wine) in that country (Hegsted & Ausman 1988). Despite claims for the particular virtues of red wine, the best evidence thus far available is that alcohol has the same effect regardless of the carrier, that is, alcohol from beer, wine, or spirits is equally protective against coronary disease.

Not all the effects of alcohol on the vascular system are positive. Alcohol has also been shown to be associated with increased risk of hypertension and hemorraghic stroke. In addition, alcohol in excessive quantities can cause alcoholic cardiomyopathy and lead to congestive heart failure and even death (Klatsky *et al* 1992).

In non-drinkers, there is little to recommend that alcohol be started. Rather, such patients should be encouraged to follow cholesterol-lowering diets, get regular exercise, and maintain ideal body weight.

VIII COFFEE AND CORONARY ARTERY DISEASE

Scores of papers have been written about whether coffee in some form or another affects LDL-C, HDL-C, or CAD. Because coffee is often associated with other habits like cigarette smoking and high levels of saturated fat intake, which may themselves promote coronary disease, it has sometimes been difficult to separate the effects of coffee itself. In a recent meta-analysis, however, many of these studies were combined and controlled for other risk factors (Grobbee *et al* 1990). In that study, coffee ingestion was found to have no increased risk of either fatal or non-fatal coronary or cerebral vascular disease. It is likely that some individuals are susceptible to coffee, either because of the arrhymogenic effects of caffeine or for some other reason. Coffee ingestion for most of us, however, even beyond four cups a day, is of no substantial danger from the point of view of CAD. On the other hand, excessive ingestion of caffeinated coffee should be regarded as at least a mild form of drug addiction and may be associated with withdrawal symptoms when suddenly stopped (Silverman *et al* 1992).

IX DIET RESPONSE

All of what has been said assumes the more or less uniform response of individuals to various dietary factors. In fact, however, that is not always the case. There is a growing body of evidence that particular groups of individuals may reveal very different responses to dietary components. For example, men and women may not respond to dietary components in the same way. In studies where men and women have been compared, lowering of saturated fat leads to greater decreases in LDL-C in men than in women. Low saturated fat diets in women, on the other hand, may lead to greater lowering of HDL-C than in men. It is not clear whether this represents any increased danger to women. However, as noted earlier (Lehtimaki *et al* 1992), there are some individuals who respond with more sensitivity to dietary cholesterol than others. This is of little practical value, however, since there are no clinically available means to identify such individuals and not even any good evidence that such a response will be consistent if measured at different times.

Age may also be a factor in dietary responsiveness. There is some indirect evidence that as older people are followed over a ten-year period, total cholesterol and LDL-C increase even as total and saturated fat intake decline in both men and women.

Finally, there is preliminary evidence that certain genetic patterns of circulating apoproteins (for example, those with the so-called apoprotein E-4 genotype) identify individuals who may be particularly sensitive to dietary cholesterol and saturated fat (Lehtimaki *et al* 1992).

Until we have ways of identifying people who are sensitive to dietary cholesterol and saturated fat, the current recommendations of the NCEP should be regarded as moderate, prudent, and safe (Summary of NCEP Expert Panel 1993). In addition, of course, the maintenance of ideal body weight and regular exercise are also important ancillary factors.

X ANTIOXIDANTS

Recent evidence suggests that the oxidation of LDL is responsible for its atherogenicity. Animal studies and human observational studies suggest that dietary antioxidants such as vitamins E, C, and beta carotene may inhibit atherosclerosis (Rimm *et al* 1993; Stampfer *et al* 1993; Steinberg *et al* 1992). Data are so far insufficient, however, to make firm clinical or public health recommendations about dietary antioxidant supplementation.

SUMMARY

In addition to elements of the diet like saturated fat, polyunsaturated fat, and cholesterol, which have been emphasized in the past, a number of other dietary constituents also influence blood cholesterol. Monounsaturated fats tend to lower LDL but preserve HDL, unlike polyunsaturates, which lower both. Trans fatty acids, on the other hand, which are monounsaturates formed from the commercial hydrogenation of polyunsaturates, act like saturated fats, raising HDL. Fish oils have mixed effects, lowering triglycerides, raising HDL, but also, in many instances, raising LDL. If they are, in fact, beneficial in preventing heart disease, their effect may be as much related to a decrease in platelet stickiness as to their effects on lipoproteins. Dietary cholesterol, by itself, is not a potent factor in raising blood cholesterol. When combined with saturated fats, however, its effect increases. In addition, an increase in dietary cholesterol has been associated with the appearance of a small, dense form of LDL, which is thought to be highly atherogenic. Dietary soluble fiber has a modest LDL-C lowering effect but insoluble fiber does not. Alcohol, while it has been associated with lower mortality rates from some forms of cardiovascular disease, is also associated with an increased risk of hypertension, hemorraghic stroke, and cardiomyopathy. Its use in non-drinkers cannot be recommended.

Coffee has not been associated with an increased risk of coronary disease. Finally, the issue of individual responsiveness to diet is one that is currently being explored. Since many populations live quite adequately on dietary fat intakes much lower than those in western societies, however, attempts to lower total and saturated fat intake need not await these findings.

REFERENCES

Bonanome A, Grundy SM 1988 Effect of dietary stearic acid on plasma cholesterol and lipoprotein levels. N Engl J Med 318: 1244–1248

Burr ML 1989 Fish and the cardiovascular system. Prog Food Nutr Sci 13: 291–316

Goto Y 1985 Serum cholesterol and nutrition in Japan. Nutr Health 3: 255–257

Grobbee DE, Rimm EB, Giovannucci E *et al* 1990 Coffee, caffeine, and cardiovascular disease in men. N Engl J Med 323: 1026–1032

Harris WS 1989 Fish oils and plasma lipid and lipoprotein metabolism in humans: a critical review. J Lipid Res 30: 785–807

Hegsted DM, Ausman LM 1988 Diet, alcohol and coronary heart disease in men. J Nutr 118: 1184–1189

Kestin M, Moss R, Clifton PM *et al* 1990 Comparative effects of three cereal brans on plasma lipids, blood pressure, and glucose metabolism in mildly hypercholesterolemic men. Am J Clin Nutr 52: 661–666

Klatsky AL, Armstrong MA, Friedman GD 1992 Alcohol and mortality. Ann Intern Med 117: 646–654

Kromhout D, Bosschieter EB, Coulander CL 1985 The inverse relation between fish consumption and 20-year mortality from coronary heart disease. N Engl J Med 312: 1205–1209

Lehtimaki T, Moilanen T, Solakivi T *et al* 1992 Cholesterol-rich diet induced changes in plasma lipids in relation to apolipoprotein E phenotype in healthy students. Ann Med 24: 61–66

Mensink RP, Katan MB 1990 Effect of dietary trans fatty acids on high-density and low-density lipoprotein cholesterol levels in healthy subjects. N Engl J Med 323: 439–445

Mensink RP, Zock PL, Katan MB *et al* 1992 Effect of dietary cis and trans fatty acids on serum lipoprotein (a) levels in humans. J Lipid Res 33: 1493–1501

Riccardi G, Rivellese AA 1991 Effects of dietary fiber and carbohydrate on glucose and lipoprotein metabolism in diabetic patients. Diabetes Care 14: 1115–1125

Rimm EB, Stampfer MJ, Ascherio A, Giovannucci E, Colditz GA, Willett WC 1993 Vitamin E consumption and the risk of coronary heart disease in men. N Engl J Med 328: 1450–1456

Silverman K, Evans SM, Strain EC *et al* 1992 Withdrawal syndrome after the double-blind cessation of caffeine consumption. N Engl J Med 327: 1109–1114

Stampfer MJ, Hennekens CH, Manson JE, Colditz GA, Rosner B, Willett WC 1993 Vitamin E consumption and the risk of coronary disease in women. N Engl J Med 328: 1444–1449

Steinberg D and Workshop Participants 1992 Antioxidants in the prevention of human atherosclerosis: Summary of the Proceedings of a National Heart, Lung, and Blood Institute Workshop: September 5-6, 1991, Bethesda, MD. Circulation 85: 2338–2344

Summary of the second report of the National Cholesterol Education Program (NCEP) Expert Panel on detection, evaluation, and treatment of high blood cholesterol in adults (Adult Treatment Panel II) 1993 JAMA 269: 3015–3023

Van Horn LV, Liu K, Parker D *et al* 1986 Serum lipid response to oat product intake with a fat-modified diet. J Am Diet Assoc 86: 759–764

Williams PT, Krauss RM, Kindel-Joyce S *et al* 1986 Relationship of dietary fat, protein, cholesterol, and fiber intake to atherogenic lipoproteins in men. Am J Clin Nutr 44: 788–797

Multiple Risk Factors in Cardiovascular Disease, ed. by A. Yamamoto, Churchill Livingstone Japan, Tokyo, pp. 53–60 (1994)

CAN LIFESTYLE CHANGES REVERSE CORONARY HEART DISEASE? THE LIFESTYLE HEART TRIAL

Dean ORNISH

*Preventive Medicine Research Institute**

Key word: diet, stress, regression, yoga, exercise

I. CAN ATHEROSCLEROSIS REGRESS?

The Lifestyle Heart Trial is a randomized, controlled clinical trial to determine if ambulatory patients can be motivated to make and sustain comprehensive lifestyle changes and, if so, whether regression of coronary atherosclerosis can occur due to lifestyle changes alone. The Lifestyle Heart Trial is in two phases: phase 1 (after one year of intervention, completed), and phase 2 (the same patients after four years, recently completed). (Gould *et al* 1992; Ornish 1990, 1991a–d, 1992a–b, 1993; Ornish *et al* 1990).

Two previous trials in 1977 and 1980 assessed the short-term effects of lifestyle changes on coronary heart disease using non-invasive endpoint measures. Those two studies measured improvements in cardiac risk factors, functional status, myocardial perfusion (Ornish *et al* 1979), and left ventricular function (Ornish 1983; Ornish *et al* 1983).

In The Lifestyle Heart Trial, patients were randomly assigned to an experimental group asked to make comprehensive lifestyle changes or to a usual-care control group who followed more conventional recommendations. The average percentage stenosis diameter (%D) decreased from 40.0 to 37.8% in the experimental group but increased from 42.7 to 46.1% in the control group ($p = 0.001$). When only lesions exhibiting a greater than 50% stenosis were analyzed, the average %D decreased from 61.1 to 55.8% in the experimental group and increased from 61.7 to 64.4% in the control group ($p = 0.03$).

Overall, 82% of the experimental group patients had an average change which was in the direction of a reduction. The degree of overall adherence was strongly related to changes in the %D in a "dose-response" manner ($r = 0.62$, $p = 0.003$). Thus, comprehensive lifestyle changes may cause significant regression of even severe coronary atherosclerosis and may start after only one year, whereas more moderate changes resulted in significant progression of atherosclerosis.

In The Lifestyle Heart Trial, patients with angiographically documented coronary artery disease at baseline, who were not taking cholesterol-lowering drugs, were randomly assigned to an experimental group or to a usual-care control group. All patients who were eligible and volunteered were accepted into the study. Experimental group patients were prescribed a lifestyle program

* 900 Bridgeway, Sausalito, CA 94965, USA.

that included a low-fat vegetarian diet, moderate aerobic exercise, stress management training, smoking cessation and group support.

Control group patients were not asked to make lifestyle changes although they were free to do so. Progression or regression of coronary artery lesions was assessed in both groups by quantitative coronary angiography at baseline and after approximately one year. Cine arteriograms made in San Francisco were sent to the University of Texas Medical School at Houston for quantitative analyses (Gould 1988).

Patients completed a three-day diet diary at baseline and after one year to assess nutrient intake and dietary adherence (Stuff *et al* 1983). Patients were asked to complete a questionnaire describing smoking behavior and the type, frequency and duration of exercise and of each stress management technique. Information from these adherence questionnaires was quantified using a formula determined a priori.

To reduce the possibility that knowledge of the group assignment may bias the outcome measurements, the technicians responsible for all medical tests remained unaware of the patient group assignment. Different personnel provided the lifestyle intervention, performed the tests, analyzed the results, and computed the statistical analyses.

Experimental-group patients were asked to consume a low-fat vegetarian diet for at least one year. The diet included fruits, vegetables, grains, legumes and soybean products without caloric restriction. No animal products were allowed except for egg whites and one cup per day of non-fat milk or yogurt. The calorific content of the diet consisted of approximately 10% fat (P/S ratio >1), 15–20% protein, and 70–75% predominantly complex carbohydrates. Cholesterol intake was limited to 5 mg/day or less and salt was restricted only for hypertensive patients. Caffeine was excluded, and alcohol was limited to no more than 2 ounces per day or equivalent. The stress management techniques included stretching exercises, breathing techniques, meditation, progressive relaxation, and imagery (Benson *et al* 1974; Ornish 1992b; Patel & North 1975; Patel *et al* 1985). Patients were asked to practice these stress management techniques for at least one hour per day. Patients were individually prescribed exercise levels (typically walking) according to their baseline treadmill test results. Patients were asked to exercise for a minimum of three hours per week and to spend a minimum of 30 minutes per session exercising within their target heart rates. The twice-weekly group discussions provided social support to help patients adhere to the lifestyle-change program (Ornish 1990, 1992b; Orth-Gomer *et al* 1988; Ruberman *et al* 1984; House *et al* 1988).

Differences between the baseline characteristics of the experimental and control group patients were tested for statistical significance using conventional *t*-tests. Comparisons of these two study groups with respect to baseline coronary artery lesion characteristics (measured by quantitative coronary angiography) and changes in lesion characteristics from pre- to post-intervention were examined via a mixed model analysis of variance with clusters of varying sizes (Dixon *et al* 1983). Mean changes in other endpoint measures were analyzed for statistical significance by repeated measures analysis of variance.

At baseline, there were no significant differences between the experimental and control groups in terms of demographic characteristics, diet and lifestyle characteristics, functional status, cardiac history, or risk factors. High density lipoprotein (HDL) and apolipoprotein (apo) A-I were significantly higher in the control group, but the ratios of total cholesterol/HDL and low density lipoprotein (LDL)/HDL were not significantly different between groups at baseline. At baseline, the experimental and control groups did not significantly differ in terms of disease severity as measured by minimum diameter (D_{min}), %D, normal diameter (D_{norm}), or stenosis flow reserve (SFR).

In the experimental group, adherence to

the diet, exercise and stress management components of the lifestyle program was excellent. Patients in the control group made more moderate changes in lifestyle consistent with more conventional recommendations, including a diet consisting of approximately 30% fat and 200 mg dietary cholesterol.

In the experimental group, total cholesterol decreased from 226.5 to 171.5 mg/dl (24.3 %) and LDL cholesterol fell from 151.4 to 94.8 mg/dl (37.4 %). These decreases occurred even although many patients already had made some dietary changes prior to baseline testing. HDL cholesterol did not change significantly in either group. In the experimental group, apoB decreased from 104.0 to 78.9 mg/dl, but did not change appreciably in the control group. Neither group exhibited significant changes in apoA-I.

Functional status improved considerably and, in many patients, dramatically. Patients in the experimental group reported a 91% reduction in the frequency of angina, a 42% decrease in its duration and a 28% decrease in its severity. In contrast, control group patients reported a 165% increase in frequency, a 95% increase in duration, and a 39% increase in severity of their angina. In our earlier studies, we found that similar improvements in functional status occurred after only one month (Ornish 1983; Ornish *et al* 1979, 1983), suggesting that improvements in angina may precede regression of coronary atherosclerosis, perhaps by altering platelet-endothelial interactions, vasomotor tone, or other dynamic characteristics of stenoses.

All detectable lesions were included in the analysis. A total of 195 coronary artery lesions were detected and quantitatively analyzed. When all lesions were included, the average %D decreased from 40.0 to 37.8% in the experimental group but increased from 42.7 to 46.1% in the control group ($p = 0.001$, two-tailed). When only lesions with a stenosis greater than 50% were analyzed, the average %D decreased from 61.1 to 55.8% in the experimental group and increased from 61.7 to 64.4 % in the control group ($p = 0.03$, two-tailed).

Eighteen of the 22 patients (82%) in the experimental group had average lesion change scores ($\%D_{post}-\%D_{pre}$) in the direction of regression of coronary atherosclerosis (including the one woman in the experimental group). In contrast, 10 of the 19 control group patients (53%) had average lesion change scores in the direction of progression of coronary atherosclerosis; in contrast, all four women in the control group had average lesion change scores in the direction of regression of coronary atherosclerosis.

Within-group secondary analyses were performed to determine if the experimental group showed "true regression" rather than simply less progression than the control group. In this analysis, the experimental group showed 2.11 ± 0.98 units in the direction of regression ($p = 0.03$, two-tailed). The control group showed 4.23 ± 2.91 units in the direction of progression ($p = 0.15$, two-tailed).

In the experimental and combined groups, overall adherence to the lifestyle changes was strongly related to changes in lesions in a "dose-response" manner, suggesting a causal relationship between lifestyle changes and coronary atherosclerosis. These differences in overall adherence are sufficient to explain the observed differences in %D. To assess whether program adherence was related to lesion changes, patients in the experimental and combined groups were divided into three equal tertiles based on overall adherence score. The degree of adherence directly correlated with changes in %D.

This clinical trial demonstrated that a heterogeneous group of patients with coronary heart disease in an ambulatory population were motivated to make comprehensive changes in lifestyle for at least one year. These lifestyle changes substantially reduced total cholesterol, LDL cholesterol, and apoB, while HDL cholesterol and apoA-I remained largely unchanged. These lipid changes are comparable with those seen in studies in which cholesterol-lowering drugs were used. This intervention appears to be safe and compatible with other treatments of coronary heart disease.

After one year, patients in the experimental group began to demonstrate significant overall regression of coronary atherosclerosis (decreased %D stenosis), as measured by quantitative coronary arteriography (QCA). Since coronary atherosclerosis occurs over a period of decades, one would not expect to find larger changes after only one year. Perfusion is a fourth power function of coronary artery diameter, so even a small amount of regression in a critically stenosed artery has a disproportionate effect on myocardial perfusion and thus on functional status and clinical significance.

In contrast, patients in the usual-care control group who were making less comprehensive changes in lifestyle demonstrated significant overall progression of coronary atherosclerosis. This suggests that conventional recommendations for patients with coronary heart disease (such as a 30% fat diet) may not be sufficient to cause regression to occur in many patients, and that more comprehensive lifestyle changes may be required.

The strong relationship between program adherence and lesion changes indicates that most patients needed to follow the lifestyle program as prescribed in order to show regression. Those who made even more changes demonstrated even greater improvement. Since the degree of lifestyle change was correlated with the degree of stenosis change across the entire range of adherence, even moderate changes in lifestyle may slow the progression of atherosclerosis, whereas substantial changes in lifestyle may be required in order to halt or reverse it.

The five women in the study were the notable exceptions. One woman was randomly assigned to the experimental group and four were randomly assigned to the control group. All five made only moderate lifestyle changes, yet all showed overall regression. All five were post-menopausal, and none was taking exogenous estrogens. The four women in the control group showed more regression than any of the men in that group, even although some men made greater changes in lifestyle. While the numbers are small, these data raise the interesting possibility that gender may influence the progression and regression of atherosclerosis.

Five men in the control group also exhibited very small changes in average %D in the direction of atherosclerosis regression. These patients exercised more often, for longer periods and consumed fewer calories and less cholesterol than the control group patients who showed progression of atherosclerosis.

The more severely stenosed lesions showed the greatest improvement. Although this is the opposite of what was expected, the finding is important since more severely stenotic lesions are of greater clinical significance. More work is needed to determine to what extent the relationship between the change and initial site of lesions are influenced by the statistical phenomenon known as regression to the mean.

Some important questions remain unanswered. Whether or not these comprehensive lifestyle changes can be sustained in larger populations of patients with coronary heart disease remains to be determined. What is optimal is not always easy. Further research will be necessary to determine the mechanisms of changes in coronary atherosclerosis. It would be especially interesting to examine the effects of lifestyle changes in a larger sample of post-menopausal women with coronary atherosclerosis. Also, direct comparisons of intensive lifestyle changes with pharmacological or surgical interventions are interesting questions needing study. The Lifestyle Heart Trial suggests that comprehensive lifestyle changes may begin to reverse coronary atherosclerosis after only one year(Gould 1988; Shekelle & Stamler 1989).

II. IF SO, WHAT CAN BE DONE TO ACHIEVE REGRESSION OF HUMAN ATHEROSCLEROSIS?

Regression of coronary atherosclerosis in humans has been reported, either in controlled clinical trials or in anecdotal reports, in response to comprehensive lifestyle changes, various cholesterol lowering drugs, partial ileal bypass surgery, or plasmapheresis. Each of these interventions may be appropriate in some circumstances, either solely or in combination with other interventions. Given these possibilities, what criteria should determine our choice of intervention? The following criteria may be helpful:

- medical effectiveness;
- cost-effectiveness;
- risk-benefit ratio;
- patient motivation/adherence.

1) Medical effectiveness

Comprehensive lifestyle changes may cause significant improvement in risk factors and regression of coronary atherosclerosis. In comparison with other interventions, The Lifestyle Heart Trial measured a greater degree of overall regression in a shorter period of time. However, one should make comparisons between studies with caution given the variations from one study to another with respect to patient populations, recruitment, endpoint methodologies and statistical methods.

2) Cost-effectiveness

Cholesterol-lowering medications are costly. Lovastatin, for example, may cost $1,500/year; these costs are considerable when multiplied by the large number of people with hypercholesterolemia. As the goals for desirable plasma cholesterol levels become lower (from 260 to 200 to below 150 mg/dl), the number of people whose plasma cholesterol levels are defined as too high increases. Partial ileal bypass surgery and plasmapheresis are expensive and invasive. In principle, at least, a vegetarian diet, moderate exercise, smoking cessation and stress management may be learned at moderate cost. While no one has tested this hypothesis, it would not be surprising if comprehensive lifestyle changes may reduce the need for medication (e.g., lipid-lowering drugs) or surgery (e.g., angioplasty or coronary artery bypass surgery), thereby lowering health care costs.

3) Risk-benefit ratio

All drugs, including lipid-lowering medication, have risks and side-effects, both known and unknown, as well as potential benefits. The same is true for plasmapheresis and partial ileal bypass surgery. In contrast, the only side-effects of lifestyle changes are generally desirable ones.

4) Patient motivation/adherence

Clearly, the major obstacle to the widespread adoption of comprehensive lifestyle changes is patient adherence. It is often easier to submit to surgery or take medication than to change one's lifestyle. Paradoxically, however, it may be easier to motivate patients to make and maintain comprehensive changes in lifestyle than more moderate ones. When a patient makes only moderate changes in diet and lifestyle, there is often a feeling of deprivation but without substantial improvements in symptoms or plasma cholesterol levels. However, comprehensive lifestyle changes often cause marked reductions in the frequency of angina and plasma cholesterol levels, so the choices and benefits become clearer. Patients who, for whatever reason, do not wish to make comprehensive changes in lifestyle should be offered cholesterol-lowering drugs or other options after a clear discussion of the relative risks and benefits of each approach.

In The Lifestyle Heart Trial, we found that adherence to lifestyle changes was strongly correlated with changes in coronary atherosclerosis in a "dose-response" manner across the entire range of adherence in both the experimental and control groups.

Regression tended to occur when adherence was high, even when plasma cholesterol did not fall below 150 mg/dl or even 200 mg/dl. Serum cholesterol is important, but coronary heart disease is a multifactorial illness. Evidence suggests that dietary cholesterol and fat may contribute to coronary atherosclerosis in part independent of the effects on plasma cholesterol (Blankenhorn *et al* 1988; Shekelle & Stamler 1989). Algorithms for treating hypercholesterolemia may tend to focus too much on plasma cholesterol; attention also should be given to dietary and lifestyle factors.

III. IS REGRESSION OF HUMAN ATHEROSCLEROSIS MEASURABLE?

Using the methods of QCA pioneered by Brown (1982), Barnedt (1977), Gould (1988), and others, it is now possible to measure the degree of coronary atherosclerosis with reasonable accuracy and reproducibility. This accuracy makes feasible clinical trials with smaller cohorts and shorter durations.

However, coronary arteriography, even when quantitatively analyzed, has some inherent limitations:

1) Atherosclerosis can be fairly widespread before it impinges into the arterial lumen. Glagov demonstrated that human coronary arteries undergo compensatory enlargement in the presence of coronary atherosclerosis to preserve the cross-sectional area of the lumen (Glagov *et al* 1987). Coronary arteries enlarge as the lesion area increases and luminal stenosis may be delayed until the lesion occupies more than 40% of the internal elastic lamina, after which the lumen diminishes markedly. This phenomenon makes it more difficult to detect regression or progression in lesions that are less than 40–50% stenosed at baseline since compensatory changes in the cross-sectional area of the lumen may occur. In contrast, there would be less compensation in more severe lesions, so progression or regression would be easier to measure. Emerging technologies such as intravascular ultrasound may give a more accurate picture of the true extent of coronary atherosclerosis.

2) It is difficult to distinguish between changes in atherosclerosis and changes in vasomotor tone. If one defines "regression" as "clinical improvement," then the question is less important, for both improvements in coronary atherosclerosis and in vasomotor tone increase myocardial perfusion. Giving nitroglycerin at the time of angiography may reduce coronary vasoconstriction; however, this may introduce another confounding variable, for nitroglycerin may not always affect vasomotor tone to the same degree each time in a given patient.

3) There is no consensus as to the best endpoint measure in QCA. Traditionally, the %D has been used, but there are limitations. The %D is a function both of D_{min} and the "normal" segment adjacent to it. However, as discussed by Glagov, even seemingly normal segments are likely to be diseased. Also, one may have an apparent improvement in %D if the proximal or distal "normal" segments narrow and D_{min} is unchanged, since %D is a relative difference between D_{min} and %D. On the other hand, up to a point, a reduction in D_{norm} may paradoxically improve perfusion, if D_{min} remains constant, due to a reduction in exit losses.

The use of the relative percentage diameter narrowing as a clinical measure of severity does not account for other important geometric characteristics of stenoses, such as length, absolute cross-sectional luminal area, multiple lesions in series, or eccentric narrowing which may be worse in one view compared with another. The concept of SFR is one way of addressing this dilemma, but it, too, has limitations. The anatomic-geometric approach utilizes all the X-ray determined geometric dimensions of a stenosis, including percentage narrowing, absolute diameter and length effects. These dimensions are integrated throughout the length of the stenosis using fluid dynamic equations to predict the pressure flow characteristics of the SFR as a single integrated measure of its severity, reflecting all the combined effects of percentage narrowing, absolute diameter and length. Determination of the SFR by this quantitative analysis of coronary arteriograms correlates well with directly measured flow reserve in animals and with perfusion effects in man. In practice, however, SFR is a strict function of %D and may not provide much additional information. Also, there is little change in SFR until a lesion becomes severely stenosed.

4) Atherosclerosis is only one of several mechanisms affecting perfusion. Changes in coronary vasomotor tone, platelet adherence and aggregation, collateral circulation, free fatty acid metabolism, local endothelial factors, preload/afterload factors, and other mechanisms may affect myocardial perfusion. Since perfusion is the "bottom line" in coronary heart disease, functional measures of perfusion (e.g., cardiac PET imaging) may be a better "gold standard" than anatomical measures such as coronary arteriography. Both anatomical and functional measures provide complementary information.

5) "Not everything that counts can be counted" (Burkitt). We focus on what is measurable, but what is measurable may not necessarily be what is most interesting or important. In the FATS study by Brown *et al*, for example, there was a 73% reduction in clinical events yet only a 0.7–0.9% regression in stenosis diameter in the experimental group (Brown *et al* 1990). Thus, mechanisms other than the regression of coronary atherosclerosis may play important roles. Psychosocial factors are more difficult to measure although these, too, may play important roles in both adherence and outcome (Blankenhorn *et al* 1988).

SUMMARY

Regression of coronary atherosclerosis in patients has been reported, either in controlled clinical trials or in anecdotal reports, in response to comprehensive lifestyle changes, various cholesterol-lowering drugs, partial ileal bypass surgery, or plasmapheresis. Criteria for determining the choice of intervention may include medical effectiveness, cost-effectiveness, risk-benefit ratio and patient motivation.

In The Lifestyle Heart Trial, patients were randomly assigned to an experimental group asked to make comprehensive lifestyle changes or to a usual-care control group who followed more conventional recommendations. The average %D decreased from 40.0 to 37.8% in the experimental group yet increased from 42.7 to 46.1% in the control group ($p = 0.001$). When only lesions decreased greater than 50% stenosed were analyzed, the average %D from 61.1 to 55.8% in the experimental group and increased from 61.7 to 64.4% in the control group ($p = 0.03$). Overall, 82% of experimental group patients had an average change which was in the direction of regression. The degree of overall adherence was strongly related to changes in the %D in a "dose-response" manner ($r = 0.62$, $p = 0.003$). Thus, comprehensive lifestyle changes may produce significant regression of even severe coronary atherosclerosis apparent after only one year, whereas more moderate changes result in significant progression of atherosclerosis.

Using QCA, it is now possible to measure coronary atherosclerosis with reasonable accuracy and reproducibility. However, coronary arteriography, even when quantitatively analyzed, has some inherent limitations. Atherosclerosis can be fairly extensive before it impinges into the arterial lumen, and is only one of several mechanisms affecting myocardial perfusion. Functional measures of perfusion (e.g., cardiac PET imaging) may be a better "gold standard" than anatomical measures such as coronary arteriography. Both anatomical and functional measures provide complementary information.

REFERENCES

Barndt R, Blankenhorn DH, Crawford DW *et al* 1977 Regression and progression of early femoral atherosclerosis in treated hyperlipoproteinemic patients. Ann Intern Med 86: 139–146

Benson H, Rosner BA, Marzetta BR, Klemchuk HM 1974 Decreased blood pressure in pharmacologically treated hypertensive patients who regularly elicited the relaxation response. Lancet i: 289–291

Blankenhorn DH, Johnson RL, El Zein HA *et al* 1988 Dietary fat influences human coronary lesion formation. Circulation 78 (suppl II): 11

Brown BG, Bolson EL, Dodge HT 1982 Arteriographic assessment of coronary atherosclerosis. Review of current methods, their limitations, and clinical applications. Arteriosclerosis 2: 2–15

Brown BG, Alberts JJ, Fisher LD *et al* 1990 Regression of coronary artery disease as a result of intensive lipid-lowering therapy in men with high levels of apolipoprotein B. N Engl J Med 323: 1289–1298

Dixon WS 1983 BMDP3V statistical software, printing with additions. University of California Press, Berkeley

Glagov S, Weisenberg E, Zarins CK *et al* 1987 Compensatory enlargement of human atherosclerotic coronary arteries. N Engl J Med 316: 1371–1375

Gould KL 1988 Identifying and measuring severity of coronary artey stenosis. Quantitative coronary arteriography and positron emission tomography. Circulation 78: 237–245

Gould KL, Ornish D, Kirkeeide R *et al* 1992 Improved stenosis geometry by quantitative coronary arteriography after vigorous risk factor modification. Am J Cardiol 69: 845–853

House JS, Landis KR, Umberson D 1988 Social relationships and health. Science 241 (4865): 540–545

Ornish DM 1983 Stress, Diet, & Your Heart. New York: Holt, Rinehart and Winston 1982; New American Library (Signet Books)

Ornish D 1990 Dr. Dean Ornish's Program for Reversing Heart Disease. Random House, New York

Ornish D 1991a Can life-style changes reverse coronary atherosclerosis? Hospital Practice, May

Ornish D 1991b Can you prevent — and reverse — coronary artery disease? Patient Care 25: 25–41

Ornish D 1991c Lessons from the Lifestyle Heart Trial. Choices in Cardiology 1(5): 1–4

Ornish D 1991d Reversing heart disease through diet, exercise, and stress management. J Am Dietetic Assoc 91: 162–165

Ornish D 1992a Can atherosclerosis regress? Cardiovasc Risk Factors, 2: 274–281

Ornish D 1992b Reversing heart disease. Random House, New York, 1990; Ballantine Books, 1992

Ornish D 1993 Can lifestyle changes reverse coronary coronary heart disease? World Rev Nutr Dietetics 72: 38-48

Ornish DM, Gotto AM, Miller RR et al 1979 Effects of a vegetarian diet and selected yoga techniques in the treatment of coronary heart disease. Clinical Research 27: 720A

Ornish DM, Scherwitz LW, Doody RS et al 1983 Effects of stress management traning and dietary changes in treating ischemic heart disease. JAMA 249: 54–59

Ornish DM, Brown SE, Scherwitz LW et al 1990 Can lifestyle changes reverse coronary athcrosclerosis? The Lifestyle Heart Trial. The Lancet 336: 129–133; Yearbook of Medicine and Yearbook of Cardiology (New York: C.V. Mosby, 1991)

Orth-Gomer K, Unden AL, Edwards ME 1988 Social isolation and mortality in ischemic heart disease. Acta Med Scand 224: 205–215

Patel C, North WR 1975 Randomised controlled trial of yoga and bio-feedback in management of hypertension. Lancet. ii: 93–95

Patel C, Marmot MG, Terry DJ, Carruthers M, Hunt B, Patel M 1985 Trial of relaxation in reducing coronary risk: Four year follow up. BMJ 290: 1103–1106

Ruberman W, Weinblatt E, Goldberg JD, Chaudhary BS 1984 Psychosocial influences on mortality after myocardial infarction. N Engl J Med 311: 552–559

Shekelle RB, Stamler J 1989 Dietary cholesterol and ischemic heart disease. Lancet 1: 1177–1179

Stuff JE, Garza C, Smith EO *et al* 1983 A comparison of dietary methods in nutritional studies. Am J Clin Nutr 37: 300–306

Multiple Risk Factors in Cardiovascular Disease, ed. by A. Yamamoto, Churchill Livingstone Japan, Tokyo, pp. 61–64 (1994)

REDUCING THE BURDEN OF CORONARY HEART DISEASE THROUGH SECONDARY PREVENTION (THE CASE FOR SECONDARY PREVENTION)

Basil M. RIFKIND

*Lipid Metabolism-Vascular Research Program, National Heart, Lung, and Blood Institute, National Institutes of Health**

Key words: secondary prevention, cholesterol lowering, prospective studies, clinical trials, angiographic trials

The distinction between primary and secondary prevention is a somewhat arbitrary one so far as cholesterol lowering is concerned, since the aim of treatment is to slow the progression of the atherosclerotic lesions common to individuals with or without symptomatic disease. However, the potential for benefit in the former group may be limited by the effect prior disease has already had on the myocardium.

However, because of the myocardial consideration and the expectation that, by the time someone has manifested coronary heart disease (CHD), the underlying lesions would be large, complicated and resistant to therapy, a negative view has prevailed regarding the potential of secondary prevention through cholesterol lowering. However, it is now increasingly appreciated that, far from offering limited opportunities, secondary intervention is highly effective, and holds great promise for reducing the overall burden of CHD in the community and is likely to result in reduced health-care costs. Furthermore, it has been suggested that patients with CHD are easier to find than those without clinical manifestations so that their identification and subsequent management may be relatively efficient. It is also hoped that the prior experience of the disease and fear of its recurrence may stimulate better adherence to therapy compared with asymptomatic individuals.

The evidence suggesting that cholesterol lowering helps prevent recurrent myocardial infarction (MI) and related disease is derived from a large body of pathological, animal, genetic, metabolic, clinical, and epidemiological data. Of particular importance have been the findings of prospective observational studies and clinical trials.

PROSPECTIVE STUDIES

Prospective epidemiological studies have done much to establish that the serum cholesterol level is an important risk factor for CHD in individuals without CHD. The recognition that it also predicts further clinical events in patients with prior manifestations was delayed, however, by the findings from the placebo group of the Coronary Drug Project (CDP) which showed that the most powerful factors relating to long-term prognosis are those reflecting the status of the myocardium. What received less attention, however, was that, in this study, the serum cholesterol was still related to the

* Room 401, Federal Bldg., Bethesda, MD 20892, USA.

risk of all causes and CHD mortality, sudden death and the incidence of non-fatal MI plus coronary death. It was estimated from these findings that a 10% decrease in cholesterol should reduce CHD mortality by 6%, less than in the case of primary prevention but not inconsiderable. The cholesterol level has, in fact, been identified as a risk factor in many studies of patients with CHD, whether or not the state of the myocardium was taken into account.

The report from the Lipid Research Clinics Follow-up Study (LRCFS) focused attention on this and considerably strengthened the importance of cholesterol in the patient who has manifest CHD and extended it to low density lipoprotein (LDL-C) and high density lipoprotein (HDL-C) levels (Pekkanen *et al* 1990). The analyses was based on the ten-year follow up of 2,541 white men, with or without preexisting cardiovascular disease (CVD). Among the men with CVD at baseline, those with cholesterol levels above 260 mg/dl had a risk of CVD 3.45 times higher than that of men with levels below 200 mg/dl. Similarly, LDL-C and HDL-C levels were important predictors. These lipids were also independent predictors in the men without CHD at entry, but at a much lower level of absolute risk of death. It is also possible that these and other prospective study data understate the strength of the risk relationship, since it has been generally computed on the basis of a single cholesterol determination, an approach which is subject to the impact of the regression — dilution phenomenon due to the within-individual variability of cholesterol.

The absolute risk of death in patients with prior CHD is striking and of crucial importance in defining the potential of secondary prevention strategies for preventing large numbers of CHD events and in containing the associated costs. In the LRCFS those with cholesterol above 260 mg/dl had a 19.6% risk of dying from CVD in ten years compared with 14.9% in men whose levels were under 200 mg/dl. Similarly, in various prospective studies and in the placebo groups of several clinical trials, about 5% of subjects with prior MI reinfarcted each year over the next four to six years. In the CDP placebo group involving 2,789 men aged 30–64 at entry, with such a history, 26.2% had a recurrent infarction, 16.2% died of infarction, and 20.9% died from all causes over the next five years. In general, these rates are about five times higher than those in corresponding men without CHD.

CLINICAL TRIALS OF CHOLESTEROL LOWERING

Two groups of clinical trials are important in the assessment of the efficacy of secondary prevention of cholesterol lowering, namely those using clinical endpoints and those using angiographic endpoints.

Clinical Endpoint Studies

All but four or five of the main trials of cholesterol lowering utilizing clinical endpoints are secondary prevention studies, presumably reflecting the smaller numbers of participants that are required due to the much higher event rate in patients belonging to this group. Notwithstanding its limitations, the technique of meta-analyses has been used to explore the overall experience of treatment in such patients. Several such analyses have been reported (Holme 1993; Rossouw *et al* 1990); in general, they report significant reductions in CHD deaths and in non-fatal MI confirming the expectations raised by the prospective study data. The impact of treatment on total mortality has been also encouraging in that it shows an overall near significant reduction. This is in contrast to primary prevention trials in which total mortality has been essentially unchanged or has been (insignificantly) increased. This difference may be attributable to the much higher proportion of deaths due to CHD in secondary prevention trials, so that the reduction in CHD mortality is reflected by a reduction in total mortality.

Angiographic Endpoint Studies

Since meaningful information can only be obtained on relatively advanced lesions from coronary angiography and since many of the patients had symptomatic CHD as the basis for their angiogram, such studies can be regarded as predominantly secondary prevention trials. About ten of these studies have been recently reported and almost all of them have reported slowing in lesion progression and a presumed regression. This has often been accompanied by a reduction in clinical events and procedures such as bypass surgery although the numbers are quite small. Although the lesion changes are modest, they have been correlated with the concomitant reduction in CHD events, especially in the POSCH (Program on the Surgical Control of the Hyperlipidemias) study. It may be noteworthy that, in several studies, it is the smaller lesions which correlate best with clinical events, supporting the view that it is not the larger lesions per se that account for many CHD deaths but rather the smaller lipid-rich unstable plaques.

In summary, both sets of trials provide strong and complementary evidence of the benefits of reducing plasma cholesterol levels with little evidence of harm. It is also likely that the greater degrees of lowering that can be obtained using the statin class of drugs or combination drug therapy will be accompanied by greater reductions in risk; the POSCH study reduced cholesterol by 23% and the rate of CHD by 43%. Results from recently published studies using one of the statin drugs are encouraging in this respect.

THE NATIONAL CHOLESTEROL EDUCATION PROGRAM GUIDELINES

These and related considerations have led the Adult Treatment Panel of the National Cholesterol Education Program (NCEP), in their recently released and revised guidelines, to focus attention on patients with CHD (and other atherosclerotic diseases) as a special target group for aggressive intervention (NCEP Expert Panel 1993). In addition, this group of patients was separately categorized with respect to the cholesterol cut-off points used to determine treatment needs and goals of such treatment.

The decision to employ a separate set of cut-off points was based on the higher risk of these patients. Hitherto, it has been customary to apply the same set of cut-off points for CHD patients as for patients without CHD in determining their eligibility for treatment. This, in retrospect, is inappropriate. Cut-off points are selected, using data derived from prospective studies, because they denote (together with other measures) the level of risk that the patient carries. Patients with or without CHD have, as described above, very different levels of risk. For example, those with levels below 200 mg/dl and CHD have almost the same risk as those with levels of 240 mg/dl and no CHD.

The specific recommendations of the NCEP pertaining to secondary prevention are as follows in (outline):

- In adults with evidence of CHD, lipoprotein analyses (LDL-C, HDL-C, total cholesterol and triglycerides) should be performed.
- If the LDL-C is optimal (100 mg/dl) no aggressive measures are undertaken.
- If the LDL-C is higher than optimal (100 mg/dl) then therapy is initiated after taking into account the history and clinical status of the patient.
- Maximal dietary therapy is initially used, the goal being an LDL-C of 100 mg/dl.
- If the LDL-C remains above 130 mg/dl drug therapy should be considered.

COST IMPLICATIONS OF GUIDELINES

The cost consequences of implementing these recommendations will be considerable. Using data from the first phase of the third National Health and Nutrition Survey (NHANES III) it has been estimated that, based on the 1990 US population, approximately 52 million US adults with or without prevalent CHD or 29% of the adult population require dietary modification for high blood cholesterol. About 20% of these have CHD. Assuming that diet results in a uniform 10% reduction in cholesterol levels, it was further calculated that approximately 4 million adults with CHD might require drug treatment.

Clearly, the costs of an expanded program of cholesterol control in CHD patients involving much more drug and dietary management and other elements, are considerable. However, the resulting increased expenditures will often be compensated by increased cost savings resulting from such outcomes as a decreased volume of surgical procedures such as coronary bypass. Economic models of prevention strategies have been constructed to attempt to compute their net costs (Goldman *et al* 1992). For example, lovastatin used for the secondary prevention of recurrent events in persons with preexisting CHD was estimated to have a very favorable cost-effectiveness ratio. For men aged 35–64 years and women aged 35–54 years, intervention with 20 mg/day of lovastatin was projected to cost less than the savings from CHD events that were prevented. For older men and women, the cost-effectiveness ratio ranged from $3,300 to $15,000 per year of life saved. These estimates do not take into account the savings through the avoidance of lost earnings through death or disability. In general, the cost-effectiveness of secondary prevention can be attributed to the high risk-benefit ratios seen in such a high risk population. Of course, reductions in drug costs would greatly improve the ratio.

SUMMARY

A large body of evidence suggests that lowering the level of cholesterol offers considerable protection from a recurring event in the patient with manifest CHD. Such an approach focuses attention on a major underlying cause of the disease and is becoming increasingly effective due to the availability of potent, easily administered cholesterol-lowering drugs, with few side effects. Given that about half of all new MI occur in individuals with prior manifestations of coronary ischemia, secondary prevention could have a substantial impact on reducing the overall burden of CHD in the population. Finally, it may reduce the substantial health care costs presently associated with one of the major causes of death and disability. However, it must be emphasized that an increased emphasis on secondary prevention must not be at the cost of the concurrent implementation of primary prevention strategies to address the equally large fraction of the disease burden attributable to individuals with no prior history, many of whom die suddenly, thus providing no opportunity for secondary prevention. The revised guidelines of the NCEP provide recommendations for the selection and aggressive treatment of CHD patients.

REFERENCES

Goldman L, Gordon DJ, Rifkind BM *et al* 1992 Cost and health implications of cholesterol lowering. Circulation 85: 1960–1968

Holme I 1993 Relation of coronary heart disease incidence and total mortality to plasma cholesterol reduction in randomised trials: use of meta-analysis. Br Heart J 69(S): S42–S47

Pekkanen J, Linn S, Heiss G *et al* 1990 Ten-year mortality from cardiovascular disease in relation to cholesterol level among men with and without preexisting cardiovascular disease. N Engl J Med 322: 1700–1707

Rossouw JE, Lewis B, Rifkind BM 1990 The value of lowering cholesterol after myocardial infarction. N Engl J Med 323: 1112–1119

Summary of the Second Report of the National Cholesterol Education Program (NCEP) Expert Panel on Detection, Evaluation, and Treatment of High Blood Cholesterol in Adults (Adult Treatment Panel II) 1993 JAMA 269: 3015–3023

Multiple Risk Factors in Cardiovascular Disease, ed. by A. Yamamoto, Churchill Livingstone Japan, Tokyo, pp. 65–70 (1994)

SOY PROTEIN DIET: SUGGESTIONS ABOUT THE MECHANISM OF ITS CHOLESTEROL-LOWERING ACTIVITY

Maria R. LOVATI, Cristina MANZONI, and Cesare R. SIRTORI

*Institute of Pharmacological Sciences, University of Milano**

Key words: animal/vegetable proteins, soybean protein diet, hypercholesterolemic type II patients, plasma/LDL cholesterol, LDL-receptor, 7S/11S soybean globulins

The role of nutritional factors in the etiology of hypercholesterolemia and atherosclerosis was recognized by Ignatowski as far back as 1909, when he found that rabbits fed diets containing animal proteins developed arterial lesions resembling human atherosclerosis. Initially, the arterial lesions were ascribed to the nature of the protein in the diet, however this idea was abandoned when Anitschkow and Chalatow (1913) showed that crystalline cholesterol fed to rabbits also resulted in severe arterial lesions. Nevertheless, a number of investigators over the years clearly confirmed that in the experimental models animal proteins can play a major role in the development of hypercholesterolemia and atherosclerosis (Carroll & Hamilton 1975).

PLANT PROTEINS AND PLASMA CHOLESTEROL

Epidemiological studies have provided evidence of a clear link between the mortality from coronary heart disease (CHD) and the intake of animal proteins. Moreover, a negative correlation has been found with vegetable proteins (Connor & Connor 1972).

A study carried out in the People's Republic of China, a population with an extremely low intake of animal protein and saturated fat, revealed far lower levels of total plasma cholesterol compared with those obtained in people of a similar age living in Belgium and the Republic of Korea (Kesteloot *et al* 1985). The Chinese diet consists of about 10% of fat, 12 % protein (of which only 7% is of animal origin) and 78% carbohydrates. These results were true for both sexes and were independent of the rural or urban location of the Chinese population. Therefore, the low levels of total plasma cholesterol obtained in the Oriental populations, with a diet containing high levels of vegetable proteins, are linked to the rare appearance of cardiovascular disease.

Vegetarians have generally lower plasma lipid and lipoprotein levels compared with omnivorous individuals (Sacks *et al* 1975). This reflects several important differences, such as lower intake of fat, particularly of animal origin, and of cholesterol, as well as a larger consumption of carbohydrates and fiber from vegetables, fruits and cereals. Numerous intervention studies have compared the effects of vegetable vs animal proteins in normolipidemic individuals. Meinertz and coworkers (1988), in a crosso-

* Via Balzaretti 9, 20133 Milano, Italy.

ver study of plant vs animal proteins in normolipidemic subjects, did not observe any striking differences in the concentrations of major lipoproteins. However, the same authors obtained different results in normocholesterolemic individuals consuming the same liquid formula diet but with a cholesterol intake of 500 mg/day (Meinertz *et al* 1989). In this other study the concentration of low density lipoproteins (LDL) cholesterol was 16% lower on the soy protein diet vs the casein regimen. Increased levels (+16%) of plasma high density lipoprotein (HDL) have been also detected following a soy protein diet.

These findings suggest that cholesterol intake may have a crucial influence on the cholesterolemic response to dietary proteins of plant and animal origin.

CLINICAL STUDIES OF THE SOY PROTEIN DIET

Soybean proteins have also received wide clinical attention. The Soybean protein diet has proved, in fact, to be an effective alternative to drug treatment in *type II hypercholesterolemic patients*, as repeatedly demonstrated in controlled studies in hospitalized or outpatients. More than ten years ago Sirtori and coworkers (1977) observed that a textured vegetable protein (TVP) product from soybean produced a 14% decrease in plasma cholesterol levels after two weeks and a 21% decrease after three weeks when substituted for animal proteins in a group of 20 patients with type II hyperlipoproteinemia. In a multicenter study the same authors found a marked fall of total and LDL (–25%) plasma cholesterol after a soybean protein diet (Descovich *et al* 1980). The hypocholesterolemic effect of TVP was present with or without the daily addition of 500 mg cholesterol to the diet (Sirtori *et al* 1977). Furthermore, Sirtori *et al* (1979) underlined that the most marked reductions in plasma cholesterol were observed in patients with elevated values of cholesterol at the start of the dietary treatment. The addition of soybean protein diet to a standard low-lipid diet has also been shown to be effective in reducing cholesterol in type II hypercholesterolemia (Sirtori 1983). An interesting area for the use of the soybean protein diet has been in the treatment of the pediatric hypercholesterolemia. In an Italian multicenter study of 18 pre-puberal children a reduction of cholesterol of around 25% or more was consistently achieved (Gaddi *et al* 1987). These findings have been recently confirmed by Widhalm *et al* (1993), who evaluated the regimen in 23 children with familial or polygenic hypercholesterolemia. This study differs from the previous one, in having a cross-over design and children with far lower starting cholesterol. However, results are quite similar, with an LDL-C reduction of 22% when the TVP diet preceded the standard lipid-lowering diet and a reduction of 25%, when it was given as the second treatment.

MECHANISM OF THE HYPOCHOLESTEROLEMIC EFFECT OF VEGETABLE PROTEINS AT THE MOLECULAR LEVEL

The mechanism/s whereby the administration of animal or vegetable proteins may influence cholesterolemia remain poorly understood. In particular, differences in amino acid composition (Kritchevsky *et al* 1982), possible hormonal modulation (Forsythe 1986; Noseda *et al* 1982), and differences in the fecal excretion of bile acids and neutral sterols (Kim *et al* 1980) have been suggested as being responsible for the different actions of these proteins on cholesterol. Moreover, significant discrepancies exist between the results of animal and human studies: in fat-fed animals the introduction of vegetable proteins to the diet leads to increased fecal steroid excretion as well as to an increased turnover of circulating cholesterol (Huff & Carroll 1980). This is not the case of type II patients treated with this regimen where, in spite of the dramatic plasma cholesterol reduction, no increase in fecal neutral or acidic steroid excretion or an accelerated turnover of cholesterol can be detected (Fumagalli *et al* 1982).

In vivo and *in vitro* studies (Brown *et al* 1981) have shown that the major site of removal of lipoprotein cholesterol is at the hepatocyte level, by way of high-affinity receptors for LDL. We examined the regulation of high-affinity lipoprotein receptors in rodent liver as well as lipoprotein catabolism in rats, fed on cholesterolemic regimens with soybean protein or casein as the protein source. In these animals a casein-containing diet significantly suppressed liver LDL receptors, whereas the same regimen with soybean did not modify LDL binding to liver membranes (Sirtori *et al* 1984). An accelerated lipoprotein catabolism was also detected in rats when soybean protein was substituted for casein (Lovati *et al* 1985).

In a clinical study, the LDL receptor activity was examined in freshly isolated mononuclear cells from type II patients, receiving either a low lipid diet with animal proteins or an identical diet (in terms of cholesterol and lipid content) with TVP. The degradation of LDL by mononuclear cells was consistently elevated by the soybean protein diet, to an extent about eight fold higher than that achieved by a standard low lipid diet with animal proteins (Fig. 1) (Lovati *et al* 1987). This study confirms that some factor/s in soy protein may exert an up-regulation of LDL receptors. Indirect confirmation of these clinical findings comes from a recent study by Gaddi *et al* (1991) on differences in plasma cholesterol after TVP administration in type II patients of different apoprotein E phenotypes. It is well know that the apo E4 genotype is generally associated with higher plasma cholesterol levels, probably because of a suppressed peripheral LDL receptor activity by E4 protein, compared with lower levels of cholesterol in subjects with apo E2 genotype, where the E3 variant is an inefficient regulator of the LDL receptor (Davignon *et al* 1988). When examining the plasma cholesterol response of

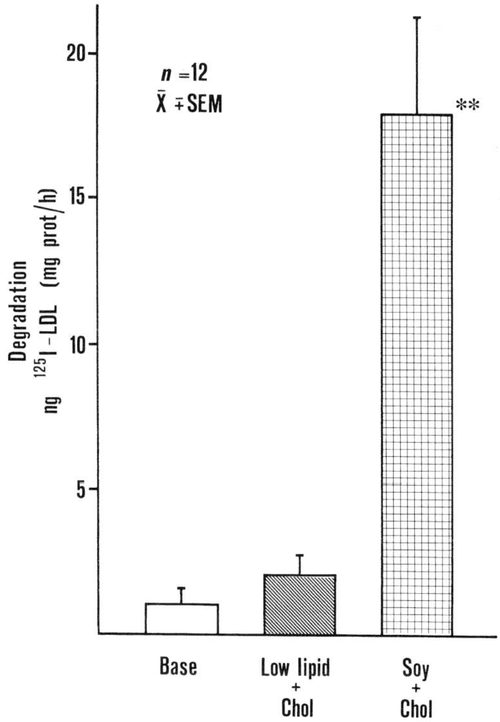

Fig. 1. Degradation of ^{125}I-LDL by freshly isolated mononuclear cells from type II hypercholesterolemic patients, before and after dietary treatment with a low lipid diet or with a soybean protein diet with an identical cholesterol content.
** $p < 0.01$ (Lovati *et al* 1987).

these individuals (Gaddi *et al* 1991), it could be readily concluded that, whereas the apo E2 carriers show a very weak or negligible response to dietary change, this is not the case for patients with E3 and E4 phenotypes. These findings support the conclusion that patients with a higher LDL receptor activity (with the E2 genotype) are less likely to show a favorable response to the regimen, compared with patients where the LDL receptor activity may be relatively suppressed (E3 and E4 genotypes).

In the last few years, after the repeated suggestions by a number of authors that some protein or peptide components of the soybean diet might be responsible for the hypocholesterolemic effect, the identification of these components and their mechanism of action has been attempted in different animal and *in vitro* models.

The effects of an ethanol-soluble extract from TVP (SPHEE) have been tested in hypercholesterolemic mice. A dose-related hypocholesterolemic response was detected, with a parallel rise in lipoprotein receptors in the liver (Lovati *et al* 1991). This study, however, left some uncertainties as to the exact identification of the component, since the SPHEE is rather heterogenous and it is not possible to totally eliminate non-protein components.

Therefore, more recent studies have been focused on isolated proteins, mostly in cell culture systems, investigating their direct activity on LDL-receptor expression.

The major storage globulins, 7S and 11S, were carefully isolated from soy proteins and their effect on cholesterol homeostasis investigated in *in vitro* and *in vivo* systems (Lovati *et al* 1992). *In vitro*, two cell types were examined, human skin fibroblasts (HSF) and human hepatoma cell line (Hep G2). In Hep G2 cells a dose-dependent increase in both the uptake and degradation of ^{125}I-LDL, is induced by 7S globulin; in this same cell line 11S globulin induced a lower, up regulation of the LDL receptor activity which was not dose-dependent. In contrast, in HSF the 11S globulin increased the uptake of ^{125}I-LDL, 3.5 fold compared with controls at the higher concentration; the 7S globulin affected LDL uptake to a lesser extent. Neither of the two globulins stimulated LDL degradation in this system (Fig. 2).

These *in vitro* findings were substantiated by an *in vivo* investigation, where rats fed a casein-cholesterol diet were treated daily with 30 mg protein/kg of 11S or 7S globulin for 2 weeks. The addition of both soy globulins significantly reduced basal total cholesterol, –35% and –34% for 7S and 11S globulin, respectively compared with controls. This is very similar to the results generally obtained with total substitution of the proteins. Isolated liver membrane preparations from the treated rats, showed an increase, not statistically significant, in the maximal binding of labeled LDL to high affinity receptors, more marked after 7S globulin administration.

These rather surprising and somewhat exciting results indicate for the first time that isolated protein components may affect cholesterolemia, most likely by a general mechanism which does not alter the absorption/elimination of other nutrients.

At present, studies have been carried out in order to evaluate the activity of isolated components of 7S and 11S on different cell systems. These studies will provide probably the definitive, or at least most biologically satisfactory, answer to the likely mechanism of action whereby soybean proteins in lowering cholesterolemia.

SUMMARY

Numerous investigations, in man and a variety of animal models support the hypothesis that animal proteins may play a major role in the elevation of plasma lipids, clearly established as major risk factors for cardiovascular disease. Over the past 20 years, our research group has carried out a series of studies starting with controlled human investigations, progressing to tissue and cellular models, examining the potential of a diet based on vegetable proteins from soybean to modify plasma lipid levels. In essentially all the studies, textured products (textured vegetable protein = TVP) have been used. Clinical studies have suggested that a complete replacement of animal proteins with TVP from soybean is most suitable for patients with clear-cut type II hyperlipoproteinemia. The soy protein diet may be particularly good for the treatment of pediatric hypercholesterolemia, since physicians wish to avoid long-term drug treatment before puberty. Different hypotheses have been put forward to explain the mechanism/s whereby animal or vegetable proteins influence cholesterol. Differences in amino acid composition, possible hormonal modulation, effects on lipoprotein high-affinity receptor regulation and the diversity

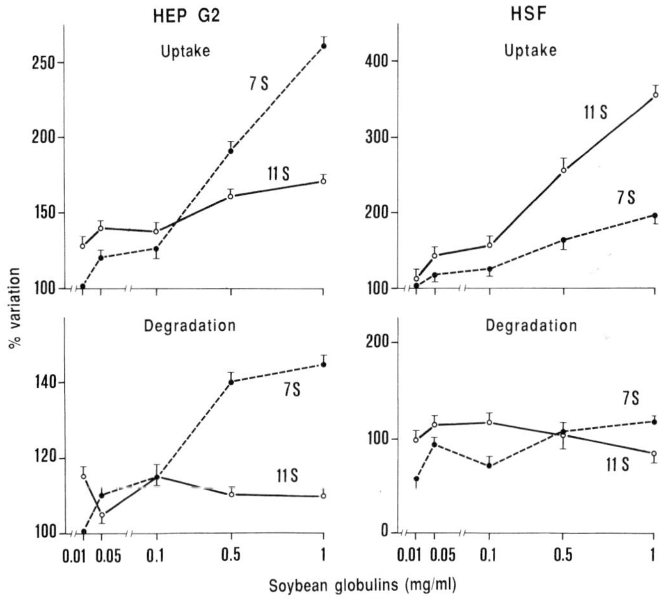

Fig. 2. Effect of soybean globulins on the uptake (binding + internalization) and degradation of ^{125}I-LDL by human hepatoma cells (Hep G2) and skin fibroblasts (HSF). Confluent monolayers of cells were preincubated for 24 h at 37°C in MEM-F11 with 5% LPDS, in the presence or absence of soybean globulins at the reported concentrations. After the addition of ^{125}I-LDL (7.5 μg lipoprotein/ml of medium), cells were incubated at 37°C for a further 5 h. Values (means ± SEM of triplicate incubations) express the percentage changes vs controls (equal to 100%). See Lovati *et al* 1992.

in the fecal excretion of bile acids and neutral sterols have all been suggested as being responsible. The results presented above clearly suggest that the mode of action of soy proteins is unlikely to be related to sterol absorption/excretion, but rather to a modulatory effect mediated by protein subunits or related peptides on cholesterol synthesis/distribution. Such an activity seems to occur predominantly in the liver, but intestinal changes in lipoprotein handling cannot be excluded. Whatever the mechanism may be, the nature of dietary proteins is an important variable in maintaining low plasma lipids, clearly established as major risk factors for the development of atherosclerotic disease.

REFERENCES

Anitschkow N, Chalatow S 1913 Uber experimentelle Cholesterinsteatose und ihre Bedeutung fur die Entstehung einiger pathologischer Prozesse. Centbl allgem Path Anat 24: 1–9

Brown MS, Kovanen PT, Goldstein JL 1981 Regulation of plasma cholesterol by lipoprotein receptors. Science 212: 628–635

Carroll KK, Hamilton RMG 1975 Effects of dietary protein and carbohydrate on plasma cholesterol levels in relation to atherosclerosis. J Food Sci 40: 18–23

Connor WE, Connor SL 1972 The key role of nutritional factors in the prevention of coronary heart disease. Prev Med 1: 49–83

Davignon J, Gregg RE, Sing CF 1988 Apolipoprotein E polymorphism and atherosclerosis. Arteriosclerosis 8: 1–21

Descovich GC, Gaddi A, Mannino G *et al* 1980 Multicentre study of soybean protein diet for outpatient hypercholesterolaemic patients. Lancet ii: 709–712

Forsythe WA 1986 Comparison of dietary casein or soy protein effects on plasma lipids and hormone concentrations in the Gerbil (Meriones unguiculatus). J Nutr 116: 1165–1171

Fumagalli R, Soleri L, Farina R *et al* 1982 Fecal cholesterol excretion studies in type ll hypercholesterolemic patients treated with the soybean protein diet . Atherosclerosis 43: 341–353

Gaddi A, Descovich GC, Noseda G *et al* 1987 Hypercholesterolaemia treated by soybean protein diet. Arch Dis Child 62: 274–278

Gaddi A, Ciarocchi A, Matteucci A *et al* 1991 Dietary treatment for familial hypercholesterolemia — differential effects of dietary soy protein according to the apolipoprotein E phenotypes. Am J Clin Nutr 53: 1191–1196

Huff MW, Carroll KK 1980 Effect of the dietary protein on turnover, oxidation and absorption of cholesterol, and on steroid excretion in rabbits. J Lipid Res 21: 546–558

Ignatowski A 1909 Über die Wirkung des tierischen Eiweisses auf die Aorta und die parenchymatosen Organe der Kaninchen. Virchows Arch Path Anat Physiol Klin Med 198: 248–270

Kesteloot H, Huang DX, Yang XS *et al* 1985 Serum lipids in the People's Republic of China. Comparison of western and eastern populations. Arteriosclerosis 5: 427–433

Kim DN, Lee KT, Reiner JM, Thomas WA 1980 Increased steroid excretion in swine fed high-fat, high-cholesterol diet with soy protein. Exp Mol Pathol 33: 25–35

Kritchevsky D, Tepper SA, Czarnecki SK, Klurfeld DM 1982 Atherogenicity of animal and vegetable protein. Influence of the Iysine to arginine ratio. Atherosclerosis 41: 429–431

Lovati MR, Allievi L, Sirtori CR 1985 Accelerated early catabolism of very low density lipoproteins in rats after dietary soy proteins. Atherosclerosis 56: 243–246

Lovati MR, Manzoni C, Canavesi A *et al* 1987 Soybean protein diet increases low density lipoprotein receptor activity in mononuclear cells from hypercholesterolemic patients. J Clin Invest 80: 1498–1502

Lovati MR, Manzoni C, Agostinelli P, Ciappellano S, Mannucci L, Sirtori CR 1991 Studies on the mechanism of the cholesterol lowering activity of soy proteins. Nutr Metab Cardiovas Dis 1:18–24

Lovati MR, Manzoni C, Corsini A *et al* 1992 Low density lipoprotein (LDL) receptor activity is modulated by soybean globulins in cell culture. J Nutr 122: 1971–1978

Meinertz H, Faergeman O, Nilausen K, Chapman MJ, Goldstein S, Laplaud PM 1988 Effects of soy protein and casein in low cholesterol diets on plasma lipoproteins in normolipidemic subjects. Atherosclerosis 72: 63–70

Meinertz H, Nilausen K, Faergeman O 1989 Soy protein and casein in cholesterol-enriched diets: effects on plasma lipoproteins in normolipidemic subjects. Am J Clin Nutr 50: 786–793

Noseda G, Fragiacomo C, Gatti E, Descovich GC, Sirtori CR 1982 Glucagon release following experimental diets in man: effects of soybean and casein enriched diets. Pharmacol Res Commun 14: 867–878

Sacks FM, Castelli WP, Donner A, Kass EH. 1975 Plasma lipids and lipoproteins in vegetarians and controls. New Engl J Med 292: 1148–1151

Sirtori CR 1983 Reply to the letter: "Soybean protein, a hypocholesterolemic drug?" Trends in Pharm and Sci 4:63

Sirtori CR, Agradi E, Conti F, Mantero O 1977 Soybean-protein diet in the treatment of type-ll hyperlipoproteinaemia. Lancet i : 275–278

Sirtori CR, Gatti E, Mantero O *et al* 1979 Clinical experience with the soybean protein diet in the treatment of hypercholesterolemia. Am J Clin Nutr 32: 1645–1658

Sirtori C R, Galli G, Lovati M R, Carrara P, Bosisio E, Galli Kienle M 1984 Effects of dietary proteins on the regulation of liver lipoprotein receptors in rats. J Nutr 114: 1493–1500

Widhalm K, Brazda G, Schneider B, Kohl S 1993 Effect of soy protein diet versus standard low fat, low cholesterol diet on lipid and lipoprotein levels in children with familial or polygenic hypercholesterolemia. J Pediatr 123: 30–34

Multiple Risk Factors in Cardiovascular Disease, ed. by A. Yamamoto, Churchill Livingstone Japan, Tokyo, pp. 71–79 (1994)

THE INFLUENCE OF CALCIUM CHANNEL BLOCKERS ON THE EVOLUTION OF CORONARY ATHEROSCLEROSIS

David WATERS*[1,2] and Jacques LESPÉRANCE*[3,4]

*[1] *Division of Cardiology, Hartford Hospital,* *[2] *the University of Connecticut School of Medicine,* *[3] *the Department of Radiology, Montreal Heart Institute, and* *[4] *the University of Montreal Medical School*

Key words: atherosclerosis, diltiazem, dihydropyridine, nifedipine, progression

Progression of coronary atherosclerosis leads to unstable angina, myocardial infarction, congestive heart failure, and sudden coronary death. Treatments aimed at these consequences of coronary disease progression have reduced morbidity and mortality; however, a more direct approach would be preferable. Interventions that could prevent the appearance of the atherosclerotic plaque, slow its progression, stabilize its fibrous cap to reduce the risk of plaque fissure, or induce regression of established lesions, would obviously have a major impact on the incidence of coronary events.

Based on the work published to date, lipid-lowering therapy appears to be the most promising intervention for accomplishing these objectives. However, favorable modifications of lipid levels do not solve the problem entirely. For example, in the Familial Atherosclerosis Treatment Study (FATS) patients treated with colestipol plus niacin, in spite of a low density lpoprotein (LDL)-cholesterol reduction of 32% and a high density liporotein (HDL)-cholesterol increase of 43%, one quarter of these patients developed coronary progression in only 2.5 years (Brown *et al* 1990). Obviously, other approaches need to be explored.

A large body of experimental evidence and three clinical trials suggest that calcium channel blockers exert a favorable effect on the development of coronary atherosclerosis. The purpose of this paper is to review the clinical studies.

CALCIUM CHANNEL BLOCKERS IN ANIMAL MODELS OF ATHEROSCLEROSIS

Kramsch *et al* (1981) reported in the early 1980's that the calcium channel blocker lanthanum suppressed experimental atherosclerosis. A beneficial effect upon the development of atherosclerosis in the cholesterol-fed rabbit was subsequently demonstrated with the dihydropyridines nifedipine (Henry & Bentley 1981), isradipine (Habib *et al* 1986), nisoldipine (Fronek 1988), nilvadipine (Nomoto *et al* 1987), and nicardipine (Willis *et al* 1985), and also with diltiazem (Sugano *et al* 1988), and verapamil (Rouleau *et al* 1983). The study of Henry and Bentley (1981) using nifedipine is typical of these reports. A 2% cholesterol diet was fed for 8 weeks to 13 placebo rabbits and 13 rabbits treated with nifedipine, 10 mg twice per day.

*[1] 80 Seymour Street, Hartford, CT 06102-5037, USA.

The aortic intimal surface covered with lipid-stainable lesions averaged 40 ± 5% in placebo-treated and 17 ± 3% in nifedipine-treated rabbits ($p < 0.001$), in spite of similar high serum cholesterol levels in both groups.

Several studies have failed to demonstrate a beneficial effect of calcium channel blockers on experimental atherosclerosis. Potential reasons for this discrepancy include an inadequate sample size, given the wide variability in atherosclerosis development among rabbits, and poor drug bioavailability (Henry 1990). Felodipine has recently been reported to retard aortic atherosclerosis in the cholesterol-fed rat (Nunnari *et al* 1993). Nifedipine (Lichtor *et al* 1989) and amlodipine (Kramsch *et al* 1993) have also been shown to suppress atherogenesis in monkeys, a model more analogous to human atherosclerosis.

MECHANISM OF ACTION

The anti-atherogenic effects of calcium channel blockers are important because they act independently from serum lipid lowering and thus provide an alternative approach to influencing the evolution of human coronary atherosclerosis. Several mechanisms of action have been advanced to account for this benefit. In many of the animal experiments, high doses were used and the benefit could thus be explained by a lowering of arterial pressure. However, Habib *et al* (1986) used low doses of isradipine, within the range used in humans, and demonstrated that the anti-atherogenic effect was still present, even in the absence of changes in arterial pressure. On the other hand, in the clinical trial using nicardipine discussed below, lowering of arterial systolic pressure and a lower systolic pressure at baseline were significant predictors of prevention of minimal lesion progression (Waters *et al* 1990).

Increased platelet aggregation is associated with coronary progression and a higher risk of coronary events (Lam *et al* 1994). Calcium channel blockers exert only a weak antiaggregatory effect on platelets; however, recent data indicate that verapamil inhibits platelet thrombus formation in humans (Lacoste *et al* 1994). Platelet-derived growth factor (and other growth factors) play a key role in atherogenesis by stimulating smooth muscle cell proliferation. Nifedipine (Jackson *et al* 1988), isradipine (Handley *et al* 1986), and verapamil (Yang *et al* 1993) have been shown to block this response. The antiatherosclerotic effect of calcium channel blockers could therefore be related to their antiplatelet activities.

Macrophages and endothelial cells do not contain voltage-dependent calcium channels; however, calcium channel blockers inhibit cholesteryl ester deposition (Daugherty *et al* 1987) and promote cholesterol efflux from macrophages (Schmitz *et al* 1988). The calcium channel blocker isradipine has been shown to partially reverse the endothelial dysfunction associated with hypercholesterolemia in rabbits (Habib *et al* 1986). In patients with risk factors including hypercholesterolemia, but without angiographic evidence of coronary atherosclerosis, endothelial function is already abnormal, as indicated by its vasoconstrictive response to acetylcholine (Vita *et al* 1990). The anti-atherogenic effects of calcium channel blockers may be related to their beneficial effects upon endothelial function.

Oxidation of LDL-cholesterol greatly increases its atherogenic potential (Steinberg *et al* 1989) and this oxidation can probably occur in the subendothelial microenvironment where antioxidant levels may be low. Several recent reports indicate that different calcium channel blockers behave as weak antioxidants in membrane systems (Henry 1991). They could thus shift the balance away from LDL oxidation and block the generation of foam cells. In a recent preliminary report (Kramsch *et al* 1993), amlodipine-treated hypercholesterolemic monkeys had less circulating oxidized LDL-cholesterol and less coronary and aortic atherosclerosis than control animals with comparable plasma levels of total and LDL-cholesterol.

Intracellular lipid accumulation is an important feature of the atherosclerotic plaque that can be favorably influenced by nifedipine (Etingin & Hajjar 1985) or verapamil (Stender *et al* 1986). As shown by Etingin and Hajjar (1985), nifedipine increases cholesteryl ester hydrolase activity and thus reduces cholesterol and cholesteryl ester levels in lipid-laden, cultured smooth muscle cells from rabbits. This mechanism has been proven to be relevant to human atherosclerosis (Etingin & Hajjar 1990): in 35 patients undergoing coronary bypass surgery, aortic tissue samples were obtained and stripped of endothelium and adventitia. In the 23 patients treated with calcium channel blockers for several months, cholesteryl ester hydrolase activity was significantly higher in the tissue samples, and cholesterol and cholesteryl ester levels significantly lower, compared with the 12 patients not pretreated with a calcium channel blocker. These differences were independent of serum cholesterol levels, age and other medications. The mechanism by which calcium channel blockers stimulate cholesteryl ester hydrolase activity is by increasing intracellular cyclic AMP (Henry 1991).

In addition to smooth muscle cell proliferation, discussed above, migration of smooth muscle cells from the media to the intima is another component of atherogenesis that is favorably influenced by calcium channel blockers. Nakao *et al* (1983) demonstrated that nicardipine can block smooth muscle cell migration. In a recent preliminary report (McMurray & Chahwala 1991), amlodipine, nitrendipine and verapamil each inhibited smooth muscle cell migration induced by platelet-derived growth factor, with amlodipine being somewhat superior to the other two drugs.

CLINICAL TRIALS OF CALCIUM CHANNEL BLOCKERS AND CORONARY ATHEROSCLEROSIS

The results of three randomized, placebo-controlled clinical trials assessing the effect of calcium channel blockers upon the evolution of coronary atherosclerosis have been reported (Waters *et al* 1990; Lichtlen *et al* 1990; Schroeder *et al* 1993) and are discussed below. An additional small study that was neither randomized nor blinded reported that nifedipine-treated patients had less coronary progression and more regression than patients treated with isosorbide dinitrate or propranolol (Loaldi *et al* 1989). These results with nifedipine were not confirmed by the much larger the International Nifedipine Trial on Antiatherosclerotic Therapy (INTACT) study.

A salutary effect of nifedipine upon the development of atherosclerosis in coronary bypass grafts, as assessed in a randomized, double-blind, placebo-controlled trial, was reported in preliminary form in 1989 (Gottlieb *et al* 1989). The Frankfurt Isoptin Progression Study (FIPS) randomized patients after coronary bypass surgery to verapamil or placebo to determine whether this drug had a favorable effect on the evolution of atherosclerosis in bypass grafts and native vessels. The trial was hampered by a very high dropout rate, and the results have not yet been published.

The effect of isradipine upon the development of carotid atherosclerosis is being assessed using ultrasonography in the Multicenter Isradipine Diuretic Atherosclerosis Study (MIDAS). This trial was recently completed, but the results have not yet been reported. The Prospective Randomized Evaluation of the Vascular Effects of Norvasc Trial (PREVENT) is currently randomizing 720 patients with mild coronary atherosclerosis to amlodipine or placebo. Patients will undergo repeat coronary arteriography after 3 years and a subset of patients are also being assessed by carotid ultrasonography. The results of these trials will help clarify the clinical role of calcium channel blockers as antiatherosclerotic therapy.

THE MONTREAL HEART INSTITUTE NICARDIPINE TRIAL

The specific purpose of this study was to determine whether chronic treatment with nicardipine could influence the progression of coronary atherosclerosis (Waters *et al* 1990). Patients aged 65 or less with stenoses less than 75% in at least 4 coronary artery segments were randomized within one month of baseline coronary arteriography to double-blind therapy with placebo or nicardipine, 30 mg 3 times per day. Excluded were those with previous or planned bypass surgery or angioplasty, those with an ejection fraction less than 0.40, severe triple vessel disease or left main stenosis and those requiring a calcium channel blocker. Of the 383 patients enrolled, 335 (87%) underwent repeat coronary arteriography at 24 months with coronary lesions measured quantitatively.

Coronary events (5 deaths, 22 myocardial infarctions, and 28 episodes of unstable angina) occurred in 28 of the 192 nicardipine patients and 23 of the 191 placebo patients ($p = 0.21$). Progression, defined as a worsening of minimum diameter by at least 0.4 mm, was detected in 44% of nicardipine and 43% of placebo patients; 23% of nicardipine and 19% of placebo patients experienced regression of one or more lesions. None of these differences approach statistical significance.

Among the 217 patients with 411 stenoses of 20% or less at the first arteriogram, such minimal lesions progressed in only 15 of 99 nicardipine patients compared with 32 of 118 placebo patients (15 vs 27%, $p = 0.046$). In this subgroup, 16 of 178 minimal lesions in nicardipine patients and 38 of 233 minimal lesions in placebo patients progressed ($p = 0.038$). Progression of a minimal lesion is illustrated in Fig. 1. By stepwise logistic regression analysis, baseline systolic blood pressure ($p = 0.04$) and the change in systolic blood pressure between baseline and 6 months ($p = 0.002$) correlated with the progression of minimal lesions. This finding suggests that blood pressure reduction might account for the beneficial effect of nicardipine upon minimal lesions.

Overall, the results of this trial indicate that nicardipine has no effect upon advanced coronary atherosclerosis but may retard the progression of minimal lesions, defined as those less than 20% in stenosis diameter on the first arteriogram. This effect of the drug is compatible with the experimental data discussed previously. Although "new" lesions, or minimal lesions that progress, are rarely severe enough to cause myocardial ischemia, they are dangerous because they increase the risk of a coronary event. Coronary lesions that rupture and cause myocardial infarction are usually in the range of 30 to 70% diameter stenosis (Taeymans *et al* 1992), and new lesions in this range are likelier to be at higher risk than older, more fibrotic stenoses.

THE INTERNATIONAL NIFEDIPINE TRIAL ON ANTIATHEROSCLEROTIC THERAPY (INTACT)

The purpose of INTACT was to assess whether treatment with nifedipine retarded the angiographic progression of coronary atherosclerosis (Lichtlen *et al* 1990). In 9 European centers, 425 patients with "mild" coronary artery disease were randomly allocated to double-blind therapy with placebo or nifedipine 80 mg per day in divided doses. Inclusion criteria included age less than 65 years and the presence of at least one coronary risk factor. Patients previously treated with calcium channel blockers for at least 6 months, those with diffuse or severe coronary disease and patients requiring extensive revascularization procedures were excluded. Repeat coronary arteriography was planned after 3 years and all films were interpreted quantitatively.

The two groups were well matched for clinical variables and 282 of the patients (82%) had repeat arteriography. Progression and regression were defined as a change of at least 20% in diameter stenosis or of at least

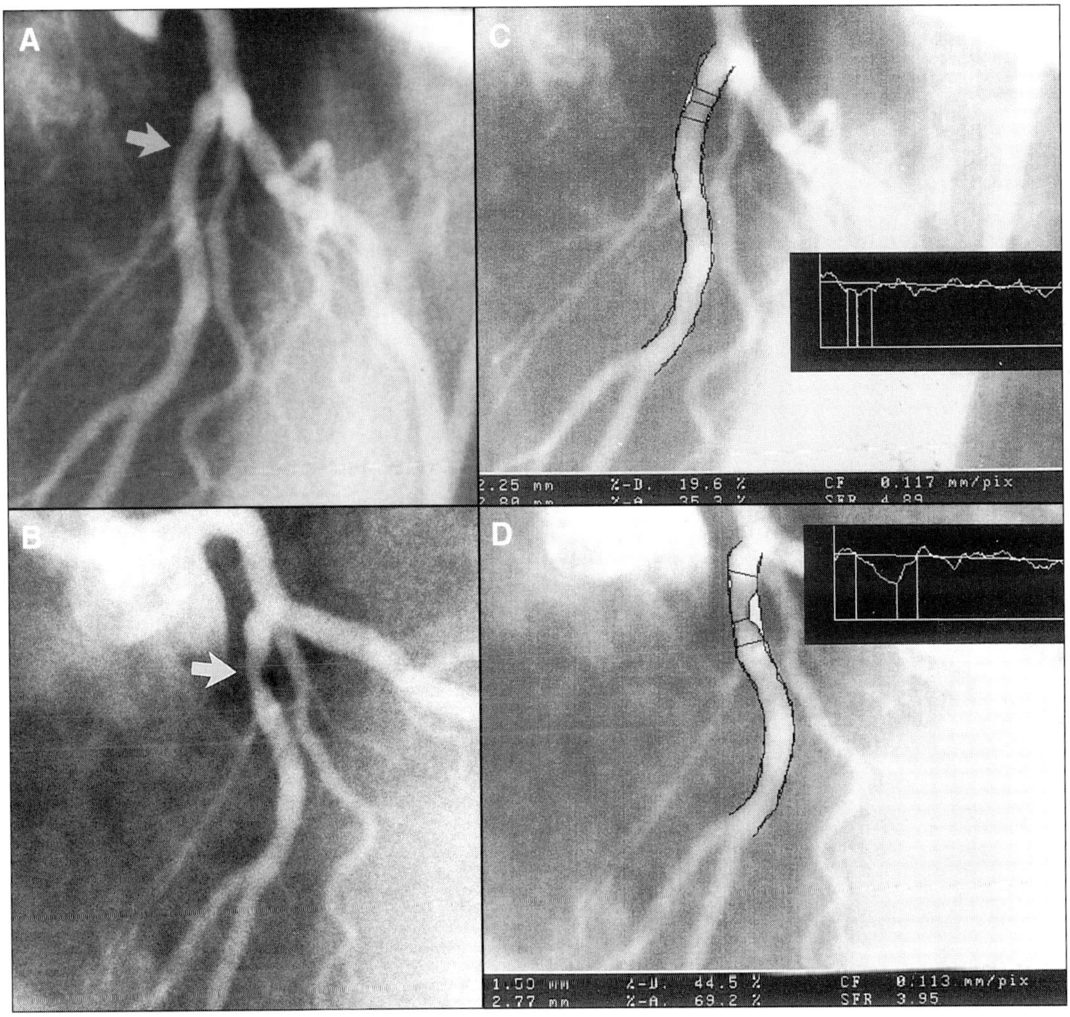

Fig. 1. Development of a new coronary lesion.
A. This segment of the left anterior descending coronary artery contains only minimal irregularities (arrow).
B. Repeat arteriography 26 months later reveals a definite lesion (arrow) at the same site.
C. The quantitative measurement system calculates a minimum lumen diameter of 2.25 mm and a diameter stenosis of 19.6% for the first film. Stenoses within this range can be classified as measurement noise.
D. The minimum lumen diameter has decreased to 1.53 mm and the diameter stenosis is now 44.5%. Although this lesion is not severe enough to cause ischemia, it could rupture and occlude, causing myocardial infarction.

0.4 mm in minimum diameter. Progression, using the latter criterion, was seen in 35% of placebo- and 29% of nifedipine-treated patients; 21% of placebo and 16% of nifedipine patients had regression; these differences were not statistically significant.

New coronary lesions, defined as stenoses of less than 20% on the first arteriogram and greater than 20% on the second, developed in 49% of placebo- and 40% of nifedipine-treated patients. This difference was not statistically significant, and represents a statistically more appropriate method for evaluating a treatment effect. However, the authors also reported new lesions on a "per patient" basis: 0.82 new lesions/patient in the placebo and 0.59 in the nifedipine group. Expressed in this way, as a 28% reduction in new lesions with active treatment, the difference was statistically significant ($p = 0.034$).

Although clinical events were not an endpoint of the trial, it is disturbing to note that mortality was higher in the nifedipine group. Two placebo- and 8 nifedipine-treated patients died from cardiac causes and 4 additional non-cardiac deaths were reported in the nifedipine group. No differences between treatment groups were seen for new myocardial infarctions or unstable angina. The pattern of mortality in INTACT is consistent with two other studies in survivors of myocardial infarction where more deaths were reported in nifedipine-treated patients compared with those receiving placebo (Muller *et al* 1984; The SPRINT Study Group 1988). Dihydropyridine calcium channel blockers can occasionally be "proischemic" (Waters 1991) and how long-term treatment with these drugs will influence coronary events and overall mortality is uncertain.

CORONARY ATHEROSCLEROSIS AFTER CARDIAC TRANSPLANTATION

A form of accelerated coronary atherosclerosis develops after cardiac transplantation and limits the long-term prognosis of these patients. This process is manifest angiographically as progressive distal vessel obliteration associated with more typical proximal atherosclerotic lesions (Gao *et al* 1988). Intracoronary ultrasound shows that, one year after transplantation, all patients have developed at least some degree of intimal thickening, the initial abnormality (St Goar *et al* 1992).

Preliminary results from an ongoing study indicate that diltiazem may prevent this type of atherosclerosis (Schroeder *et al* 1993). Coronary arteriograms have been obtained early after cardiac transplantation and at one and two years in 57 of 104 consecutive eligible patients who were randomized to unblinded treatment with or without diltiazem. The average coronary arterial diameter decreased in the control group ($p < 0.001$) but remained unchanged in diltiazem patients. Coronary stenoses >50% luminal diameter have developed in 7 untreated and in 2 diltiazem-treated cases. Coronary death or retransplantation has occurred in 5 patients, none of whom were in the diltiazem group. Further follow-up will reveal whether the small improvements in coronary dimensions seen within 2 years will presage a reduction in future coronary events in these patients.

The importance of immunological mechanisms in the pathogenesis of post-transplant atherosclerosis and its similarity to ordinary atherosclerosis in terms of etiology have not been well defined. The mechanism by which diltiazem appears to prevent post-transplant atherosclerosis and the mechanism by which dihydropyridines appear to prevent the development of new lesions may be similar, but are as yet undefined.

FUTURE DIRECTIONS

A major limitation of angiographic trials is that coronary arteriography provides limited information. Although quantitative techniques can more accurately assess changes in the severity of arterial narrowings than could older methods (Waters *et al* 1993), the arterial wall and its pathology are not directly visualized. Newer techniques, specifically angioscopy and intravascular ultrasound, circumvent this limitation and will eventually yield data on lesion changes to complement coronary arteriography. Although both of these techniques are now in their infancy, intravascular ultrasound is superior to angioscopy because it does not require a blood-free field of vision and displays the entire thickness of the vessel wall, not just the surface. Intracoronary ultrasound is particularly likely to be more useful than coronary arteriography in the assessment of early coronary lesions.

In spite of these limitations, the clinical trials completed to date demonstrate that calcium channel blockers do not influence the evolution of established coronary atherosclerosis but appear to prevent the progression of early lesions. This conclusion is tentative, pending completion of ongoing clinical trials. Whether this beneficial effect is a feature of all calcium channel blockers, or whether some of these drugs are more potent than others in this regard, is as yet unknown.

The combined effect of lipid lowering therapy and a calcium channel blocker upon human coronary atherosclerosis has not yet been investigated. In the recently published Canadian Coronary Atherosclerosis Intervention Trial (CCAIT), lovastatin significantly reduced the appearance of new coronary lesions (Waters *et al* 1994). Adding a calcium channel blocker to an HMG CoA reductase inhibitor might add no additional benefit with respect to the development of new lesions, or the combination might produce an additive or synergistic effect because the mechanisms of action of the two classes of drugs differ. Further studies are likely to yield on array of drugs that exert a favorable influence upon the evolution of coronary atherosclerosis, by acting upon different components of the atherosclerotic process.

SUMMARY

Although lowering blood cholesterol levels slows the progression of coronary atherosclerosis, other approaches to stabilizing atherosclerosis should be explored, because in many patients coronary atherosclerosis will continue to progress in spite of an improvement in blood lipids. A beneficial effect on the development of atherosclerosis in the cholesterol-fed rabbit has been demonstrated with many calcium channel blockers. Nifedipine and amlodipine have also been shown to suppress atherogenesis in monkeys, a model more analogous to human atherosclerosis. Three clinical trials have examined the effect of calcium channel blockers on the angiographic evolution of coronary atherosclerosis.

In the Montreal Heart Institute Nicardipine Trial, 335 patients underwent repeat coronary arteriography after 2 years of treatment with either nicardipine or placebo. The drug had no effect on the overall progression or regression of coronary atherosclerosis; however, minimal coronary lesions, (≤20% at the first angiogram), progressed in 15 of 99 nicardipine patients compared with 32 of 118 placebo patients with reference to such lesions at baseline (15 vs 27%, $p = 0.046$). Similar results were found in INTACT: nifedipine had no influence on the progression or regression of established coronary atherosclerosis but reduced the appearance of new coronary lesions. In spite of this angiographic benefit, the mortality rate was higher in the nifedipine group than in controls. Preliminary results from an ongoing trial at Stanford University indicate that diltiazem prevents the development of coronary atherosclerosis in the transplant heart.

Further studies are required to confirm these findings and to determine how calcium channel blockers affect the incidence of coronary events.

REFERENCES

Brown G, Albers JJ, Fisher LD *et al* 1990 Regression of coronary artery disease as a result of intensive lipid-lowering therapy in men with high levels of apolipoprotein B. N Engl J Med 323: 1289–1298

Daugherty A, Rateri DL, Schonfeld G, Sobel BE 1987 Inhibition of cholesteryl ester deposition in macrophages by calcium entry blockers: an effect dissociable from calcium entry blockade. Br J Pharmacol 91: 113–118

Etingin OR, Hajjar DP 1985 Nifedipine increases cholesteryl ester hydrolytic activity in lipid-laden rabbit arterial smooth muscle cells. J Clin Invest 75: 1554–1558

Etingin OR, Hajjar DP 1990 Calcium channel

blockers enhance cholesteryl ester hydrolysis and decrease total cholesterol accumulation in human aortic tissue. Circ Res 66: 185–190

Fronek K 1988 Effect of nisoldipine on diet-induced atherosclerosis in rabbits. Ann NY Acad Sci 522: 525–526

Gao SZ, Alderman EL, Schroeder JS, Silverman JF, Hunt SA 1988 Accelerated coronary vascular disease in the heart transplant patient: Coronary arteriographic findings. J Am Coll Cardiol 12: 334–340

Gottlieb SO, Brinker JA, Mellits ED *et al* 1989 Effect of nifedipine on the development of coronary bypass graft stenoses in high-risk patients: A randomized, double-blind, placebo-controlled trial. Circulation 80 (suppl II): Abstract II-228

Habib JB, Bossaller C, Wells S, Williams C, Morrisett JD, Henry PD 1986 Preservation of endothelium-dependent vascular relaxation in cholesterol-fed rabbit by treatment with the calcium blocker PN 200110. Circ Res 58: 305–309

Handley DA, Van Valen RG, Melden MK, Saunders RN 1986 Suppression of rat carotid lesion development by the calcium channel blocker PN 200-110. Am J Pathol 124: 88–93

Henry PD 1990 Calcium antagonists as anti-atherosclerotic agents. Arteriosclerosis 10: 963–965

Henry PD 1991 Antiperoxidative actions of calcium antagonists and atherogenesis. J Cardiovasc Pharmacol 18 (suppl 1): S6–S10

Henry PD, Bentley KI 1981 Suppression of atherogenesis in cholesterol-fed rabbit treated with nifedipine. J Clin Invest 68: 1366–1369

Jackson LJ, Bush RC, Bowyer DE 1988 Inhibitory effect of calcium antagonists on balloon catheter-induced arterial smooth muscle cell proliferation and lesion size. Atherosclerosis 69: 115–122

Kramsch DM, Aspen AJ, Rozler LJ 1981 Atherosclerosis: prevention by agents not affecting abnormal levels of blood lipids. Science 213: 1511–1512

Kramsch DM, Sharma RC, Hodis HN 1993 Amlodipine suppresses in vivo low-density lipoprotein oxidation, hyperinsulinemia and atherosclerosis in primates. Circulation 88 (suppl I): Abstract I-562

Lacoste LL, Lam JYT, Hung J, Waters D 1994 Oral verapamil inhibits platelet thrombus formation in men. Circulation 89: 630–634

Lam JYT, Latour JG, Lespérance J, Waters D 1994 Platelet aggregation, coronary artery disease progression, and future coronary events. Am J Cardiol 73: 333–338

Lichtlen PR, Hugenholtz PG, Rafflenbeul W *et al* 1990 Retardation of angiographic progression of coronary artery disease by nifedipine. Lancet 335: 1109–1113

Lichtor T, Davis HR, Vesselinovitch D, Wissler RW, Mullan S 1989 Suppression of atherogenesis by nifedipine in the cholesterol-fed rhesus monkey. Appl Pathol 7: 8–18

Loaldi A, Polese A, Montorsi P *et al* 1989 Comparison of nifedipine, propranolol and isosorbide dinitrate on angiographic progression and regression of coronary arterial narrowings in angina pectoris. Am J Cardiol 64: 433–439

McMurray HF, Chahwala SB 1991 Amlodipine exerts a potent antimigratory effect on aortic smooth muscle cells in culture . J Am Coll Cardiol 17: Abstract 194A

Muller JE, Morrison J, Stone PH *et al* 1984 Nifedipine therapy for patients with threatened and acute myocardial infarction: A randomized, double-blind, placebo-controlled comparison. Circulation 69: 740–747

Nakao J, Ito H, Ooyama T, Chang WC, Murota S 1983 Calcium dependency of aortic smooth muscle cell migration induced by 12-L-hydroxy-5,8,10,14-eico-satetraenoic acid. Atherosclerosis 46: 309–319

Nomoto A, Hirosumi J, Sekiguchi C, Mutoh S, Yamaguchi I, Aoki H 1987 Antiatherogenic activity of FE34235 (Nilvadipine), a new potent calcium antagonist: effect on cuff-induced intimal thickening of rabbit carotid artery. Atherosclerosis 64: 255–261

Nunnari JJ, White SDT, Cuénoud HF 1993 The effect of felodipine on lipid deposition in the rat aorta. Circulation 88 (suppl I): Abstract I-522

Rouleau JL, Parmley WW, Stevens J *et al* 1983 Verapamil suppresses atherosclerosis in cholesterol-fed rabbits. J Am Coll Cardiol 1: 1453–460

Schmitz G, Robenek H, Beuck M 1988 Ca^{++} antagonists and ACAT inhibitors promote cholesterol efflux from macrophages by different mechanisms. Arteriosclerosis 8: 46–56

Schroeder JS, Gao SZ, Alderman EL 1993 A preliminary study of diltiazem in the prevention of coronary artery disease in heart transplant recipients. N Engl J Med 328: 164–170

The SPRINT Study Group 1988 The secondary prevention re-infarction Israeli nifedipine trial (SPRINT) II: results. Eur Heart J 9 (suppl I): Abstract I-350

St Goar FG, Pinto FJ, Alderman EL *et al* 1992 Intracoronary ultrasound in cardiac transplant recipients. *In vivo* evidence of "angiographically silent" intimal thickening. Circulation 85: 979–987

Steinberg D, Parthasarathy S, Carew TE, Khoo JC, Witztum JL 1989 Beyond cholesterol. Modifications of low-density lipoprotein that increase its atherogenicity. N Engl J Med 320: 915–924

Stender S, Ravn H, Haugegaard M, Kjeldson K 1986 Effect of verapamil on accumulation of free and esterified cholesterol in the thoracic aorta of cholesterol-fed rabbits. Atherosclerosis 61: 15–23

Sugano M, Nakashima Y, Tasaki H, Takasugi M, Kuroiwa A, Koide O 1988 Effects of diltiazem on suppression and regression of experimental atherosclerosis. Br J Exp Pathol 69: 515–523

Taeymans Y, Théroux P, Lespérance J, Waters D 1992 Quantitative angiographic morphology of the coronary artery lesions at risk for thrombotic occlusion. Circulation 85: 78-85

Vita JA, Treasure CB, Nabel EG *et al* 1990 Coronary vasomotor response to acetylcholine relates to risk factors for coronary artery disease. Circulation 81: 491–497

Waters D 1991 Proischemic complications of dihydropyridine calcium channel blockers. Circulation 84: 2598–2600

Waters D, Lespérance J, Francetich M *et al* 1990 A controlled clinical trial to assess the effect of a calcium channel blocker on the progression of coronary atherosclerosis. Circulation 82: 1940–1953

Waters D, Lespérance J, Craven TE, Hudon G, Gillam LD 1993 Advantages and limitations of serial coronary arteriography for the assessment of progression and regression of coronary atherosclerosis: Implications for clinical trials. Circulation 87 (suppl II): II-38–II-47

Waters D, Higginson L, Gladstone P *et al* 1994 Effects of monotherapy with an HMG CoA reductase inhibitor upon the progression of coronary atherosclerosis as assessed by serial quantitative arteriography: The Canadian Coronary Atherosclerosis Intervention Trial (CCAIT). Circulation 89: 959–968

Willis AL, Nagel B, Churchill V *et al* 1985 Antiatherosclerotic effects of nicardipine and nifedipine in cholesterol-fed rabbits. Atherosclerosis 5: 250–255

Yang Z, Noll G, Luscher TF 1993 Calcium antagonists differently inhibit proliferation of human coronary smooth muscle cells in response to pulsatile stretch and platelet-derived growth factor. Circulation 88: 832–836

Multiple Risk Factors in Cardiovascular Disease, ed. by A. Yamamoto, Churchill Livingstone Japan, Tokyo, pp. 81–84 (1994)

WOMEN OF MENOPAUSAL AGE AND HYPERLIPIDEMIA — EFFECTS OF ESTROGENS AND AN HMG-CoA REDUCTASE INHIBITOR[§]

Hideo HONJO,[*1] Kazunori TANAKA,[*1] Tomohiro KASHIWAGI,[*1] Hiroji OKADA,[*1] Kaori TAKANASHI,[*2] and Itsuo YOSHIZAWA[*2]

[*1] *Department of Obstetrics and Gynecology, Kyoto Prefectural University of Medicine, and*
[*2] *Hokkaido Institute of Pharmaceutical Sciences*

Keywords: women of menopausal age, lipid, estrogen, 2 hydroxy estradiol 17-sulfate, HMG-CoA reductase inhibitor

Recently, the life expectancy of Japanese women has become the longest in the world, 82.5 years in 1993. In 1993 the primary cause of death in women was heart disease (25%), and the third was cerebral vascular disease (17%) (Ministry of Health and Welfare, Japan); both of these are closely related to hyperlipidemia. Hyperlipidemia increases around menopause, when endogenous estrogens decrease. We investigated the serum lipids, estrogens, postheparin plasma lipase activities, and lipid peroxides in outpatients of menopausal age as well as examining the effects of pravastatin.

SERUM LIPIDS AT THE MENOPAUSE

Hypercholesterolemia [total cholesterol (TC) ≥220 mg/dl] was identified in 10 out of 30 female outpatients without gynecological problems (Honjo *et al* 1992a). The serum TC in men and women in the general population in 1990 has been reported by the Japanese Ministry of Health and Welfare (1993) and hypercholesterolemia was more frequently seen in women, especially after menopause, than men. Hypercholesterolemia was detected in 46.2% of women age of between 50 and 59 years (29.3% in men), 52.6% between 60 and 69 years (26.2% in men), and 42.0% in those over 70 years (22.2% in men).

Hypertriglyceridemia [triglyceride (TG) ≥150 mg/dl] was noted in 5 out of 30 female outpatients. Also according to the above report, hypertriglyceridemia was more frequently seen in women than men. Hypertriglyceridemia was detected in 22.2% of women aged between 50 and 59 years (24.6% in men), 22.0% of women between 60 and 69 years (14.3% in men), and in 17.2% of women over 70 years(13.3% in men). Low serum high-density lipoprotein cholesterol (HDL-C ≤40 mg/dl) was detected in only one out of outpatients (Honjo *et al* 1992a).

Serum TC in women before menopause has been compared with that after menopause, every year as part of a mass screening by Yamada *et al* (Honjo 1991). The TC levels before menopause were significantly ($p < 0.05$) lower than those after menopause, at 50, 51, and 52 years of age.

[*1] Kawaramachi, Hirokoji, Kamigyo-Ku, Kyoto 602 Japan.
[*2] Otaru, 047-02, Japan
[§] This study was supported in part by a Research Grant for Intractable Diseases (Primary hyperlipidemia), from the Ministry of Health and Welfare and Works of Scientific Research and Technical Development, Public Health Department of Kyoto Prefectural Government.

SERUM LIPIDS, LIPOPROTEINS, AND ESTROGENS

Among 34 women who did not receive estrogen treatment, a significant negative correlation ($r = -0.337$, $p < 0.05$) was found between serum TC levels and estradiol-17β (E_2) levels.

Serum HDL-C levels tended to increase with serum E_2 levels ($r = 0.213$, $p < 0.05$). Serum apolipoprotein A-I (apo A-I) is the main component of HDL and concentrations of apo A-I and HDL-C were strongly correlated ($r = 0.837$, $p = 0.001$). The concentration of apo A-I increased slightly with serum E_2 ($r = 0.306$, $p < 0.1$). Intestinal and/or hepatic production of apo A-I may be stimulated by estrogen, and HDL and HDL-C may increase.

In a later study of serum lipid levels involving 74 women around menopause, twelve received conjugated estrogen (0.625 to 1.25 mg daily for 21 days followed by 7 days without drugs, cyclically) for the treatment of climacteric syndrome (Honjo *et al* 1992a). In postmenopausal women, HDL-C levels were significantly higher and low-density lipoprotein cholesterol (LDL-C) levels were significantly lower in the estrogen-treated women than in the untreated women.

HTGL, LpL AND ESTROGENS

Tikkanen *et al* (1985) have reported the suppression of hepatic triglyceride lipase (HTGL) following estrogen treatment. Recently, we measured HTGL, lipoprotein lipase (LpL) (10 min value, postheparin inj.), lipids and E_2 in 82 women (37–70 years) including some receiving estrogen replacement therapy (ERT). HTGL decreased inversely with E_2 ($r = -0.244$, $p < 0.05$). LpL also decreased inversely with serum E_2 ($r = -0.288$, $p < 0.05$). The effects of ERT in the postmenopausal group were analyzed. There was no difference in LpL between ERT(+) women and ERT(–) women. The mean HTGL in ERT(–) women was 0.198 μM/ml/min and the corresponding figure in ERT(+) women was significantly ($p < 0.05$) lower at 0.145 μM/ml/min.

HTGL was correlated with both LDL-C ($r = 0.41$, $p = 0.0003$) and TC ($r = 0.409$, $p = 0.0002$).

Estrogens (moderate or low dose) produce mostly ameliorative effects on lipid metabolism. Figure 1 shows a tentative schema of the mechanisms of the effects of estrogen on HTGL, LpL and lipids. Estrogens suppress HTGL which accelerates conversion of HDL_2-C to HDL_3-C and induces

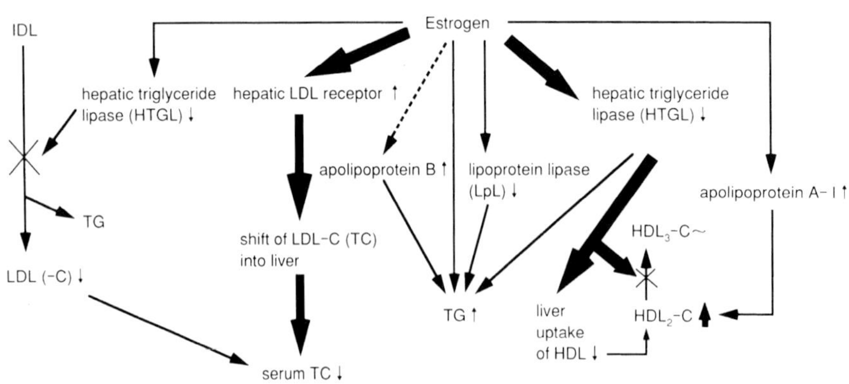

Fig. 1. A tentative schema of the mechanism of estrogen effects on lipid metabolism.
Moderate or low dose or level of estrogens induce mostly ameliorative effects on lipid levels. -C and C, cholesterol; TG, triglyceride.

the uptake of HDL by the liver. Thus, HDL-C may increase with apo A-I.

In addition, estrogen also increases the number of hepatic LDL receptors and accelerates the transfer of LDL-C (and TC) from serum to the liver. Consequently, serum TC decreases. Additionally, HTGL may also accelerate conversion of intermediate density lipoprotein (IDL) to LDL while the suppression of HTGL by estrogen may lower LDL-C (and TC).

LIPID PEROXIDES AND ESTROGENS — 2 HYDROXY ESTRADIOL 17-SULFATE

The relationship between serum lipid peroxides and estrogens were investigated. A correlation ($r = 0.41$, $p = 0.02$) was observed between serum lipid peroxides and TG.

In 1992, human serum estradiol 17-sulfate (E_2-17-S) was measured for the first time (Honjo *et al* 1992b). E_2-17-S can easily be converted to 2 hydroxy (-OH) or 4-OH E_2-17-S.

These catecholized E_2-17-S (= 2-OH E_2-17-S, 4-OH E_2-17-S) are more stable than the free catechol estrogens (= 2-OH E_2, 4-OH E_2) and suppress lipid peroxidation very strongly. In normal pregnancy, when serum E_2-17-S is low, lipid peroxides are high. When E_2-17-S increased, lipid peroxides decrease. Pregnant women with pregnancy-induced hypertension and/or diabetes mellitus exhibit low levels of E_2-17-S and high levels of lipid peroxides. Some discordances were speculated in these diseases. In our *in vitro* study, using endothelial cells from the human umbilical vein, 2-OH E_2-17-S was found to protect these cells from oxidative stress. In a subsequent *in vitro* study, endothelial cells from the human artery were studied. ^{51}Cr release assay was used to determine whether and how 2-OH E_2-17-S could protect the cells from oxidative stress by *t*-BuOOH. E_2-17-S strongly suppressed ^{51}Cr release, while 2-OH E_2-17-S suppressed it even more strongly (Fig. 2). Thus, these estrogens are able to protect human arterial endothelial cells from oxidative stress. These estrogens may also inhibit oxidation (oxidizing degeneration) of LDL-C and suppress atherosclerosis of the vascular endothelium.

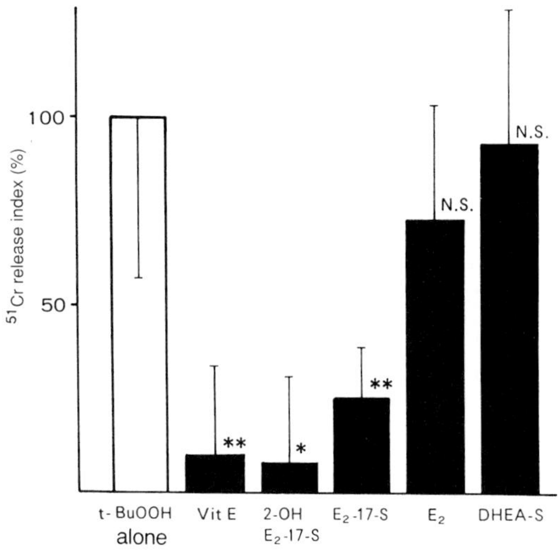

Fig. 2. Suppression of oxidative stress by various steroids.
t-BuOOH induced oxidative stress on endothelial cells from human arteries. 2-OH E_2-17-S and E_2-17-S suppressed oxidative stress compared to vitamin E. Mean ± SD. $^*p < 0.02$; $^{**}p < 0.02$. HEDA-S, dehydroepiandrosterone sulfate.

Recently, Rosano *et al* (1993) reported the rapid direct beneficial effects of estrogen on the coronary artery.

Because of the above three beneficial effects of estrogens on 1) lipids, 2) antioxidation, and 3) vascular walls, ERT (and hormone replacement therapy, HRT) may become more widely used.

HMG-CoA REDUCTASE INHIBITOR

The HMG-CoA reductase inhibitor, pravastatin, is a new drug. It is hydrophilic and tissue-selective and very effective in reducing serum TC (Honjo *et al* 1992a). The effect on TC (LDL-C) is more rapid than that of estrogens. Pravastatin affects the pathway leading from acetate to cholesterol by inhibiting the action of HMG-CoA reductase. Concern has been expressed, however, that pravastatin may reduce levels of endogenous estrogen (a further metabolite of cholesterol) .

Pravastatin was given to 25 women of menopausal age with hyperlipidemia. Before and during pravastatin therapy, serum lipids and estrogens were measured. Two weeks after pravastatin therapy, serum TC had decreased significantly ($p < 0.01$). LDL-C had also decreased significantly ($p < 0.05$) two weeks later, while serum TG and HDL-C levels were unchanged. Serum levels of E_2 and estrone (E_1) showed no marked changes during treatment. Serum estrone sulfate (E_1-S) was measured by direct radioimmunoassay (Honjo *et al* 1986, 1987), and was unchanged. Consequently, endogenous estrogens, which may have beneficial effects on lipids, were not suppressed during pravastatin therapy.

SUMMARY

Hyperlipidemia and cardiovascular diseases increase around the menopause, when endogenous estrogens decrease. The serum lipids, estrogens, postheparin plasma lipase activity, and lipid peroxides in outpatients of menopausal age were investigated. The effects of pravastatin (an HMG-CoA reductase inhibitor) were also examined.

Serum TC, TG, HDL-C, LDL-C, E_1, E_2, E_1-S, postheparin plasma lipase activity and lipid peroxides were analyzed. The effects of estrogens (2-OH E_2 17-S and others.) on lipid peroxides were studied *in vitro*, using human aortic endothelial cells.

Many women (10/30) showed raised total cholesterolemia (≥220 mg/dl). TC was negatively correlated with E_2 ($r = -0.337$, $p < 0.05$). Exogenous estrogen elevated HDL-cholesterol and suppressed LDL-cholesterol, especially after menopause (both, $p < 0.05$). Lipid peroxides correlated with TG ($r = 0.41$, $p < 0.05$). In addition 2-OH E_2 17-S strongly suppressed ^{51}Cr release (lipid peroxidation) in endothelial cells *in vitro*.

Pravastatin, 5–30 mg/day, was given to 25 women of menopausal age with hyperlipidemia. Two weeks after therapy, serum TC had decreased significantly ($p < 0.01$), LDL-C had also decreased two weeks later ($p < 0.05$), while serum levels of E_2, E_1, and E_1-S were unchanged.

Conclusion: Estrogens (moderate or low dose or level) produce mostly ameliorative effects on lipid metabolism and may protect endothelial cells from oxidative stress. Pravastatin effectively lowers lipid levels without decreasing endogenous estrogens.

Acknowledgments
We express our sincere thanks to Professor Toshio Nambara, Sendai, for giving us the antibody for E_1-S and also to Sankyo Co., Ltd., Japan for their cooperation.

REFERENCES

Honjo H 1991 Clinical data of Mevalotin: Its usefulness in hypercholesterolemia around menopause. JAMA (Jpn Ed) 10: Append 26–29

Honjo H, Kitawaki J, Itoh M *et al* 1986 Serum and urinary oestrone sulphate in pregnancy and delivery measured by a direct radioimmunoassay. Acta Endocrinol 112: 423–430

Honjo H, Kitawaki J, Itoh M *et al* 1987 Serum and urinary etrone sulfate during the menstrual cycle measured by a direct radioimmunoassay, and fate of exogenously injected estrone sulfate. Horm Res 27: 61–68

Honjo H, Tanaka K, Urabe M *et al* 1992a Menopause and hyperlipidemia: Pravastatin lowers lipid levels without decreasing endogenous estrogens. Clin Ther 14: 699–707

Honjo H, Tanaka K, Yasuda J *et al* 1992b. Serum estradiol 17-sulphate and lipid peroxides in late pregnancy. Acta Endocrinol 126: 303–307

Rosano GMC, Sarrel PM, Poole-Wilson PA *et al* 1993 Beneficial effect of oestrogen on exercise-induced myocardial ischaemia in women with coronary artery disease. Lancet 342: 133–136

Tikkanen MJ, Kuusi T, Nikkilä EA *et al* 1985 Very low density lipoprotein triglyceride kinetics during hepatic lipase suppression by estrogen: Studies on the physiological role of hepatic endothelial lipase. FEBS Lett 181: 160–164

Multiple Risk Factors in Cardiovascular Disease, ed. by A. Yamamoto, Churchill Livingstone Japan, Tokyo, pp. 85–89 (1994)

STRESS AND HEART DISEASE: INVOLVEMENT OF CATECHOLAMINES

Pallab K. Ganguly and Robert E. Beamish

*Division of Cardiovascular Sciences, St. Boniface General Hospital Research Centre**

Key words: catecholamines, stress, Ca^{2+} overload, oxidative products

It is generally accepted that stress influences the hormonal and metabolic equilibrium of an individual and it becomes operative when the individual can no longer cope with the demands of the internal or external environment, or both. This is due to excessive mental, emotional, physical or social demands which in turn may be aggravated or alleviated by the psychosocial environment impinging on the stressed person. Thus the situation is complex with psychological, psychiatric, psychosocial and pathophysiological overtones.

In recent decades it has been postulated that stress plays a role in the genesis of heart disease and also serves to aggravate or complicate existing heart disease. The consequences may manifest themselves in cardiac symptoms (palpitations, dyspnea, or cardiac pain), angina pectoris, myocardial infarction, or sudden death. Although the mechanisms by which this occurs are somewhat obscure and incompletely understood, catecholamines are clearly implicated. The purpose of this chapter is to emphasize the relationship between stress and heart disease and examine the evidence that catecholamines and their oxidation products are involved.

STRESS AND HEART DISEASE

Although its definition is somewhat difficult, everyone knows or thinks they know what stress is, even if the perception is highly individual. It is generally believed that what is stress for one person could be a stimulus for another. However, the majority of people are aware of the fact that stress is often associated with uncomfortable sensations such as tachycardia, epigastric discomfort, perspiration, tremor, muscular tension and a sense of fear, at times of danger, frustration, anxiety or excessive physical or psychological demands. This syndrome is commonly accepted as stress. The question remains: how does stress induce heart disease?

Olsson and Rehnquist (1982) described the following in a case report: "A 70-year-old man, taking part in a post-infarction study, died suddenly out of the hospital while Holter-monitored. Death was preceded by immediate major psychological stress (loss of wallet containing important documents) but there were no cardiac symptoms. Electrocardiogram showed a 15 min period of sinus tachycardia with increased ventricular

* 351 Tache Avenue, Winnipeg, Manitoba R2H 2A6, Canada.

ectopic activity prior to the initiation of ventricular fibrillation. There were no signs of myocardial infarction at autopsy. It is proposed that increased catecholamine stimulation due to psychologic stress, in combination with myocardial ischemia, may have precipitated the fatal arrhythmia."

Scientists have long been aware of the link between emotions and the heart. In 1628, Sir William Harvey (1628) in his excellent description of the heart and circulation wrote "Every affection of the mind that is attended with either pain or pleasure, hope or fear, is the cause of an agitation whose influence extends to the heart." This perceptive observation went unheeded until the present century when Cannon (1929), Raab (1953), and Selye (1982) laid the foundations for the present postulates of stress and its physiological and pathophysiological effects in health and disease.

In the Framingham study (Haynes *et al* 1980), 1674 event-free individuals were followed for eight years for evidence of the development of coronary heart disease (CHD). Women (aged 45 to 64) who developed CHD scored significantly higher in terms of type A behavior, suppressed hostility, tension and anxiety symptom scales than women remaining free of CHD. Type A women developed twice as much CHD and three times as much angina as type B women. Men exhibiting Framingham type A behavior, work overload, suppressed hostility, and frequent job promotions were also at increased risk of CHD. Boman (1982) reported that "anxiety and depression have both been shown to predict the development of CHD in studies covering follow-up spans of up to 40 years, and that in patients who have suffered an infarct, neurotic symptoms may worsen their prognosis."

Gecele *et al* (1992) have taken into account the relationships among type A and other risk factors and the possible biological mechanisms through which type A behavior may promote CHD. Type A behavior consists of a variety of psychological, behavioral and cognitive features and represents an important risk factor for CHD. Vogele and Steptoe (1993) have reported that anger inhibition and family history are modulators of cardiovascular responses to mental stress in adolescent boys. Their results suggest that the tendency to inhibit anger expression interacts with familial factors (blood pressure) in determining reactivity patterns that may be indicative of a raised risk of future cardiovascular disease. Denollet (1993) also suggested that inhibited individuals (characterized by the nonexpression of anger) may be particularly coronary prone which may indicate that research should focus on the interaction of global traits that may define subtypes of patients with CHD.

Social and economic forces create an environment in which disordered lipid metabolism and deranged endocrine metabolism combine to produce harmful cardiovascular effects. The relationship between stress and lipid derangements has been well documented but strangely underestimated in the issue of stress-induced heart disease. It is believed that disturbed lipid metabolism is the direct result of abundant food, higher calorie and fat intake, less physical activity, decreased energy consumption and, finally, disturbed endocrine function (catecholamines and free radicals). These factors are well correlated with social and economic forces, a high standard of living and stress. Dimsdale and Herd (1982) in a review of 60 studies of the effect of short-term emotional arousal on plasma lipids observed that free fatty acids were almost invariably elevated and that most studies showed cholesterol to be increased from 8 to 65% above baseline. It must be emphasized that some individuals exhibit more marked endocrine and metabolic reactions to stress and it may well be that they are more prone to cardiovascular disease.

CATECHOLAMINES AND HEART DISEASE

A significant increase in the levels of catecholamines has been reported in a variety of stressful conditions (Beamish *et al* 1991). Severe emotional stress, racing-car driving, sexual arousal, acute physiological stress, and simulated battle conditions are all accompanied by an increase in plasma catecholamines. The onset of chest pain and acute myocardial infarction are also known to be accompanied by a significant increase in plasma and urine catecholamines.

A variety of social and environmental stresses are frequently associated with increased levels of circulating catecholamines (Beamish *et al* 1991). Although the cardiotoxic properties of high doses of catechol amines have been known for many years, the role of catecholamines in the development of stress-associated cardiomyopathy has only been recognized recently. It has been proposed that excessive amounts of catecholamines are responsible for myocardial pathology in stressful situations similar to that found in patients with pheochromocytoma. Animals injected with high doses of isoproterenol, a synthetic catecholamine, have been shown to exhibit myocardial cell damage, and this is considered to be a good experimental model for studying the structural, biochemical and functional alterations in the heart during the development of cardiomyopathy (Rona 1985). The time course of cardiac ultrastructural changes, following high doses of isoproterenol in rats, have been studied extensively. The earliest changes, evident within 4 to 6 minutes, are disorientation of myofilaments, irregular sarcomere length, occasional regions of contracture or rupture of myofilaments and some slight dilatation of the sarcoplasmic reticulum. By 10 minutes, mitochondrial swelling is evident, with the occasional occurrence of electron-dense bodies. Within 30 minutes to an hour, electron-dense granular deposits are frequently noted within mitochondria and numerous lipid droplets are also seen. Over the course of the next few hours, all of these changes become progressively widespread and more severe throughout the myocardium.

One important aspect in this regard is the involvement of abnormal movements of Ca^{2+}, which is required to activate biochemical processes during cardiac contraction. Ca^{2+} transport systems in different membranes adapt to high doses of administered catecholamines by initially increasing Ca^{2+} fluxes but thereafter these mechanisms deteriorate (Panagia *et al* 1985). However, the occurrence of intracellular Ca^{2+} overload (at a later period) due to membrane defects initiates a variety of events, including excessive utilization of high-energy phosphates and alteration in cellular integrity leading to cell death.

OXIDATION PRODUCTS OF CATECHOLAMINES

The normal catabolism of catecholamines proceeds through enzymatic pathways (monoaminooxidase, catechol-o-methyltransferase, and phenolsulphotransferase). In addition, nonenzymatic oxidative pathways may also be involved since catechols are readily oxidized. The oxidation of catecholamines is a complex process in which quinones, hydroquinones, and semiquinone free-radical intermediates are formed. Any alteration in the metabolism of catecholamines or disruption of their transport mechanisms may lead to anomalously high concentrations of these substances and consequently the enzymes dealing with their catabolism may be unable to cope efficiently. Therefore, catecholamines may undergo autooxidation in those cell compartments where their concentration has increased, giving rise to potentially toxic products such as free radical, ortho-quinones and indolic catechols (Bindoli *et al* 1992).

A new hypothesis has been advanced concerning the pathological mechanism of catecholamine-induced myocardial injury, whereby adrenochrome and free radicals or other catecholamine oxidation products may be regarded as possible candidates for cardiotoxicity when excess levels of catecholamines are present in the circulation (Ganguly 1991). The accumulation of the oxidation products of catecholamines in the myocardium could directly or indirectly, acting by themselves or in conjunction with other effects of catecholamines, initiate processes leading to myocardial necrosis. In fact, adrenochrome has been shown to impair the contractile function of the heart and this deleterious action is clearly a dose- and time-dependent phenomenon. The toxic influence of adrenochrome on the myocardium and its modification by various cationic and pharmacological agents support the participation of this oxidation product in the pathogenesis of catecholamine-induced cardiomyopathy.

Recently, an HPLC assay for the measurement of plasma adrenolutin has been developed (Dhalla *et al* 1989) and relatively high levels of adrenolutin have been found in the plasma of the rat, dog, rabbit, and pig. Furthermore, these levels were increased by the administration of different catecholamines, suggesting the presence of an efficient mechanism for the oxidation of catecholamines *in vivo*. Adrenochrome, unlike adrenolutin, was not detected in plasma by this method.

SUMMARY

From this discussion, it is evident that stress-induced increases in the sympathetic drive with resultant excess catecholamines in the blood can result in arrhythmias, myocardial cell damage and even sudden death. Increase in intracellular calcium, indicating altered membrane permeability, has been considered to be an important determining factor in catecholamine-induced cardiomyopathy. It is our belief that cardiac injury is mediated by the oxidation products of catecholamines. However, the contribution of the other pharmacological actions of catecholamines to the toxic effects of these oxidation products cannot be ruled out.

REFERENCES

Beamish RE, Singal PK, Ganguly PK 1991 Stress, catecholamines and heart disease. *In*: Ganguly PK (Ed) Catecholamines and heart disease. CRC Press, Boca Raton, Fl, p 231

Bindoli A, Rigobello MP, Deeble DJ 1992 Biochemical and toxicological properties of the oxidation products of catecholamines. Free Radic Biol Med 13: 391–405

Boman B 1982 Psychosocial stress and ischemic heart disease. Aust N Z Psychiatry 16: 265–275

Cannon WB 1929 Bodily changes in pain, hunger, fear and rage. Appleton and Co., New York

Dhalla KS, Ganguly PK, Rupp H, Beamish RE, Dhalla NS 1989 Measurement of adrenalin as an oxidation product of catecholamines in plasma. Mol Cell Biochem 87: 85–92

Denollet J 1993 Biobehavioral research on coronary heart disease: where is the person? J Behav Med 16: 115–141

Dimsdale JE, Herd JA 1982 Variability of plasma lipids in response to emotional arousal. Psychosom Med. 44: 412–427

Ganguly PK 1991 Antioxidant therapy in congestive heart failure: is there any advantage? J Intern Med 229: 205–209

Gecele M, Grossi S, Franceletti G, Meluzzi A 1992 Relationship between type A behaviour and the other risk factors in chronic disease. Minerva Psychiatr 33: 33–43

Harvey W 1628 Exercile de motu cordis et sanguinis; cited by Hackett TP, Rosenbaum JF, Tesor GE. *In*: Braunwald E (Ed) Heart disease, WB Saunders, Philadelphia 1984 p 1883

Haynes SG, Feinleib M, Kannel WB 1980 The relationship of psychosocial factors to coronary heart disease in the Framingham study III. 8 year incidence of CHD. Am J Epidemiol III: 37–49

Olsson G, Rehnquist N 1982 Sudden death precipitated by psychological stress — a case report. Acta Med Scand 212: 437–451

Panagia V, Pierce GN, Dhalla KS, Ganguly PK, Beamish RE, Dhalla NS 1985 Adaptive changes in subcellular calcium transport during catecholamine induced cardiomyopathy. J Mol Cell Cardiol 17: 411–420

Raab W 1953 Hormonal and neurogenic cardiovascular disorders. Williams and Wilkins, Baltimore

Rona G 1985 Catecholamine cardiotoxicity. J Mol Cell Cardiol 17: 291–306

Selye H 1982 History and present status of the stress concept. *In*: Goldberger L, Breznitz S (Eds) Handbook of stress. The Free Press (Mcmillan), New York

Vogele C, Steptoe A 1993 Anger inhibition and family history as modulators of cardiovascular responses to mental stress in adolescent boys. J Psychosom Res 37: 503–514

SECTION 3.
HYPERTENSION & STROKE

Multiple Risk Factors in Cardiovascular Disease, ed. by A. Yamamoto, Churchill Livingstone Japan, Tokyo, pp. 93–97 (1994)

BLOOD PRESSURE IN ACUTE STROKE

John L. REID

*Department of Medicine and Therapeutics, University of Glasgow**

Key words: blood pressure, acute stroke, risk and benefits, cerebral blood flow

Stroke is closely associated with hypertension. Not only is hypertension a well established risk factor for all stroke sub-types (MacMahon *et al* 1990; Shaper *et al* 1991) but, as discussed later, reduction of blood pressure at least in primary prevention studies reduces the relative risk of atherothrombotic and hemorrhagic strokes (Collins *et al* 1990). In addition, acute transient elevation of blood pressure has been reported in patients presenting to hospital with an acute stroke (Wallace & Levy 1981; Carlberg *et al* 1991; Lees *et al* 1992). This brief review addresses the profile of blood pressure in acute stroke sub-types and discusses current views on the management of hypertension complicating acute stroke syndromes. In addition, the benefit of reducing blood pressure in primary and secondary prevention (in the absence or presence of a previous stroke/transient ischemic attacks) are reviewed as is the current performance in implementing prevention in clinical practice.

BLOOD PRESSURE IN ACUTE STROKE

Many studies have identified the importance of autoregulation in control of brain perfusion and the interference with autoregulation of cerebral blood flow that occurs during acute stroke (Barry *et al* 1984). Most of the earlier antihypertensive drugs lowered blood pressure with catastrophic effects on cerebral blood flow and brain perfusion. Some more recent drugs may have little or no effect on cerebral blood flow and may be more suitable for use in acute stroke (Waldemar *et al* 1989). A review of acute strokes admitted to hospital revealed that blood pressure is increased in most patients and falls over 24–48 hours (Wallace & Levy 1981; Carlberg *et al* 1991); blood pressure may remain elevated for longer in patients with hemorrhagic stroke. In patients with pre-existing hypertension, the blood pressure rise may be quantitatively greater but will usually fall to the pre-stroke levels over 3–5 days. A systematic study of blood pressure during acute stroke admissions by Carlberg *et al* (1991) suggested that this short-lived rise in blood pressure is not primarily related to the stroke but is associated with hospital admission. These workers reported that the profile of blood pressure in patients who were admitted to hospital within a few hours of stroke was very similar to that of those whose admissions were delayed for up to a week.

* Glasgow, Scotland.

It is generally agreed that the transient increase in blood pressure should not be treated with antihypertensive agents unless blood pressure persists at very high levels (diastolic pressures >120–130 mmHg), or features of hypertensive encephalopathy are present. The co-existence of other cardiac or vascular urgencies. such as aortic aneurysm, heart failure, myocardial infarction is also an indication for active treatment (Yatsu & Zivin 1985; Spence & Del Maestro 1985). Proposed objectives of treatment of hypertension in stroke patients are presented in Table I. In the future, however, there are likely to be other situations in which it is advisable to lower blood pressure in a controlled manner in the patient with an acute stroke. These could include patients with intracerebral hemorrhage and also those patients who have been given thrombolytic drugs in whom the risk of extension of hemorrhage or hemorrhagic transformation of the infarct may be considered to outweigh the risk of compromising cerebral blood flow. On any occasion when blood pressure is lowered in acute stroke the emphasis should be on cautious controlled blood pressure reduction. Unfortunately, there is little systematic experience of blood pressure modification in acute stroke. Most reports are anecdotal or uncontrolled and no agreed ideal drug exists. Older agents were given intravenously and caused unpredictable large and long-lasting falls in blood pressure associated with paralysis of sympathetic reflex mechanisms. There is a current need for further study of short-acting drugs with predictable, reversible effects on blood pressure.

TABLE I. Proposed Objectives of Treatment of Hypertension in Stroke Patients

1. Avoidance of hypertensive encephalopathy, fits and cerebral hemorrhage in patients with malignant hypertension or severe hypertension.
2. Secondary prevention of other fatal or non-fatal cardiovascular events including aortic aneurysm, cardiac failure, arrhythmias, myocardial infarction or sudden death.
3. Secondary prevention of further stroke by control of blood pressure and other anti-atherogenic strategies.
4. Prevention of short-term extension of stroke by a further bleed in hemorrhagic stroke or hemorrhagic transformation in thrombotic stroke (especially after thrombolytic or other anticoagulant therapy).

There is a need to define the optimal blood pressure profile in acute stroke and for the opportunity to combine the optimal hemodynamic profile with the most useful neuroprotective mechanisms. It is likely that only when optimal hemodynamics are combined with appropriate delivery of the neuroprotective drug will the full potential for protection be achieved.

RISK OF STROKE AND BLOOD PRESSURE

Raised blood pressure has been clearly identified as a major risk factor for subsequent stroke in all the classic prospective epidemiological studies (MacMahon *et al* 1990; Shaper *et al* 1991). The relative risk of stroke is directly and linearly related to blood pressure. In a meta-analysis of prospective studies, this increased risk extended even into 'normal' levels of diastolic blood pressure (MacMahon *et al* 1990). On the basis of these prospective studies it was calculated that patients with a 6–7 mmHg fall in diastolic blood pressure would have a 42% lower relative risk of stroke.

BENEFITS OF BLOOD PRESSURE REDUCTION

There is good evidence that reduction of blood pressure by antihypertensive drugs can successfully lower stroke risk (Collins *et al* 1990). As noted above, prospective trials indicate a 42% increased risk for those with higher diastolic blood pressure. In intervention trials, a consistent benefit has been shown in reduction of stroke. A meta-analysis of unconfounded controlled intervention trials suggested that, for a 5- to 6-mmHg reduction in diastolic blood pressure, there was a 38% reduction in the relative risk of stroke (Collins *et al* 1990). This is very similar to the theoretical benefit calculated from prospective studies and indicates that treatment can achieve almost the full benefit of a reduction in stroke risk.

It appears that elderly patients at increased risk of stroke would be particularly likely to benefit from a blood pressure reduction. Earlier studies by the European Working Party on High Blood Pressure in the Elderly (Amery *et al* 1985; Coope & Warrender 1986) indicated a reduction in stroke risk of 35 and 42% respectively (Table II). Three recently published studies on older patients confirm the magnitude of the benefit (Dahlof *et al* 1991; MRC Working Party 1992; SHEP Co-operation Research Group 1991). In particular, the Systolic Hypertension in the Elderly Programme on patients with isolated systolic hypertension confirmed that even in this patient group there was a substantial potential for improvement in stroke risk with antihypertensive therapy.

EFFECTIVENESS OF ANTIHYPERTENSIVE TREATMENT IN PRACTICE

Although the benefits of antihypertensive therapy in primary prevention of stroke are now well established and unchallenged, the potential benefits may not always be translated into practice. It is widely recognized that even in 1994 many hypertensive patients are either not identified or, more commonly, not on effective treatment. The potential loss of benefit is not limited to stroke but, given the size of the benefit and the costs of caring for patients who survive a stroke, it appears worthwhile to target antihypertensive therapy at these older hypertensive patients who are at risk.

To determine the frequency of antihypertensive treatment of patients with a history of hypertension, we reviewed the admissions to the Western Infirmary Acute Stroke Unit for 1991–1992. This unit serves a population of 230,000 and admits all patients with stroke referred to the hospital service for intensive investigation and assessment (Morris *et al* 1993). Of 351 consecutive admissions, 132 were known to be hypertensive before presentation with stroke. This information was obtained from the patient, relatives or the family doctor. Of the patients with known hypertension, 53% were not on any recognized antihypertensive therapy at the time of their stroke (Lees *et al* 1992). We have not investigated the reasons why these patients were not on treatment, but it was not related to their age, as the percentage of patients on treatment who were over 80 years was similar to that of those aged under 70 years (Table III). In addition, the presence or absence of other cardiovascular risk factors did not influence whether the patients were treated or not. These findings, while not unexpected, emphasize the need for continued education of general practitioners and patients about the benefits of antihypertensive therapy, particularly in high-risk groups.

TABLE II. Reduction in Relative Risk of Stroke in Prospective Placebo-

Controlled Trials of antihypertensive Therapy in Older Patients	
European Working Party on Hypertension in the Elderly	35%
Coope and Warrender	42%
Swedish Trial in Old Patients with Hypertension	47%
Medical Research Council Trial of Hypertension in Older Adults	25%
Systolic Hypertension in the Elderly Program	36%

(from Reid 1993.)

PRIMARY VERSUS SECONDARY PREVENTION OF STROKE

Although the evidence supporting primary prevention of stroke in hypertensive patients

TABLE III. Influence of Patient Age on Antihypertensive Treatment States Prior to Acute Stroke in 351 Consecutive Admissions

Age (years)	Number of patients	Known hypertensives	Treated hypertensives	%on treatment
< 70	154	58	27	47
70–79	117	47	23	49
> 80	80	27	12	44

(from Lees *et al* 1992.)

is overwhelming, relatively little controlled trial information is available on the benefits of secondary prevention, let alone the benefits of alternative drug strategies. Placebo-controlled clinical trials performed over 20 years ago with a range of active drugs including methyldopa, diuretics, reserpine, and guanethidine came to contradictory conclusions (Carter 1970; Hypertension-Stroke Comparative Study Group 1974). These studies recruited patients who were stable after a completed stroke. The smaller of the studies concluded that there was significant benefit in secondary prevention of further stroke (Carter 1970). The other, larger, study did not show any significant reduction in cardiovascular endpoints apart from a reduction in congestive cardiac failure in the actively treated group. There appear to be good grounds for considering a new prospective controlled trial of secondary prevention in patients with previous transient ischemic attacks or completed minor strokes. A case could be made for including all patients, including those with normal (especially high-normal) blood pressures, and for basing treatment strategies on some of the newer drug groups, which may be less likely to affect cerebral blood flow adversely (Waldemar *et al* 1989) or for which neuroprotective or anti-ischemic properties have been claimed.

It has been proposed that in patients with transient ischemic attacks or completed stroke the benefit of antihypertensive therapy may be outweighed by the risk of provoking cerebral hypoperfusion and infarction, if significant stenosis of carotid or vertebral arteries is present. This issue could be directly addressed in the trial proposed. Alternatively, non-invasive Doppler ultrasound imaging of the main extracerebral vessels can easily identify these patients (Grosset 1992) and they can be excluded from the study.

SUMMARY

Raised blood pressure is not only a risk factor for all stroke types but blood pressure may be further elevated during admission to hospital with acute stroke. Blood pressure rises tend to be greater and more sustained in patients with hemorrhagic stroke compared with atherothrombotic stroke. In the latter patients the blood pressure falls over 48 to 72 hours to pre-stroke levels. It appears that the transient rise in blood pressure is more dependent on hospital admission than consequences of acute cerebral ischaemia. Acute hypertension in stroke is presently only treated pharmacologically if the rise is substantial (diastolic over 120–130 mmHg) and sustained or if associated with other major cardiac or vascular disease.

Primary prevention of stroke with antihypertensive therapy is a consistent and effective approach to reducing stroke risk. The evidence of the benefit of antihypertensive treatment after stroke is less well established. While prevention of stroke is possible and accepted there is evidence that many patients who might benefit are receiving sub-optimal treatment or none at all.

REFERENCES

Amery A, Birkenhager W, Brixko P *et al* 1985 Mortality and morbidity results from the European Working Party on High Blood Pressure in the Elderly Trial. Lancet i: 1349–1345

Barry DI, Lassen NA 1984 Cerebral blood flow autoregulation in hypertension and the effect of antihypertensive drugs. J Hypertens 5: 519–526

Carlberg B, Asplund K, Hagg E 1991 Factors influencing admission blood pressure levels in patients with acute stroke. Stroke 22: 527–530

Carter AB 1970 Hypotensive therapy in stroke survivors. Lancet i: 485–489

Collins R, Peto R, MacMahon S *et al* 1990 Blood pressure, stroke and coronary heart disease, Part 2: Short term reductions in blood pressure; overview of randomised drug trials in their epidemiological context. Lancet 335: 827–838

Coope J, Warrender TS 1986 Randomised treatment of hypertension in the elderly in primary care. BMJ 293: 1145–115

Dahlof B, Lindholm LH, Hanssonn L, Schersten B, Ekhom T, Wester PO 1991 Morbidit and mortality in the Swedish trial in old patients with hypertension (STOP). Lancet 385: 1281–1285

Grosset DG 1992 Clinical, radiological and functional evaluation following acute stroke. Br J Clin Pharmacol 34: 477–485

Hypertension-Stroke Comparative Study Group 1974 Effects of antihypertensive therapy on stroke recurrence. JAMA 299: 409–418

Lees KR, McInnes GT, Reid JL, Semple PF, Squire IB 1992 Managing hypertension. BMJ 304: 713

MacMahon S, Peto R, Cutler J *et al* 1990 Blood pressure, stroke and coronary heart disease, Part I: Prolonged differences in blood pressure; prospective observational studies corrected for regression dilution bias. Lancet 335: 765–774

Morris AD, Grosset DG, Squire IB, Lees KR, Bone I, Reid JL 1993 The experiences of an acute Stroke Unit — implications for multicentre acute stroke trials. J Neurol Neurosurg Psychiatry 56: 352–355

MRC Working Party 1992 Medical Research Council trial of hypertension in older adults: Principal results. BMJ 304: 405–412

Reid JL 1993 Hypertension and stroke: opportunities for prevention and prospects for protection. J Hypertens 11 (Suppl 5): 52–56

Shaper AG, Philips AN. Pocock SJ, Walker M, MacFarlane PN 1991 Risk factors for stroke in middle aged British men. BMJ 302: 1111–1115

SHEP Cooperative Research Group 1991 The prevention of stroke by anti-hypertensive drug treatment in older persons with isolated systolic hypertension. Final results of the systolic hypertension in the elderly programme (SHEP). JAMA 265: 3255–3264

Spence JD, Del Maestro RF 1985 Hypertension in acute ischaemic stroke – Treat. Arch Neurol 42: 1000–1002

Waldemar G, Vorstrup S, Anderson AR, Pedersen H,. Paulson OB 1989 Angiotensin converting enzyme inhibition and regional cerebral blood flow in acute stroke. J Cardiovasc Pharmacol 14: 722–729

Wallace JD. Levy LL 1981 Blood pressure after stroke. JAMA 246: 2177–2180

Yatsu FN, Zivin J 1985 Hypertension in acute ischaemic strokes — Not to treat. Arch Neurol 42: 999–1000

Multiple Risk Factors in Cardiovascular Disease, ed. by A. Yamamoto, Churchill Livingstone Japan, Tokyo, pp. 99–105 (1994)

HYPERTENSION AND OTHER RISK FACTORS FOR CEREBRAL STROKE: LONG-TERM OBSERVATIONS IN A JAPANESE COMMUNITY[§]

Kazuo UEDA,[*1,2] Teruo OMAE,[*3] and Masatoshi FUJISHIMA[*2]

[*1] *School of Health Science, Kyushu University,* [*2] *Second Department of Internal Medicine, Faculty of Medicine, Kyushu University, and* [*3] *National Cardiovascular Disease Center, Osaka*

Key words: epidemiology, cerebral stroke, hypertension, diabetes mellitus, lacunar infarction

A study of health statistics in Japan reveals that the age-adjusted mortality from intracerebral hemorrhage (ICH) has sharply and consistently decreased during the last several decades, while that from cerebral infarction (CI) has shown a slow declining trend up to date in the form of a convex curve, the peak of which was reached in the mid-1970's. We can offer several reasons for this trend: development of therapeutic procedures and managing or caring for patients in ways that might prolong their survival; advances in diagnostic methods such as imaging techniques which might have resulted in the improvement of antemortem diagnosis and have influenced the accuracy of diagnosis on death certificates. Our greatest concern, however, is to discover whether the incidence of cerebral stroke has actually decreased or not, and whether this has been related to the management of hypertension. This is because the Japanese environment and lifestyle have greatly changed and because hypertension is a well known risk factor for cerebral stroke. The ideal method of providing this evidence from an epidemiological standpoint is a long-term prospective study, even although the study population is only a selected sample of the whole country. The Hisayama study is a prospective population survey which has been carried out since 1961, and the most outstanding feature of this study is that causes of death were verified by autopsy in almost all the deceased from the cohort population. We refer to the results obtained from a long-term follow-up of this study to investigate the relationship between cerebral stroke and important risk factors, including hypertension.

OUTLINE OF THE HISAYAMA STUDY

In Hisayama, a prospective community study was begun in 1961 with emphasis on detecting the incidence of cerebrovascular disease. The 1960 census figures indicated that the number of residents aged 40 and over was 1,841 or 27.6% of the population, almost identical to the Japanese average (28.0%). The annual variation in the population has remained small (less than 4%). Of a

[*1] 3-1-1 Maidashi, Higashi-ku, Fukuoka 812, Japan.
[§] This study was partially supported by cardiovascular research grants from the Japanese Ministry of Health and Welfare and facilitated by the Japan-US Cooperative Agreement in Cardiovascular Area by the National Cardiovascular Disease Center, Osaka, and National Heart, Lung, and Blood Institute, Bethesda.

total of 1,841 persons aged 40 and over, 1,658 (90.1%) were recruited from town registries and subjected to the initial screening examination. At that time 25 residents were found to have hemiplegia due to stroke. By October 31, 1961, 12 persons had died or moved out of the area. Since November 1, 1961, excluding these 37 cases, 1,621 persons (707 men and 914 women) over 40 years of age have been under observation which includes a biennial recording of blood pressure, electrocardiogram (ECG), examination of the ocular fundi, and other tests (first cohort). The study has the following features.

Members of our study group visited the town at least once weekly to maintain contact with physicians and the administrative staff of the town hall. Whenever a stroke occurred each patient was carefully evaluated as soon as possible and the type of cerebrovascular disease was determined by a member of our cerebrovascular research group. At times a consultation was indicated and ancillary diagnostic studies were made. Some patients with doubtful diagnosis were brought to the university hospital for further examination and diagnostic evaluation including cerebrospinal fluid examination, cerebral angiography, radioisotope brain scanning and, recently, computerized tomography (CT). When a person died, an effort was made to obtain permission for autopsy from the family. Autopsies were performed at the Department of Pathology of Kyushu University. The total autopsy rate was 82.4% on average during the follow-up period.

In 1973, two thirds of the study population had entered the geriatric age group and 20% had died. A new group of 1,156 persons aged 40 or over was added to the original cohort, resulting in a second cohort of 2,135 subjects. This cohort comprised 80% of all residents aged 40 years or over in the town in 1993. Excluding the 82 subjects who died during the period of examination or who had already had a cerebral stroke, a total of 2,053 subjects (second cohort) has been followed since November 1974 without losing any subjects to follow-up. We compared the stroke incidence between two cohorts over 13 years and analyzed changes in risk factors for cerebral stroke from the two cohort populations.

HYPERTENSION AND OTHER RISK FACTORS FOR CEREBRAL STROKE

Figures 1 and 2 show the incidence of ICH and CI in our study in terms of both systolic and diastolic blood pressures at entry after age-adjustment. Results obtained from the first cohort are given in the lower half of the figure, and those from the second cohort in the upper half. Although ICH was considerably reduced in hypertensives from the second cohort, the incidence increased stepwise with elevation in both systolic and diastolic pressures, and there seemed to be no critical level of blood pressure beyond which the incidence of ICH suddenly increased. The higher the blood pressure, the greater the incidence of ICH. It is interesting that the

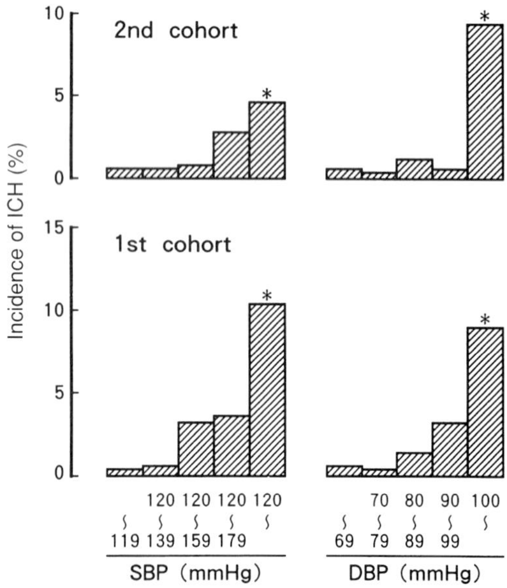

Fig. 1. Incidence of intracerebral hemorrhage (ICH) according to systolic or diastolic blood pressures (SBP or DBP), in those not taking antihypertensive drugs, Hisayama, 10 years of follow-up.
* $p < 0.05$ (χ^2 slope).

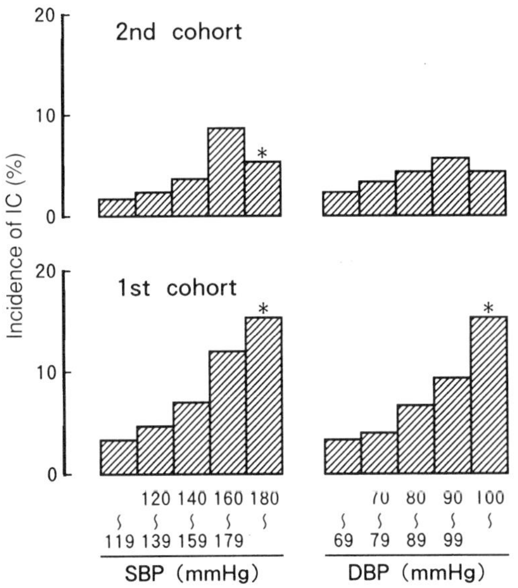

Fig. 2. Incidence of cerebral infarction (CI) according to systolic or diastolic blood pressures, in those not taking antihypertensive drugs, Hisayama, 10 years of follow-up.
* $p < 0.05$ (χ^2 slope).

boundary of diastolic pressure, at which the incidence increased abruptly was much clearer in the second cohort. The incidence of CI also increased stepwise with elevation of both systolic and diastolic pressures in the first cohort, however, there was no linear association between CI and blood pressure in the second cohort. Kagan *et al* (1980) noted in Japanese immigrants to Hawaii that the factors associated with increased risk of intracranial hemorrhage (ICH and subarachnoid hemorrhage, SAH) were: elevated blood pressure, ECG evidence of left ventricular hypertrophy (LVH) or strain, alcohol intake, and low total cholesterol. Two long-term follow-up studies conducted in Kochi (Tanaka *et al* 1982) and Akita (Shimamoto *et al* 1989), reveal a similar pattern of risk factors for ICH. Long-term persistence of hypertension is associated with LVH and an association of alcohol intake with high blood pressure is also well known. In Japanese immigrants to Hawaii, the total intake of animal protein and saturated fat were significantly lower in patients with intracranial hemorrhage than in controls (Takeya *et al* 1984). Based on the results of an 18-year follow-up, the Honolulu Heart program (Yano *et al* 1989) revealed a significant inverse association between serum cholesterol and the risk of ICH. This inverse association was nonlinear, with a higher incidence rate only for men with serum cholesterol in the lowest quintile (<189 mg/dl). There was no evidence of an interaction between blood pressure and serum cholesterol, although the inverse association was stronger for normotensive than for hypertensive men. This evidence suggests that low serum cholesterol may be a manifestation of inadequate nutrition, especially a low intake of animal protein and fat.

Table I shows the risk factors for CI analyzed by Cox's proportional hazard model based on the results from a 22-year follow-up of the Hisayama study (Ohmura *et al* 1993). Significant and independent risk factors were age, hypertension and abnormal ECG (LVH or ST depression) for men and age, hypertension and glucose intolerance for women. In the Framingham study (Kannel *et al* 1976), various components of blood pressure, including systolic and diastolic pressures, pulse pressure, lability of pressure, mean arterial pressure, and tension time index, were analyzed in relation to the incidence of atherothrombotic brain infarction (ABI). While all measures were associated with ABI incidence, the simple casual systolic pressure emerged as a good predictor of ABI incidence, as good as any other component of the pressure. The other factors made very little contribution to risk. The role of blood pressure is considered not only as a risk factor for the development of atherosclerosis but also as an accelerating factor for small arterial lesions. Diabetes mellitus is a common risk factor for CI, especially in western countries . And diabetics may be at increased risk of hypertension. Figure 3 shows the cumulative incidence of CI during a 22-year follow-up of the Hisayama study for four groups of female subjects stratified by the presence or absence of glucose intoler-

TABLE I. Relative Risks for the Incidence of CI in Terms of 9 Variables, Hisayama, 1961–1983, Using Cox's Proportional Hazards Model

	Male		Female	
	R.R.[a)]	95% C.I.[b)]	R.R.[a)]	95%C.I.[b)]
Age (years)	2.40**	1.88–3.06	2.43**	1.90–3.11
Glucose intolerance[c)]	1.50	0.91–2.47	2.71**	1.39–5.28
Hypertension[d)]	2.35**	1.51–3.67	2.62**	1.63–4.22
Proteinuria (1+ or more)	0.96	0.38–2.45	0.86	0.44–1.70
Abnormal ECG[e)]	1.83**	1.20–2.80	1.47	0.88–2.46
Quetelet index (kg/m^2)	0.93	0.75–1.16	1.02	0.82–1.26
Total cholesterol (mg/dl)	1.05	0.87–1.27	1.02	0.82–1.26
Drinking[f)]	1.39	0.89–2.17	—	—
Smoking[g)]	0.87	0.56–1.34	0.91	0.33–2.49

** $p < 0.01$.
[a)] Relative risk; [b)] 95% confidence interval; [c)] Group N = 0. Group D = 1; [d)] SBP ≥ 160 mmHg and/or DBP ≥ 95 mmHg; [e)] High R (Minnesota Code III–1) or ST depression (Minnesota Code IV-1,2,3); [f)] ethanol 33 g or more daily; [g)] 10 cigarettes or more daily.

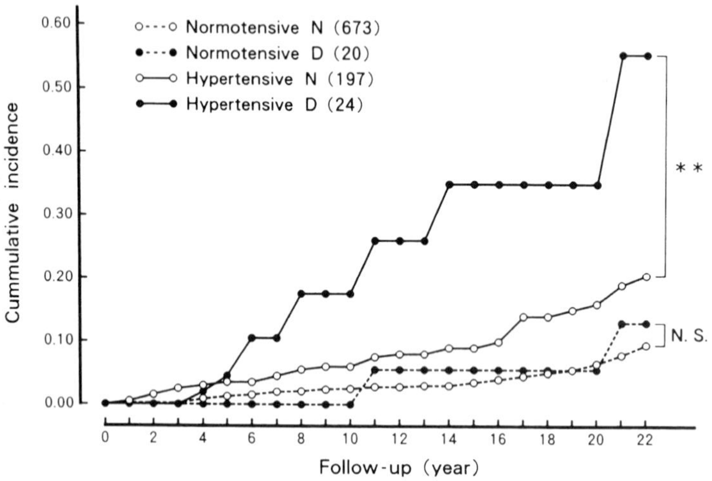

Fig. 3. Cumulative incidence of CI according to the presence or absence of glucose intolerance and hypertension, Hisayama, females, 1961–1983, Cox's Proportional Hazard Model. (from Ohmura *et al* 1993)
D, diabetics; N, nondiabetics; ( ), cases, age-adjusted. ** $p < 0.01$. Relative risk = 3.05.

ance or hypertension (Ohmura *et al* 1993). Hypertensives had a higher cumulative incidence of CI than normotensives, and hypertensive diabetics (D) clearly suffered a higher incidence of CI than normotensive nondiabetics (N) even after confounding factors were corrected using Cox's proportional hazard model. A similar trend was also observed in male subjects, but a difference in the cumulative incidence of CI between hypertensive D and hypertensive N failed to reach statistical significance. In the Framingham study (Kannel & McGee 1979), diabetes was a more important risk factor for stroke in women. It can be speculated that diabetes leads more advance atherosclerosis

TABLE II. Comparison of Risk Factors for CI by Subtypes, Hisayama

	Perforating	Cortical	Embolism
Hypertension	3.7*	2.3*	0.8
LVH on ECG	1.4	1.8	1.2
Glucose intolerance	2.3*	2.1	0.9
High hematocrit	0.4	1.0	2.2
Atrial fibrillation	3.2*	0.8	18.2*
Cholesterol	1.0	1.8	1.1
Obesity	0.9	1.9	0.8
Smoking	1.0	1.5	1.3
Alcohol	1.0	1.3	1.2

Number: relative risks, age-adjusted. * $p < 0.05$.
LVH, left ventricular hypertrophy.

in women through insulin-resistant hypertension, since hyperlipidemia or obesity is more prevalent in women than in men after middle age.

Table II demonstrates the risk factors for CI by subtypes such as perforators (lacunar infarction), cortical infarction (ABI) or embolic infarction based on the results from a 22-year follow-up of the Hisayama study; these are presented according to the relative risks of each subtype of CI compared with those without cerebral stroke after only age-adjustment. Hypertension, diabetes mellitus, and atrial fibrillation (AF) were strong predictors of lacunar infarction. Using Cox's proportional hazard model to take the interaction of each variable into account, age, hypertension and diabetes were independent and significant risk factors for lacunar infarction especially for men, although the impact of hypertension and diabetes on lacunar infarction for women was reduced in the later period of follow-up. Lacunes are generally believed to be caused by a combination of hypertension and characteristic vascular lesions involving single perforating arteries. The lesion can be accentuated by the existence of diabetes. The frequency of lacunar infarction in the Hisayama study was surprisingly higher than previously reported values (Ueda 1991a). This leads us to assume that hypertensive arteriolopathy could be important as a cause of CI in the Japanese. The Harvard Cooperative Stroke Registry (Mohr *et al* 1978) revealed that more patients with hypertension had lacunar infarcts than large artery thrombosis, and atherosclerosis was common in patients with large artery thrombosis. The Oxfordshire Community Stroke Project Group (Lodder *et al* 1990), however, failed to find a difference between patients with lacunar infarcts and those with carotid artery-distribution infarcts involving the cortex in the presence of prestroke hypertension or in the presence of markers of sustained hypertension.

CHANGING PATTERN IN CEREBRAL STROKE AND RELATED FACTORS DURING LONG-TERM FOLLOW-UP

Table III shows the age-specific incidence of ICH, CI, and SAH in two cohort populations over 13 years and during each 13-year follow-up (1961 to 1974 and 1974 to 1987). The incidence of ICH decreased in the second cohort especially in those less than 70 years of age. The age adjusted incidence for all age groups decreased significantly in the

TABLE III. Comparison of Incidence of Cerebral Stroke between Two Cohort Populations in Hisayama

Age decades†	First cohort (1961–1974)			Second cohort (1974–1987)		
	ICH	CI	SAH	ICH	CI	SAH
40–49	0.8	0.8	0.3	0.4	0.9	—
50–59	2.3	4.7	0.8	0.8	2.8	0.5
60–69	2.3	11.1	0.9	1.7	7.8	1.0
70+	2.0	15.5	1.0	1.9	9.5	1.3
Total	1.8	6.3	0.7	1.1	4.5	0.6
Age adjusted††	1.8*	6.3*	0.7	1.0	4.0	0.6

rates/1000/year. †, age at entry; ††, adjusted to first cohort; *, $p < 0.05$ (vs 2nd, M-H-χ^2)
SAH, subarachnoid hemorrhage.

second cohort. CI tended to decrease in the second cohort in all age groups, and the age-adjusted incidence of CI significantly declined. There was no difference in the incidence of SAH between the two populations. The prevalence of relevant risk factors was compared between the two cohorts at the start of follow-up. The frequency of hypertension and its manifestations on ECG, as shown by high R wave and ST depression in the precordial leads, significantly decreased in men in the second cohorts; the frequency of hypercholesterolemia (total cholesterol ≥200 mg/dl) and obesity significantly increased for both sexes in the second cohort (Ueda & Omae 1985). It is generally accepted that stroke can be prevented by antihypertensive treatment. It is difficult, however, from an ethical standpoint to confirm the efficacy of drug therapy for hypertensives in community-based, double-blind, case-control studies. We compared the prognosis and outcome for mild hypertensives (90 mmHg ≤ diastolic pressure < 105 mmHg) and hypertensives (diastolic pressure ≥ 105 mmHg) between the first and second cohort populations (Ueda *et al* 1988). During each follow-up which lasted 10 years in both cases, systolic and diastolic pressures significantly decreased for both hypertensives and mild hypertensives from the second cohort compared with those from the first. Morbidity from both ICH and CI declined significantly in mild hypertensives and hypertensives in the more recently recruited cohort population. The management of hypertension was considered more likely to be effective in reducing stroke. We compared the incidence of CI in terms of the three subtypes between the two Hisayama cohort populations (Ueda 1991a). Lacunar infarction significantly decreased in the second cohort, but other types of CI did not. A pathological study also found less fibrinoid necrosis in small intracerebral arteries on the putamen in the more recent autopsy series than in the earlier one (Masuda *et al* 1983). It seems from the evidence that the decreased incidence of cerebral stroke in the recent Hisayama population is due mostly to the successful management of hypertension. However, cross-sectional examination in 1988 revealed that prevalence of hypercholesterolemia (≥ 220 mg/dl), diabetes and obesity increased considerably for both sexes in the Hisayama population, compared with data in 1961 and 1973–74 (Ueda 1991b). This may partially be related to changes in nutritional intake among the population. We have again studied the relationship between serum lipids and CI in the recent population (1983–89). The incidence of CI, especially non embolic, increased with increasing atherosclerotic index [(total cholesterol − HDL cholesterol)/total cholesterol] Since increased serum total cholesterol was not associated with an increased risk of CI in the previous cohort population, the profile of risk factors for cerebral stroke may be changing in the recent population, probably related to changes in nutritional intake or lifestyle.

SUMMARY

We have described the risk factors for cerebral stroke in epidemiological terms based on the experience from the long-term prospective study, conducted in the town of Hisayama, Japan, since 1961. The most important risk factor for both ICH and CI in the Japanese was hypertension, and low cholesterol may have been associated with the occurrence of ICH in the 1960's due to a low intake of animal protein or fat. Diabetes mellitus was also a strong precursor for CI, and it conferred an excess risk of hypertension on CI. Both ICH and CI decreased in the recent Hisayama population and this may be related to the successful management of hypertension, since both lacunar infarction and hypertensive arteriolopathy in the autopsy series also decreased. The increased prevalence of metabolic disorders such as hypercholesterolemia, diabetes or obesity is considered a warning sign that the underlying etiology of cerebral stroke in the Japanese will change from a hypertensive arteriolosclerotic type to an atherosclerotic type in the future.

REFERENCES

Kagan A, Popper JS, Rhoads GG 1980 Factors related to stroke incidence in Hawaii Japanese men. The Honolulu Heart Study. Stroke 11: 14–21

Kannel WB, McGee DL 1979 Diabetes and cardiovascular disease: the Framingham study. JAMA 241: 2035–2038

Kannel WB, Dawber TR, Soline P, Wolf PA 1976 Components of blood pressure and risk of atherothrombotic brain infarction: the Framingham study. Stroke 4: 327–331

Loder J, Bamford JM, Sandercock PAG, Jones LN, Warlow CP 1990 Are hypertension or cardiac embolism likely causes of lacunar infarction? Stroke 21: 375–381

Masuda J, Tanaka K, Omae T, Ueda K, Sadoshima S 1983 Cerebrovascular disease and their underlying vascular lesions in Hisayama, Japan. A pathological study of autopsy cases. Stroke 14: 934–940

Mohr JP, Caplan LR, Melshi JW, Goldstein RJ, Duncan GW, Kistler JP 1978 The Harvard cooperative stroke registry: a prospective registry. Neurology 28: 754–762

Ohmura T, Ueda K, Kiyohara Y *et al* 1993 The impact of glucose intolerance on stroke incidence in a 22-year follow-up study of the general population, the Hisayama study. J Jpn Diabetes Soc 36: 17–24 (in Japanese with English abstract)

Shimamoto T, Komachi Y, Inada H *et al* 1989 Trends for coronary heart disease and stroke and their risk factors in Japan. Circulation 70: 503–515

Takeya Y, Popper JS, Shimizu Y, Kato H, Rhoads GG, Kagan A 1984 Epidemiologic studies on coronary heart disease and stroke in Japanese men living in Japan, Hawaii and California: incidence of stroke in Japan, Hawaii. Stroke 15: 15–23

Tanaka H, Ueda Y, Hayashi M *et al* 1982 Risk factors for cerebral hemorrhage and infaction in a Japanese rural community. Stroke 13: 62–73

Ueda K 1991a Change in the frequency and type of cerebrovascular disease in Japan. Angiotensin Convert Enzyme Rep 75: 5–8

Ueda K 1991b Atherosclerosis and cardiovascular diseases observed in a Japanese rural community, Hisayama. J Jpn Atheroscler Soc 19: 705–715 (in Japanese with English abstract)

Ueda K, Omae T 1985 Control of hypertension in a Japanese community. *In*: Bulpitt CJ (Ed) Handbook of Hypertension, Vol 6, Epidemiology of Hypertension. Elsevier Science Publisher, Amsterdam, pp 412–423

Ueda K, Omae T, Hasuo Y *et al* 1988 Prevalence and long-term prognosis of mild hypertensives and hypertensives in a Japanese community, Hisayama. J Hypertens 6: 981–989

Yano K, Reed DM, Maclean CJ 1989 Serum cholesterol and hemorrhagic stroke in the Honolulu Heart Program. Stroke 20: 1460–1465

Multiple Risk Factors in Cardiovascular Disease, ed. by A. Yamamoto, Churchill Livingstone Japan, Tokyo, pp. 107–110 (1994)

EFFECTS OF THE LONG-TERM CONTROL OF BLOOD GLUCOSE AND BLOOD PRESSURE ON THE INCIDENCE OF STROKE IN DIABETES MELLITUS

Hisako FUSHIMI, Toru INOUE, Yuya YAMADA, and Masakuni KAMEYAMA

*Department of Medicine, Sumitomo Hospital**

Key words: blood glucose, blood pressure, cerebral infarction, prevention of strokes, diabetes mellitus

Cerebrovascular disease (CVD) and coronary heart disease (CHD) have similar risk factors. However, the mortality from CVD is decreasing significantly worldwide, while CHD is decreasing slowly. In addition, the incidence of nonfatal cerebral infarction (CI) in diabetes mellitus (DM) is increasing (Kameyama *et al* 1971) and the incidence of small- or medium-sized infarcts (nonfatal CI) appears to be a serious problem as a cause of dementia in those patients. This is attracting close attention especially in a society where the elderly population is growing.

CVD IN DM AND VARIOUS FACTORS

Arteriosclerosis, which is associated with various factors, such as hypertension, obesity, poor control of blood glucose levels, hyperinsulinemia, and hyperlipidemia, plays an important role in the pathogenesis of CVD in DM. Although in Japan, obesity and hyperinsulinemia are not so common as in Western countries, the control of blood glucose and hypertension for the prevention of strokes are considered important. Most large cohort studies including the Framingham study (Kannel & McGee 1979), have revealed a greater incidence of CVD in diabetics. In Japan, there is also a long follow-up study of the entire Hisayama district, also revealing a greater incidence in diabetics (Ohmura *et al* 1993).

DIFFERENCES IN CVD IN PATIENTS WITH OR WITHOUT DM

It has been reported that the ratio of cases of infarction and hemorrhage is higher in diabetics than in nondiabetics. We analyzed a total of 287 strokes occurring over a 15-year period (1977–1991), 111 of which were in diabetics. Out of the 287 cases of CVD studied, 253 cases (87%) (66 ± 1 years) had CI and 34 cases (13%) had cerebral hemorrhage. In the population with DM ($n = 111$) 106 cases (95.5%) suffered from CI and 5 cases (4.5%) from cerebral hemorrhage. Cerebral hemorrhage was significantly ($p < 0.05$) less frequent than CI in patients with DM. The age at the onset of CI was not significantly different between the diabetic ($n = 111$) and nondiabetic groups ($n = 176$). All 5 diabetics with hemorrhage had hypertension.

A diagnosis of stroke was made by computed tomography (Shimazu STCT-3000T)

* 5-2-2 Nakanoshima, Kita-ku, Osaka 530, Japan.

or magnetic resonance imaging (Shimazu SMT-150, 1.5 tesla).

CVD cases with atrial fibrillation were omitted from our study because of the difficulties in making a differential diagnosis between cerebral thrombosis and embolism in some cases. Cerebral hemorrhage occurred significantly less frequently than CI in DM. This critical condition seems to be triggered by hypercoagulation in the diabetic stage with angionecrosis. Moreover, 5 diabetics with hemorrhage had no diabetic neuropathy as we reported previously (Kashiwagi *et al* 1989). Catecholamine response is markedly reduced in diabetic patients and experimental diabetic rats (Fushimi *et al* 1984), both with neuropathy. A decrease in catecholamine levels in diabetic neuropathy may play a role in reducing the incidence of hemorrhage.

BLOOD GLUCOSE CONTROL AND CI

DM is an important risk factor for CI and a current problem is how strictly to control blood glucose in order to prevent or reduce CI. So far, no answers have been given to this question. Therefore we studied 202 control diabetics free from CVD and 106 diabetics whose clinical records were examined over a period of more than 3 years. Blood glucose levels were used to divide them into P (HbA1c > 9.0% or fasting blood sugar (FBS) > 180 mg/dl), F (between P and G), and G (<7.5% or 140 mg/dl) groups. Out of a total of 106, cases 44, 34, and 28 fell into groups P, F, and G, respectively, according to the classification using blood glucose control (observed distribution, O) (Table I). The non-CVD diabetics consisted of 202 cases, of whom 23, 51, and 128 cases were classified as group P, F, and G, respectively. Supposing that the number of cases as 106 instead of 202, the distribution can be calculated as 12.1, 26.8, and 67.1 in group P, F, and G, respectively. These values are the expected distribution (E). Accordingly, the O/E ratio is 3.7, 1.3, and 0.4. Control of HbA1c less than 7.5% is recommended to prevent CI.

TABLE I. Incidence of CI and Blood Glucose for a Period of over 3 Years Prior to CI in Diabetics

Blood glucose control group	No. of diabetics with CI(O)	No. of subjects without CI	Value expected (E)	O/E
P	44	23	12.1	3.7
F	34	51	26.8	1.3
G	28	128	67.1	0.4
Total	106	202	106.0	

CI, cerebral infarction; P, HbA1c > 9.0% or fasting blood sugar (FBS) > 180 mg/dl; G, HbA1c < 7.5% or FBS < 140 mg/dl; F, between P and G.

BLOOD PRESSURE AND CI

Long-term follow-up of hypertensive patients, with or without DM prior to the development of strokes, has seldom been carried out and there are still conflicting views as to the modality of strict blood pressure (BP) control for stroke prevention in DM. In this study, we have evaluated the effects of the long-term control of hypertension, particularly on the incidence of CI.

The 295 subjects, who served as controls, consisted of 202 diabetics and 93 nondiabetics, all free of CVD, for whom clinical records covering more than 3 years were available. They were selected from our outpatients as having good activities in daily life and hypertension, treated or untreated with hypotensive drugs, during a randomly chosen period for 1 week.

The number of the cases of CI with DM and hypertension was 66. Of these, 20, 38 and 8 cases could be classified as group A (systolic blood pressure (SBP) > 160 mmHg or distolic blood pressure (DBP) > 95 mmHg), B (between A and C), and C (SBP < 140 mmHg and DBP < 90 mmHg), respectively (Table II). The non-CVD population with DM and hypertension consisted of 199 cases (68 ± 1 years.), of whom 39, 89, and 71 cases could be classified as group A, B, and C, respectively, and the distribution was calculated as before to be 12.9, 29.5, and 23.5 in group A, B, and C,

TABLE II. Incidence of CI and Hypertension Control for a Period of over 3 Years Prior to CI in Diabetics and Nondiabetics with Hypertension

Hypertension group		No. of diabetics with CI (O)	No. of subjects without CI	Value expected (E)	O/E
Diabetics	A	20	39	12.9	1.6
	B	38	89	29.5	1.3
	C	8	71	23.5	0.3
	Total	66	199	65.9	
Nondiabetics	A	32	39	18.8	1.7
	B	49	89	42.9	1.1
	C	15	71	34.2	0.6
	Total	96	199	95.9	

Hypertension group: A, SBP > 160 mmHg or DBP > 95 mmHg; C, SBP < 140 mmHg or DBP < 90 mmHg; B, between A and C.

respectively. The observed distribution of BP in cases with infarction was 20, 38, and 8 for A, B, and C, respectively. Accordingly, the corresponding O/E ratios were 1.6, 1.3, and 0.3, in the diabetics, and those for non-diabetics with CI were 1.7, 1.1, and 0.6, respectively (Table II).

However, appropriate control of hypertension is the most important factor for the prevention of cerebral hemorrhage. The incidence of infarction is increased in both DM and non-DM patients, if BP control is poor. The O/E ratios determined by us suggest that it is vitally important to keep SBP and DBP below 140 and 90 mmHg, especially in diabetics. Although the difference in the O/E ratios between diabetics and nondiabetics was not statistically significant due to the small numbers of hypertensive diabetics with CI, this difference (O/E ratios 1.3 in diabetics and 1.1 in non-diabetics) suggests that diabetics are more susceptible to even borderline hypertension. In addition, BP fluctuates over a 24 h period and it may not be sufficient to measure BP at only a periodical physical examination usually taking place every month or two.

Too strict control of BP is known to increase the risk of vascular events in the elderly. Therefore, special care, must be exercised not to lower BP too much in the patients in question. A medical care system in which all patients with CVD can undergo serial BP measurement for more than 24h, at least occasionally, should be established as soon as possible.

SUMMARY

To study how to control blood glucose and hypertension, and to prevent strokes, 287 patients with CVD including 111 diabetics and 176 nondiabetics, all of whom were admitted to Sumitomo Hospital during the period from 1977 to 1991, were investigated together with 202 diabetics and 93 nondiabetics who were free from CI, as controls Clinical records covering more than 3 years were available in all these subjects. To prevent CI blood glucose and BP should be maintained under 7.5% (as HbA1c) and under 140/90 mmHg, respectively, especially in diabetics.

REFERENCES

Fushimi H, Inoue T, Kishino B *et al* 1984 Abnormalities in plasma catecholamine response and tissue catecholamine accumulation in streptozotocin diabetic rats. A possible role for diabetic autonomic neuropathy. Life Sci 35: 1077–1081

Kameyama M, Endo T, Murati T 1971 Diabetes mellitus and cerebral vascular disease (CVD). Tonyobyo 14: 345–351 (in Japanese)

Kannel WB, McGee DL 1979 Diabetes and cardiovascular disease; The Framingham Study. JAMA 241: 3035–3038

Kashiwagi H, Fushimi H, Horie H, Kishino B, Inoue T, Kameyama M 1989 Cerebrovascular incidence in diabetes mellitus and catecholamines. Domyakukoka 17: 695–698 (in Japanese)

Ohmura T, Ueda K, Kiyohara Y *et al* 1993 The impact of glucose intolerance on stroke incidence in a 22-year follow-up study of the general population, the Hisayama study. Tonyobyo 36: 17–24 (in Japanese)

Multiple Risk Factors in Cardiovascular Disease, ed. by A. Yamamoto, Churchill Livingstone Japan, Tokyo, pp. 111–116 (1994)

MULTIPLE DIETARY FACTORS INFLUENCING BLOOD PRESSURE

Paul ELLIOTT

*Environmental Epidemiology Unit, Department of Public Health and Policy, London School of Hygiene and Tropical Medicine**

Key words: blood pressure, diet, sodium, potassium, alcohol

The cardiovascular diseases (CVDs), mainly coronary heart disease and stroke, are major causes of adult morbidity, disability, and premature/excess mortality worldwide. Raised blood pressure (BP) is the single most important risk factor for stroke as well as an established risk factor for coronary heart disease. An unfavorable pattern of BP is found in most populations around the world. Current strategies for dealing with this BP problem are directed almost entirely at those at highest risk, through the detection and pharmacological treatment of individuals with established hypertension. The relationship of BP, both systolic and diastolic, to CVD risk is not, however, confined to hypertensive individuals; rather it is continuous, graded, and strong for the (typically) 80% or so of the population with BPs above optimal levels, i.e., for adults, systolic BP ≥ 120 and diastolic BP ≥ 80 mmHg (Stamler *et al* 1989a).

A pharmacological approach to BP control implies a program of continuous screening to detect, diagnose, and treat new hypertensive individuals; in isolation, it can deal with only a fraction of the BP problem as risks are ignored for the majority with BPs above optimal, but who are not frankly hypertensive. Because of the large numbers of people involved, this group contributes a substantial proportion of all cases of CVD attributed to raised BP in a population. Thus, for an effective preventive strategy to lower BP, a population-wide approach is also required, with its emphasis on primary prevention. The aims of such a combined strategy are to lower the average BP in populations, stem the increase in BP with age, and hence reduce the high prevalence of hypertension in older people that results from this increase in BP with age.

Improved diet and nutrition are crucial to these aims. Four nutritional/hygienic factors are considered established risk factors for high BP in populations: high salt intake, low potassium intake, high body mass index (indicative of calorie intake chronically in excess of energy needs), and high alcohol intake (Stamler 1992). The purpose of the present paper is to review, with respect to these four variables, results mainly from INTERSALT, a multicenter epidemiological study of urinary electrolyte excretion and other factors in relation to BP, carried out in 32 countries and 52 centers worldwide. Other dietary and nutritional factors possibly associated with BP are also briefly discussed.

* Keppel Street, London WC1E 7HT, U.K.

THE INTERSALT STUDY

Details of INTERSALT methods and its main results have been published (Elliott & Stamler 1988; INTERSALT 1988, 1989). Data were collected from around 200 men and women aged 20–59 in each of the 52 centers, based on a highly standardized protocol (Elliott & Stamler 1988) with central training of investigators, a data coordinating center and a central laboratory for all urine analyses. BP was measured in a standard fashion using a random-zero sphygmomanometer, and a timed and supervised 24-hour urine collection was obtained from all participants for the measurement of urinary sodium and potassium excretion. A random 8% of participants made a second urine collection, for the estimation of the within-subject variability in electrolyte excretion.

Relationships with BP were examined using multiple regression, both across the 52 centers of the study and among the 10,079 eligible individuals within centers. The analysis of individuals was carried out separately within each of the 52 centers. Regression coefficients from each of the centers were then pooled, weighted according to the inverse of the variance, to give study-wide estimates of relationships among individuals of urinary electrolyte excretion and other factors to BP. However, misclassification of individuals due to large intra-individual variability in daily electrolyte excretion leads to problems of 'regression dilution,' i.e., where estimates of association are biased towards the null (no effect) value. Data from the repeat collections were used to correct for that bias, at least to some extent (INTERSALT 1988, 1989; Dyer *et al* 1994a, b).

SODIUM AND POTASSIUM

For sodium, evidence from animal studies, clinical observations, therapeutics (e.g., with diuretics), controlled clinical trials and epidemiological observations is largely concordant in showing that lower BPs are associated with lower sodium (Elliott 1989). Evidence for an inverse association of potassium with BP is also strong, but less extensive (Stamler 1992). Results of an overview of all eligible randomized controlled clinical trials of sodium reduction and BP (Cutler *et al* 1991) are summarized in Table I. Data were analyzed separately for trials of hypertensive individuals (18 trials) and of normotensive individuals (6 trials), and were then pooled from all trials, to give data for a total of 1,536 people. Sodium reductions averaging around 70 mmol per day reduced BP among hypertensive individuals on average by 4.9 mmHg systolic and 2.6 mmHg diastolic; the corresponding reductions for normotensive individuals were 1.7 mmHg systolic and 1.0 mmHg diastolic. Pooling the data from all trials, the BP was lower by an average of 2.9 mmHg systolic and 1.6 mmHg diastolic. All these results were highly significant (Table I).

Consistent results were obtained from a formal overview of all eligible within-population studies of salt and BP (excluding INTERSALT) that used a 24-hour urine collection to estimate salt intake (Elliott 1991). As regression coefficients are underestimated because of the high ratio of intra- to inter-individual variability in daily sodium

TABLE I. An Overview of Randomized Controlled Trials of Sodium Reduction and Blood Pressure[†]

	BP change (SE) (mmHg)	
	SBP	DBP
Hypertensive individuals	−4.92**	−2.64**
(n = 18 trials)	(0.65)	(0.42)
Normotensive individuals	−1.70**	−0.97*
(n = 6 trials)	(0.50)	(0.33)
All trials	−2.91**	−1.60**
(n = 1,536 people)	(0.39)	(0.25)

* $p < 0.01$; ** $p < 0.001$. SBP, systolic blood pressure; DBP, diastolic blood pressure.

[†] Adapted from Cutler *et al.* Pooled estimates were obtained by weighting according to sample size.

excretion, results are corrected for 'regression dilution.' Fourteen studies of 16 populations fulfilled the entry criteria; data were available only for simple (unadjusted) regression. Sex-specific regression analyses were carried out, and also analyses for both sexes combined; sample sizes for the three analyses were 7,099 men, 6,136 women, and 12,503 men and women combined (Elliott 1991). Regression slopes were pooled by weighting inversely according to their variance. Positive and highly significant relationships were seen in all analyses; regression coefficients were somewhat larger in women than in men. Overall, for men and women combined, the regression coefficients corrected for 'regression dilution' using new estimates from INTERSALT (Dyer *et al* 1994a) indicate a systolic pressure lower by 4.5 mmHg and a diastolic pressure lower by 2.5 mmHg for a sodium lower by 100 mmol.

In INTERSALT, median sodium excretion ranged from less than 1 mmol/day (Yanomamo Indians of Brazil) to 242 mmol/day (Tianjin, China) and potassium excretion from 23 mmol/day to 81 mmol/day (INTERSALT 1988). There were four isolated and distinctive populations with sodium excretion at or below 50 mmol/day. They also had low BPs, low or absent prevalence of hypertension and little or no upward change in BP with age; among these four centers, there was a perfect rank correlation between the mean sodium excretion and mean systolic BPs (Mancilha Carvalho *et al* 1989). Among the remaining 48 centers, there was a highly significant association between the upward change in BP with age and the median sodium excretion of the centers, such that, over a 30 year period, rise in systolic BP was estimated to be on average 9 to 10 mmHg less for a median daily urinary sodium excretion lower by 100 mmol (INTERSALT 1988).

Estimates of the size of the multiple regression coefficients of BP to sodium and potassium excretion, among the 10,000 + individuals in INTERSALT, have recently been revised (Dyer *et al* 1994b). A simple estimate made previously of the degree of 'regression dilution' of electrolyte-BP coefficients (INTERSALT 1988) did not take into account other variables in the multiple regression model, nor did it allow for correlated errors between sodium and potassium resulting from their measurement in the same 24-hour urine collection. The revised regression coefficients relating individual BP to individual urinary sodium or potassium excretion are some 40–50% larger than those estimated previously, and 150–200% larger than the uncorrected coefficients (Dyer *et al* 1994b). They indicate, for example, that with full adjustment for confounding variables, 100 mmol lower sodium excretion is associated with a systolic BP lower by 3.1 mmHg (Table II, first row).

BODY MASS AND ALCOHOL

There is a large volume of evidence to indicate that both body mass index and excess alcohol intake are positively associated with BP (Stamler 1992). In INTERSALT, a positive association between body mass index and BP was found in 51 of the 52 centers for systolic BP and all 52 centers for diastolic BP (INTERSALT 1988). Overall, a 10 kg difference in body weight was associated on average with a 3.0 mmHg difference in systolic BP and a 2.2 mmHg difference in diastolic BP (Dyer & Elliott 1989). Recent analyses indicate that sodium and body mass index appear to act independently on BP with no evidence of their interaction (Dyer *et al* 1994c). However, adjustment for body mass index in the multiple regression models had a large impact on the size of the coefficients relating sodium and BP. This may represent statistical over-adjustment for body mass index which can be measured on a single occasion essentially without error, in contrast to the large variability in daily sodium excretion noted above. When the relationship of sodium to systolic BP in individuals was examined with adjustment for age, sex, urinary potassium, and alcohol intake, but not for body mass index, the resulting coefficient for

TABLE II. Predicted Effect of Changes in 24-hour Urinary Sodium and Potassium Excretion, Body Mass Index (BMI), and High Alcohol Intake on Systolic Blood Pressure (SBP) in the INTERSALT Study

Variable	Coefficient*	Change	Predicted SBP difference (mmHg)
Sodium (mmol/24 h)	0.31†	170 → 70	−3.1
Potassium (mmol/24 h)	−0.67†	55 → 70	−1.0
BMI (kg/m^2)	0.73‡	25 → 22	−2.2
Alcohol (% 300+ ml/week)	3.54§	14 → 0	−0.5

* Multivariate adjusted for 'regression dilution' (sodium and potassium); † mmHg/10 mmol/24 h; ‡ mmHg/unit body mass index (BMI); § 300+ ml/week vs zero ml/week.

BP-sodium was 6.0 mmHg per 100 mmol, compared with the 3.1 mmHg noted above (when body mass index was included in the regression model).

INTERSALT also reported a highly significant positive association between heavy alcohol drinking (≥300 ml alcohol per week) and BP (INTERSALT 1988). Recent analyses have extended these findings to examine the shape of the alcohol-BP relationship in men and women (Marmot *et al* 1994). The results are summarized in Fig. 1. The figure shows the mean difference in systolic pressure between alcohol drinkers, at each level of intake, and non-drinkers within each center, pooled across all centers contributing to that analysis. For both men and women, there was a tendency for these BP differences to be positive at levels of intake above 50 ml/week, significantly so above 300 ml/week. Further analyses found no evidence to suggest that either withdrawal from alcohol in the 24 hours prior to BP measurement, or an acute effect of alcohol intake, were dominant explanations for the alcohol-BP findings, implying a sustained effect of chronic alcohol consumption on BP (Marmot *et al* 1994).

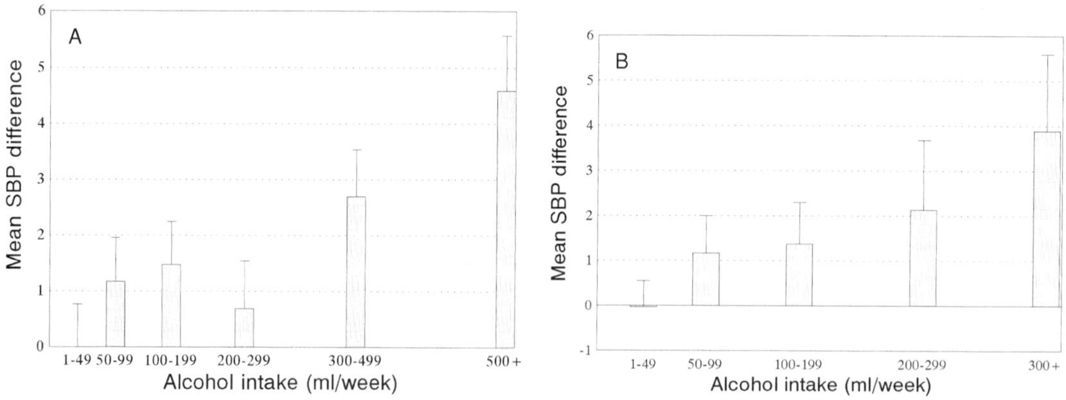

Fig. 1. Association of levels of alcohol intake (ml/week) to systolic blood pressure (SBP, mmHg) in INTERSALT, adjusted for age, urinary sodium and potassium excretion, body mass index and cigarette smoking. Results are mean differences in SBP (SE bars) compared to non-drinkers, pooled over all centers: A) men, B) women.

Table II summarizes the predicted effect on systolic BP of various interventions, based on independent multiple regression coefficients in INTERSALT, adjusted for regression dilution. As can be seen, favorable changes in population average levels of these four risk factors for high BP, could result in large changes in the population average BP. These could be expected to lead to sizable reductions in the adult risks of CVD and all-cause mortality (Stamler *et al* 1989b).

OTHER FACTORS

In addition to the four established risk factors for high BP summarized above, there are other dietary and nutritional factors, both macro- and micro-nutrients, that are implicated in the etiology of high BP, although research data are currently insufficient to lead to firm judgments about causality (Stamler 1992). These factors include the amount and type of dietary protein and fat, carbohydrate and fiber, and the dietary intakes of calcium, magnesium, and the antioxidant vitamins. Recent results for dietary protein from INTERSALT and other population studies may be especially relevant; they indicate significant inverse associations with BP of (markers of) dietary protein intake, of a magnitude that could be of public health importance (Dyer *et al* 1992; Elliott *et al* 1992). These associations were found independent of, and in addition to, the effects of urinary sodium and potassium excretion, body mass index and alcohol intake.

SUMMARY

Results, mainly from INTERSALT, of analyses relating four lifestyle factors to BP are reviewed. These factors are high sodium intake, low potassium intake, high body mass index and high alcohol intake. For sodium, the quantitative results from INTERSALT are similar to those obtained from an overview of randomized controlled trials of sodium reduction and BP, and from an overview of within-population epidemiological studies. The INTERSALT results were previously underestimated because of insufficient correction for the 'regression dilution' bias. New multiple regression estimates indicate a systolic BP lower by 3.1 mmHg for a sodium lower by 100 mmol, and lower by 1.0 mmHg for a potassium higher by 15 mmol. The sodium effect is probably over-adjusted for the association with body mass index; without body mass index in the multiple regression model, the regression estimate for systolic BP and sodium is increased to 6.0 mmHg/100 mmol. A positive, but non-significant, effect of alcohol on systolic BP is seen below 300 ml/week; intakes above that level are positively and significantly related to BP in both men and women. Combining the effects of favorable changes in these four risk factors for high BP suggests that it may be possible to lower mean systolic BPs in populations by 6 mmHg or more. BP changes of that order are associated with large differences in adult risks of CVDs and all-cause mortality. Further research in population studies is needed to investigate the possible effects on BP of a number of other dietary and nutritional variables, especially the macronutrients.

REFERENCES

Cutler J, Follman D, Elliott P, Suh I 1991. An overview of randomised trials of sodium reduction and blood pressure. Hypertension 17 (suppl 1): I-27–I-33

Dyer AR, Elliott P 1989 The INTERSALT Study: Relations of body mass index to blood pressure. J Hum Hypertens 3: 299–308

Dyer A, Elliott P, Kesteloot H *et al* 1992 Urinary nitrogen excretion and blood pressure in INTERSALT. J Hypertens 10 (suppl 4): S122 Abstract p 95

Dyer AR, Shipley M, Elliott P 1994a Urinary electrolye excretion in 24 hours and blood pressure in the INTERSALT Study: I. Estimates of reliability. Am J Epidemiol 139: 927–939

Dyer AR, Elliott P, Shipley M 1994b Urinary electrolye excretion in 24 hours and blood pressure in the INTERSALT Study: II.

Estimates of electrolyte-blood pressure associations corrected for regression dilution bias. Am J Epidemiol 139: 940–951

Dyer AR, Elliott P, Shipley M, Stamler R, Stamler J 1994c Body mass index and associations of sodium and potassium with blood pressure: *In* INTERSALT. Hypertension 23:729–736

Elliott P 1989 The INTERSALT Study: An addition to the evidence on salt and blood pressure, and some implications. J Hum Hypertens 3: 289–298

Elliott P 1991 Observational studies of salt and blood pressure. Hypertension 17 (suppl 1): I-3-I-8

Elliott P, Stamler R 1988 Manual of operations for INTERSALT, an international cooperative study of the relation of sodium and potassium to blood pressure. Controlled Clin Trials 9 (suppl): 1–118S

Elliott P, Freeman J, Pryer J, Brunner E, Marmot M 1992 Dietary protein and blood pressure: A report from the Dietary and Nutritional Survey of British Adults. J Hypertens 10 (suppl 4): S141 Abstract p 105

INTERSALT Co-operative Research Group 1988 INTERSALT: An international study of electrolyte excretion and blood pressure. Results for 24-hour urinary sodium and potassium. BMJ 297: 319–328

INTERSALT Co-operative Research Group 1989 The INTERSALT Study. An international co-operative study of electrolyte excretion and blood pressure: Further results (Ed Elliott P). J Hum Hypertens 3: 279–408

Mancilha Carvalho JJ, Baruzzi RG, Howard PF *et al* 1989 Blood pressure in four remote populations in the INTERSALT Study. Hypertension 14: 238–246

Marmot MG, Elliott P, Shipley MJ *et al* 1994 Alcohol and blood pressure: The INTERSALT Study. BMJ 308: 1263–1267

Stamler J, Neaton JD, Wentworth DN 1989a Blood pressure (systolic and diastolic) and risk of fatal coronary heart disease. Hypertension 13 (suppl I): I-2 – I-12

Stamler J, Rose G, Stamler R, Elliott P, Dyer A, Marmot M 1989b INTERSALT study findings. Public health and medical care implications. Hypertension 14: 570–577

Stamler R 1992 The primary prevention of hypertension and the population blood pressure problem. *In*: Marmot M, Elliott P (Eds) Coronary heart disease epidemiology: From aetiology to public health. Oxford University Press, Oxford, pp 415–434

Multiple Risk Factors in Cardiovascular Disease, ed. by A. Yamamoto, Churchill Livingstone Japan, Tokyo, pp. 117–121 (1994)

SALT INTAKE, ALCOHOL CONSUMPTION, BODY WEIGHT AND BLOOD PRESSURE

Eduardo FARINARO,[*1] Salvatore PANICO,[*2] Antonio ASTI,[*2] Paola RESCIGNO,[*2] Rocco GALASSO,[*2] and Camilla AMBROSCA[*2]

[*1] *Institute of Hygiene and Preventive Medicine — Community Medicine, and* [*2] *Institute of Internal Medicine and Metabolic Diseases, School of Medicine, University "Federico II", Naples*

Key words: cardiovascular disease, salt, alcohol, body weight, blood pressure

Non-optimal blood pressure levels in populations are quite frequent and account for a large number of deaths in many societies (Stamler 1994). This phenomenon is amenable to preventive measures by nutritional and hygienic means, most of which are related to diet (Stamler 1994).

A number of characteristics of life in modern societies (e.g. means of transportation, food storage and preservation, structure of social networks) have contributed to cardiovascular risk through mass exposure to unfavorable lifestyles, particularly with respect to dietary habits and physical activity. These are the main reasons why the epidemiology of blood pressure and hypertension identify a major determinant role for salt consumption, alcohol intake, and body weight. As a consequence, the prevention of cardiovascular diseases due to hypertension is essentially based on the modification of these determinants in populations.

SALT

A number of experimental, clinical and epidemiological studies have shown that excess salt intake increases blood pressure (Muntzel & Druecke 1992). However, some uncertainties still exist, due to the complex effect of sodium on the vascular system and blood pressure regulation. Renal function, sympathetic activity, calcium and potassium metabolism, and natriuretic hormone have been claimed to be responsible for the effect of sodium intake on blood pressure (Muntzel & Druecke 1992)

Cross-sectional and ecological studies have shown that populations and individuals with low sodium intake (less than 100 mmol/day) are virtually hypertension-free (Hunt 1983; INTERSALT 1988). Nutritional confounding factors cannot be definitively ruled out in the case of these findings, since low-fat consumption, low-alcohol intake, high-potassium intake, low incidence of obesity, and high levels of physical activity are also typical of these populations. A sodium intake ranging from 100 to 200 mmol/day does not affect blood pressure significantly.

The results of experimental trials carried out to evaluate the long-term effect of sodium restriction on blood pressure are conflicting but suggest an effect which, although modest per se, may be of great value at a population level (MacGregor *et al* 1989;

[*1,2] via S. Pansini, 5, 80131 Naples, Italy.

Stamler 1989). In contrast to animal experiments, studies on humans are not conclusive as far as a reduction of blood pressure is concerned in the young after long-term sodium restriction; however, trials in hypertensives tend to show that sodium restriction decreases blood pressure and allows a reduction of the number of antihypertensive pills and, consequently, their dosage (Muntzel & Druecke 1992).

A crucial role in the association between salt intake and blood pressure is played by salt-sensitivity. There are individuals more sensitive to salt intake as far as an increase in blood pressure is concerned, due to genetic or physiological factors; they are also more responsive to dietary sodium restriction. All the supposed pathophysiological mechanisms reported to explain the relationship between salt intake and blood pressure have been claimed to be enhanced in salt-sensitive individuals. Elderly and black people have been found to be more salt-sensitive (Law *et al* 1991); weight reduction in the obese is associated with a reduction in salt-sensitivity (Tuck *et al* 1981). However, the identification of salt-sensitive individuals is not an easy task due to the poor reproducibility of the testing procedure; therefore, more research is needed to evaluate conclusively this phenomenon.

BODY WEIGHT

In 1969 Chiang published a review of the relationship between obesity and hypertension in which he suggested that an increase in body weight is a determinant of high blood pressure and hypertension (Chiang 1969). He also pointed out the importance of a genetic predisposition in this phenomenon. Thirty-one studies carried out in 15 countries were reviewed: an increase in body weight with age was associated with an increase in blood pressure, and the association between body weight and pressure tended to be higher in those populations with a greater prevalence of obesity. Populations with a lower increase in blood pressure had been previously reported as having a lower mean body weight. The association between body weight and blood pressure has been reported to be rare in primitive societies, where no positive association between age and blood pressure has been found. In modern industrialized societies body weight is found to be positively associated with blood pressure and evidence is available from both cross-sectional and longitudinal investigations (Harriet & Dustan 1991). The most recent information on obesity and hypertension in large populations comes from NHANES Il (Van Itallie 1985). The risk of developing hypertension in overweight individuals has been found to be three times that in non-overweight individuals. In younger age groups the relative risk has been found to be even greater (more than five-fold), whereas in older age groups the relative risk is 1.9. Socio-economic factors play an important role in modifying the relationship between body weight and blood pressure. The lower the socio-economic level, the higher the incidence of overweight, obese and hypertensive individuals.

From the pathophysiological point of view obesity is correlated with hypervolemia and an increase in cardiac output (Messerli *et al* 1981). Obesity is also associated with endocrine disorders found to be associated also with hypertension (Van Itallie 1985). Hyperinsulinemia has been recently reported as being responsible for obesity-related hypertension (Landsberg *et al* 1989). Cell metabolism, renal, cardiac and hemodynamic functions, and small-vessel reactivity are believed to explain this relationship.

Blood pressure reduction may be achieved by reducing body weight both in normotensive and hypertensive individuals (Stamler 1980). Interestingly, mild hypertensives may benefit from body weight reduction, thus providing an important and safe means of treatment (Stamler 1989). Moreover, a decrease in body weight can reduce the dose of anti-hypertensive drugs required, and is effective in maintaining favorable blood pressure if drug treatment is stopped (Harriet & Dustan 1991).

In agreement with the pathophysiological hypotheses for the relationship between overweight, obesity and hypertension, a reduction in body weight produces a beneficial effect on glucose tolerance (Farinaro *et al* 1977), plasma renin activity (Tuck *et al* 1981), cardiac output and peripheral resistance (Alexander & Peterson 1972).

ALCOHOL

The relationship between alcohol and blood pressure was established at the beginning of this century (Lian 1915). A large number of cross-sectional, cohort studies and intervention trials have analyzed this relationship and it has been estimated that chronic alcohol consumption ranks second after overweight among the non-genetic risk factors for hypertension (Keil *et al* 1993).

Cross-sectional studies have shown that the association between alcohol and blood pressure is independent of some confounding factors (age, smoking, body weight, physical activity), and that an alcohol intake above 30–60 g/day increases blood pressure in both men and women (Keil *et al* 1993). European and North-American studies have shown that non-drinkers have blood pressures higher than or equal to those individuals consuming 10–20 g alcohol/day: data thought to be compatible with a mixing of information and selection biases.

Prospective cohort studies and intervention trials are consistent with these data; however, problems with data interpretation have been claimed such as the accuracy of the alcohol intake estimates, confounding and effect modification control.

In general, all these investigations suggest that an increase of 10 g alcohol/day (defining 30g alcohol/day as a threshold) influences systolic blood pressure by 1–2 mmHg and diastolic by 1 mmHg. Some studies suggest a threshold of 60 g alcohol/day. There has been no consistent finding of a different threshold for women compared with men in the few studies reporting data in both sexes.

Some methodological problems have to be taken into account when interpreting the results of all these studies, especially those involving cross-sectional investigations.

Alcohol intake is generally based on written or oral information and, therefore, the correct identification of "true" non-drinkers and those underreporting their intake may not be easy. The "non-drinkers" are a heterogeneous group including true abstainers, those drinkers who deny alcohol consumption and those individuals who have alcohol-related health problems.

Some confounding factors or effect modifiers (age, sex, body weight, smoking), affecting the relationship between alcohol consumption and blood pressure, have generally been controlled in most studies, whereas others (diet, electrolyte intake, drugs, physical activity) have not. Stress is another confounding factor often not evaluated: individuals who do not drink are more responsive to stressful events than drinkers. Moreover, self-selection, genetic factors and observer blinding are frequently not taken into account and may cause misclassification. The methodological problems raised may help explain the J- or U- shaped curve of the change in mortality rate with increasing levels of alcohol intake reported virtually for all the populations studied.

Neurohormonal and vascular factors have been reported as responsible for the association between alcohol and blood pressure, sympathetic activity, plasma renin activity, and an increase in circulating cortisol are reported as responsible for blood pressure elevation, especially in the acute phase of alcohol intake (Keil *et al* 1993). Cell membrane fluidity changes and the sodium-potassium ATP-ase-dependent pump are affected by chronic alcohol consumption and may possibly be responsible for blood pressure elevation.

From a public health point of view the excess risk due to alcohol consumption is crucial. In particular, the estimated amount of hypertension in the community that could be avoided by a reduction in alcohol intake (e.g. less than 40 g alcohol/day) has been calculated as about 7% in Germany and 11% in the US and Australia (Keil *et al* 1993).

THE ITALIAN EXPERIENCE

Raised blood pressure in Italy still represents an important public health problem. National data based on randomised samples of the adult population have indicated that in the age range 20–59 the prevalence of hypertension was 19% in the late 70s and somewhat less in the mid-80s; for the years between 1978 and 1984, a slight decrease in the mean level of both systolic and diastolic blood pressures was found (Menotti *et al* 1992). These findings together with a sizable improvement in the detection and treatment of hypertension may well have had an effect on the decline in the mortality rates for cardiovascular diseases, particularly stroke. However, there is a tremendous burden on the health system since 85,000 men per year still suffer from a myocardial infarction between the ages of 40 and 75 years, 37,000 men and women develop a stroke before the age of 59 and 66,000 men and women have a transient ischemic attack between 40 and 69 years.

According to our analyses of data from the 4 Italian centers participating in the INTERSALT Study, we estimate that a reasonable modification of salt (net average sodium reduction of 100 mmol/day, with an increase of 15 mmol/day in the potassium intake) and alcohol intake (the change from heavy drinking — 25% of the population — to a more acceptable level) and of body mass index (reduction of 2.5 units, i.e. about 10 kg) in the Italian population might substantially affect cardiovascular risk through an average reduction of 6 mmHg in the systolic blood pressure (Farinaro *et al* 1991).

SUMMARY

Salt and alcohol intake are involved in blood pressure regulation and their control may have a beneficial effect in reducing blood pressure in individuals and populations. Body weight is an established determinant of blood pressure. Reduction of excess body weight is of great value in individuals (particularly hypertensives) and populations in reducing cardiovascular risk (including the component due to raised blood pressure). The overall impact on morbidity and mortality rates for cardiovascular diseases is dramatic across different cultures.

REFERENCES

Alexander JK, Peterson K 1972 Cardiovascular effect of weight reduction. Circulation 65: 310–318

Chiang BN, Perlman LB, Epstein FH 1969 Overweight and hypertension. Circulation 39: 403–421

Farinaro E, Stamler J, Upton M *et al* 1977 Plasma glucose levels: Long-term effect of diet in Chicago Coronary Prevention Evaluation Program. Ann Intern Med 86: 147–154

Farinaro E, Trevisan M, Jossa J *et al* 1991 INTERSALT in Italy: Findings and community health implications. J Hum Hypertens 5: 15–19

Harriet P, Dustan MD 1991 Obesity and hypertension. Diabetes care 14: 488–503

Hunt JC 1983 Sodium intake and hypertension: a cause for concern. Ann Intern Med 98: 724–728

INTERSALT Cooperative Research Group 1988 An international study of electrolyte excretion and blood pressure. Results for 24-hour urinary sodium and potassium excretion. BMJ 297 :319–328

Keil U, Swales JD, Grobbee DE 1993 Alcohol intake and its relation to hypertension. *In*: Verschuren PM (Ed) Health issues related to alcohol consumption, ILSI Press, pp 17–42

Landsberg L, Krieger DR 1989 Obesity, metabolism and the sympathetic nervous system. Am J Hypertens 2: 125S–132S

Law MR, Frost CD, Wald NJ. 1991 By how much does dietary salt reduction lower blood pressure? I. Analysis of observational data among populations. BMJ 302: 811–815

Lian C 1915 L'alcoholisme, cause d'hipertension arterielle. Bull Acad Natl Med 74: 525–528

MacGregor GA, Sagnella GA, Markandu ND *et*

al 1989 Double-blind study of three sodium in-takes and long-term effects of sodium restriction in essential hypertension. Lancet i: 1244–1247

Menotti A, Scanga M, Responsible Investigators of the RF2, OB43, MICOL Research Group 1992 Recent trends in selected coronary risk factors in Italy. Int J Epidemiol 21: 883–892

Messerli FH, Christie B, De Carvalho SG *et al* 1981 Obesity and essential hypertension: Hemodinamics, intravascular volume, sodium excretion, and plasma renin activity. Arch Intern Med 141: 81–85

Muntzel M, Druecke T 1992 A comprehensive review of the salt and blood pressure relationship. Am J Hypertens 5: 1s–42s

Stamler J 1994 Assessing diets to improve world health: nutritional research on disease causation in populations. Am J Clin Nutr 59 (suppl): 146S–156S

Stamler J, Farinaro E, Moonier L, Holl J, Moss D, Stamler R 1980 Prevention and control of hypertension nutritional hygienic means. Long-term Experience of the Chicago Coronary Prevention Evaluation Program. JAMA 243: 1819–1823

Stamler R, Stamler J, Gosch FC *et al* 1989 Primary prevention of hypertension by nutritional-hygienic means. JAMA 262: 1801–1807

Tuck ML, Sowers J, Dornfeld L *et al*.1981 The effect of weight reduction on blood pressure, plasma renin activity, and plasma aldosterone levels in obese patients. N Engl J Med 304: 930–933

Van Itallie I 1985 The problem of obesity: health implication of overweight and obesity in the United States. Ann Intern Med 103: 983–988

SECTION 4.

LIPOPROTEIN & ATHEROSCLEROSIS

Multiple Risk Factors in Cardiovascular Disease, ed. by A. Yamamoto, Churchill Livingstone Japan, Tokyo, pp. 125–130 (1994)

THE ROLE OF APOLIPOPROTEINS IN ATHEROGENESIS[§]

Gert M. Kostner

*Institute of Medical Biochemistry, University of Graz**

Key words: apolipoproteins, atherogenesis, risk factors, cholesterol, lipoproteins

Numerous studies in the past have documented the multifactorial etiology of atherogenesis. Many of the well recognized risk factors seem to affect directly the normal physiological function of 4 main cell systems: endothelial cells, smooth muscle cells, blood platelets, and monocytes/macrophages. They do so by interfering with cell adhesiveness, aggregation, proliferation, foam cell- and clot-formation. In all these events, plasma lipids and hemostatic factors are intimately involved. Concerning plasma lipids, there is no doubt that free and esterified cholesterol play a key role in the pathophysiology of atherosclerosis. Cholesterol is synthesized in almost all body cells and transported in the plasma by 5 main lipoprotein fractions: very low density lipoproteins (VLDL), intermediate density lipoproteins (IDL), low density lipoproteins (LDL), lipoprotein (a) (Lp(a)), high density lipoproteins (HDL_2), and HDL_3 (Reviewed by Kostner 1983). Although, all these lipoproteins contain cholesterol, their characteristic features involve their apolipoproteins (apo-Lp).

Apo-Lp have three main physiological functions: i) transport of lipids out of the cell; ii) activation and inactivation of enzymes; iii) binding to specific cell-surface receptors. Thus, it becomes evident that apo-Lp affect the whole intravascular lipid metabolism and play a key role in determining plasma lipid levels. Following Kostner and Alaupovic (1972), apo-Lp are grouped into families and named with capital letters in alphabetical order as apoA, apoB, . . . apoJ. In addition apo-a, which is probably not a classical apo-Lp, is a component of a very atherogenic plasma fraction. Of great interest today are the genetic isoforms of apo-Lp with impaired metabolic functions such as the apoB-3500 variant or truncated forms apoB, which may be linked to an increase or decrease in plasma apoB. Another protein whose isoforms reflect the concentration in plasma is apo-a; there is an inverse relation between the molecular weight of apo-a isoforms and their plasma concentrations.

From all these well accepted facts it seems clear that a complete picture of the lipoprotein metabolism in a given individual may only be obtained by determining genetic variants and the metabolic features of different plasma apo-Lp and lipids. A more feasible approach may be to measure

* Harrachgasse 21, A-8010 Graz, Austria.
[§] This study was supported by a grant from the Austrain Research Foundation (Project S07104-Med).

the plasma concentrations of certain lipoprotein subfractions since the latter are strongly affected by genetic factors determining lipoprotein turnover. With these facts in mind, we tested the hypothesis that measuring plasma apo-Lp concentrations in combination with lipids and lipoprotein lipids may predict the risk for various forms of atherosclerosis. In essence, we performed 3 independent studies on patients suffering from peripheral vascular diseases (PVD), myocardial infarction (MI), and cerebrovascular diseases (CVD) or stroke. All three studies had a case-control design aimed at evaluating the optimal discriminators by univariate and by stepwise multivariate discriminant analysis.

PVD-STUDY

In this study, 49 male patients and 39 male controls, between 40–60 years of age, were investigated (Pilger *et al* 1983). Patients represented a consecutive series of subjects referred to the clinic because of intermittent claudication. The diagnosis of PVD was based on the results of Doppler ultrasound examination and on angiography. A total of 11 patients were classified as Stage 1 and 38 patients as Stage 2 according to Fontains criteria. The controls were selected randomly from individuals referred to the clinic for medical checkup. In the control group, PVD was excluded by ultrasound examination of the ankle arteries. Hypertension, diabetes mellitus, hyperuricemia, and smoking were considered as risk factors.

Laboratory analyses were obtained after the individuals had fasted for 12–14 h. Serum lipids were measured enzymatically (Boehringer/Mannheim), LDL-C and HDL-C were measured after polyanion precipitation, apolipoproteins AI (apoA-I), apoA-II, apoB, and Lp(a) were quantified immunochemically using antibodies prepared in our own laboratories and standards from Immuno A.G./Vienna.

Statistical analyses were performed by the Wilcoxon rank sum test assuming that the rank sum is normally distributed. Cut-off points were defined as the minimum or maximum level, where error rates reached a minimum. By stepwise linear discriminant analysis a better classification of patients was achieved. For the selection of the best discriminant function, the *t*-values, error rates, sensitivities and specificities were used. The error rate is defined as the number of falsely negative plus falsely positive classified patients and controls as a percentage of the total individuals studied. Table I summarizes the results of this PVD study. Significant discriminators from univariate analysis were total cholesterol (TC), triglycerides (TG), LDL-C, apoB, apoA-II and some ratios of these. The lowest error rate of 25% was obtained with the apoA-I/apoB ratio. By multivariate analysis, including LDL-C/HDL-C and the apoA-I, apoA-II, and apoB, an error rate of some 13% was achieved. These results indicate that measurement of plasma lipids or lipoprotein-lipids by themselves does not allow an optimal discrimination between patients and controls. By including the apo-Lp of the A and B family a refinement of the discrimination has been achieved.

MI-STUDY

The lipoproteins and apo-Lp concentrations in 92 male survivors of MI aged < 60 years were measured and compared with that of a control group matched for age, sex and socio-economic status (the results are displayed in Table II). Here again, the ratio of apoA-I/apoB had a much greater discriminant power than LDL-C/HDL-C. In addition, Lp(a) was found to be a significant independent risk indicator. At a cut-off of 35 mg/dl Lp(a) an error rate of 36% was achieved.

STROKE-STUDY

A total of 45 male and 27 female consecutive cases of cerebrovascular arteriopathy, between 35–70 years of age, were compared

TABLE I. Discriminators for Peripheral Vascular Disease

Parameters	Median values PVD (mg/dl)	Controls (mg/dl)	Cut-off points (mg/dl)	ER (%)
TG	176*	145	154	34
TC	222**	177	192	31
HDL-C	37	40	40	44
LDL-C	141**	100	117	40
C/HDL-C	6	4	5	34
LDL-C/HDL-C	4*	3	3	34
apoB	136**	107	117	29
LDL-apoB	110*	97	99	39
apoA-I	104	109	108	40
apoA-II	38**	44	40	40
TC/apoB	2	2	2	45
apo A-I/apoB	1**	1	1	25
apo A-II/apoB	0**	0	0	27

Multivariate analysis

Independent variables	Sensitivity	Specificity	ER (%)
apoA-II, apoB, apoA-I/apoB	0.78	0.79	21.3
LDL-C/HDL-C, TC, apoA-I, apoA-I/apoB	0.84	0.89	13.4

Univariate analyses were performed by Wilcoxon-U test and multivariate analysis by stepwise discriminant regression. * $p < 0.01$, ** $p < 0.001$. ER, error rate = sum of false positives and false negatives in %. TG, triglycerides; TC, total cholesterol.

TABLE II. Discriminators for Myocardial Infarction

Risk indicators for myocardial infarction

Parameters	Cut-off points (mg/dl)	ER (%)
TG	> 184.0	41
TC	> 284.0	35
HDL-C	< 33.0	38
LDL/HDL-C	> 3.5	31
Lp (a)	> 35.0	36
apoA-I/apoB	< 0.8	23

Multivariate analysis

Independent	Sensitivity	Specificity	ER(%) Variables
LDL-C/HDL-C, Lp(a) apoA-I, apoA-II, apoB	0.92	0.94	7.6

Univariate analyses were performed by Wilcoxon-U test and multivariate analysis by stepwise discriminant regression.

TABLE III. Discriminators for Stroke

Parameters	Median values Patients (mg/dl)	Controls (mg/dl)	Cut-off point (mg/dl)	ER(%)
Males				
TC	185.00	201.40	201.80	41.30
FC	43.60	50.50	50.70	45.50
LDL-C	128.70	134.60	138.30	42.80
HDL-C	29.30**	48.30	37.60	26.90
TG	135.00	119.70	117.70	48.20
apoA-I	81.20**	122.40	98.50	9.10
apoA-II	29.20***	44.70	33.40	15.80
apoB	86.10	91.40	90.70	43.90
Lp(a)	13.70	10.30	11.80	45.40
LDL-C/HDL-C	4.25*	3.14	3.37	37.50
apoA-I/apoB	0.96**	1.34	1.09	33.70
Females				
TC	166.00	198.50	182.30	42.60
FC	47.40	46.30	46.70	48.80
LDL-C	104.10	131.10	112.60	43.50
HDL-C	33.70***	50.20	37.90	32.10
TG	142.00	128.80	144.20	49.50
apoA-I	86.40***	129.40	105.20	11.80
apoA-II	28.20***	42.50	34.40	22.40
apoB	75.90	84.60	76.10	43.30
Lp(a)	15.70	10.80	12.40	39.10
LDL-C/HDL-C	3.33	2.84	3.25	47.90
apoA-I/apoB	1.09*	1.50	1.24	35.20

Models of stepwise discriminant analysis for estimating the CVD risk

Mod. No.	Independent variables	Sensitivity	Specificity	ER(%)
Males				
1	FC, TG, HDL-C, HDL_2, DHL_3	0.95	0.93	4.40
2	TG, HDL-C, apoA-I, apo-A-II, systolic BP	0.98	0.97	2.60
Females				
1	TC, HDL-C, PL, apoA-I, apoA-II	0.93	0.89	7.40
2	HDL-C, apoA-I, apoA-II, BMI, diastolic BP	0.96	0.97	3.60

Univariate analyses were performed by Wilcoxon-U test and multivariate analysis by stepwise discriminant regression. * $p < 0.05$; ** $p < 0.01$; *** $p < 0.001$. FC, free cholesterol; PL, phospholipids; BP, blood pressure; BMI, body mass index.

immediately after the cerebral attack with a control group matched for age and sex (Kostner *et al* 1986). CVD was diagnosed by EEG, cerebral angiograms and brain scan and classified into grades-I to grades-III. A total of 4 cases of brain infarction caused by cerebral embolism or subarachnoid hemorrhage and intracerebral hemorrhage were excluded from the study. Table III lists the parameters measured individually for the male and female groups. Whereas plasma lipids were not significantly different between patients and controls, HDL-C and even more apoA-I and apoA-II were significantly lower in the patient group. It was of particular interest to note that patients had lower TC and apoB values than controls which is at variance with the findings in PVD and MI patients. Males and females behaved almost identically. By multiple regressional discriminant analysis, CVD could be predicted with an error rate of only 3–7%. CVD-patients with different grades of diseases showed very similar changes in their lipid and lipoprotein patterns.

In a final study the role of Lp(a) as an independent risk indicator for MI was evaluated (Hoefler *et al* 1988). A total of 1486 young male soldiers were examined and their plasma lipids, lipoproteins and Lp(a) determined. The volunteers were divided into probands whose parents had no MI (control group, $n = 1434$) and probands whose mothers or fathers suffered from MI (patient group, $n = 52$). This kind of approach is particularly suitable for the assessment of Lp(a) as a discriminator because Lp(a) is inherited in an autosomally dominant fashion. Individuals with Lp(a) > 25 mg/dl were labeled Lp(a)$^+$, those with Lp(a) < 25 mg/dl as Lp(a)$^-$. In the control group, 13.4% of the children were Lp(a)$^+$ whereas 32% in the patient group were Lp(a)$^+$. This difference was statistically highly significant ($p < 0.01$). In addition, we observed a significant difference in the LDL-C/HDL-C ratio. The data from this study, which comes close to the validity of a prospective study, suggests that individuals with plasma Lp(a) levels > 25 mg/dl have an approximately 2.5-fold higher risk of MI, independent of other plasma lipids and lipoproteins.

A causal relationship between elevated plasma cholesterol, and also TG, and premature vascular diseases has been documented in numerous prospective studies as well as case control studies. Since these lipids are transported in plasma by different classes of lipoproteins, some of them being recognized as antiatherogenic, it seems plausible that measuring the cholesterol content of lipoprotein subfractions will allow a better discrimination between patients and controls, in comparison with TC measurements. This has also led to the term "atherosclerosis index," i.e. LDL-C/HDL-C or TC/HDL-C.

Because the lipid metabolism is governed by different apo-Lp, we tried to push this concept even further by asking three basic questions: i) are apo-Lp better discriminators of atherosclerotic diseases than lipids?; ii) can the atherosclerotic risk be better evaluated by measuring several risk factors and combining them into a mathematical model?; and iii) do patients with different forms of atherosclerosis have different risk profiles? To answer these questions, we have chosen a case control design which can be performed cheaply and quickly and may be considered as the basis for further, more sophisticated, studies. The three above questions may be answered as follows:

By univariate analysis, apo-Lp and, in particular apoA-I and apoB, are better risk discriminators than lipids or lipoprotein lipids. In addition we found that the measurement of several parameters including apoA-I, apoB, TG, LDL-C and HDL-C greatly improves the analytical discrimination power. By combining these parameters in a multivariate model, sensitivities of up to 95% with high specificities could be achieved. Lp(a) turned out to be an independent risk factor for atherosclerosis, at a cut-off level of approx. 25 mg/dl. Most importantly, however, it was found that atherosclerosis in different vessels of the body may be predicted by measuring individual apo-Lp and lipids. PVD was mainly associated with high TG, low HDL-C and high apoB/apoA-I ratios; MI was best predicted by assessing LDL-C/HDL-C, apoB/apoA-I, in addition to Lp(a); stroke and CVD were not accompanied by abnormal TC, LDL-C or apoB values but by low HDL-C, apoA-I and apoA-II values.

These models have now been tested thoroughly in our laboratory and proved to be valid for broad populations of different ages, sex and socio-economic status. After standardization of all the proposed laboratory parameters, we believe that this could become the basis of a large-scale health care screening program.

SUMMARY

Atherosclerosis is a multifactorial disease with many causes involving the dysfunction of endothelial cells, smooth muscle cells, platelets and macrophages. Despite other factors plasma lipids and in particular, cholesteryl esters are causally linked to this disease. Lipids are transported in the plasma together with apo-Lp, which, in turn, greatly influence lipid metabolism. We therefore tested the possibility of predicting the atherosclerosis risk in several areas of the body by measuring apo-Lp, in addition to lipids. The best risk indicators were assessed by multiple regressional discriminant analysis.

It was found that the apoA-I/apoB ratio and Lp(a) are optimal discriminators for MI whereas, in peripheral atherosclerosis, TG and LDL-C/HDL-C in combination with apo-Lp resulted in a good separation of patients from controls. Patients suffering from stroke had low normal cholesterol and apoB but extremely low HDL-C and apoA-I and apoA-II. For all three forms of atherosclerosis discriminant functions could be calculated which allowed to segregate patients at high risk to be identified with error rates of less than 10%. Lp(a) values >25 mg/dl were linked to a 2.5-fold risk of MI.

REFERENCES

Hoefler G, Harnoncourt F, Paschke E, Mirtl W, Pfeiffer KH, Kostner GM 1988 Lipoprotein Lp(a): A risk factor for myocardial infarction. Arteriosclerosis 8: 398–401

Kostner GM 1983 Apolipoproteins and lipoproteins of human plasma: Significance in health and in disease. Adv Lipid Res 20: 1–43

Kostner G, Alaupovic P 1972 Studies on the composition and structure of plasma lipoproteins: Separation and quantitation of the lipoprotein families occurring in the high density lipoproteins of human plasma. Biochemistry 11: 3419–3428

Kostner GM, Marth E, Pfeiffer KP, Wege H 1986 Apolipoproteins AI, AII and HDL phospholipids but not Apo-B are risk indicators for occlusive cerebrovascular disease. Eur Neurol 25: 346–354

Pilger E, Pristautz H, Pfeiffer KP, Kostner GM 1983 Risk factors for peripheral atherosclerosis: Retrospective evaluation by stepwise discriminant analysis. Arteriosclerosis 2: 57–63

Multiple Risk Factors in Cardiovascular Disease, ed. by A. Yamamoto, Churchill Livingstone Japan, Tokyo, pp. 131–135 (1994)

LIPOPROTEIN PARTICLES AND ATHEROSCLEROSIS

J.C. Fruchart and C. Fievet

*SERLIA et INSERM U325, Institut Pasteur**

Key words: coronary heart disease, lipoprotein particles, immunological methods, epidemiological study, clinical study

Results of many clinical and epidemiological studies have demonstrated that impairment in the metabolism of plasma lipoproteins is one of the most important risk of factors for coronary heart disease (CHD). Lipoproteins are usually separated according to their physicochemical properties, such as their density. Using this classification system, it has been proven that cholesteryl ester-rich low-density lipoproteins (LDL) are a major risk factor for CHD and that the high-density lipoproteins (HDL) possess a certain degree of antiatherogenic potential.

However, the use of physicochemical properties for lipoprotein identification does not take into account the protein component (apolipoproteins) of these entities, which plays a crucial role in lipoprotein metabolism. The purpose of this paper is to illustrate how apolipoproteins may be used as specific markers of lipoproteins, and how this lipoprotein-family concept may help to assess the magnitude of atherosclerotic risk in various clinically defined subpopulations and individual patients.

*1 rue du Pr Calmette, 59019 Lille cédex, France.

METABOLIC AND FUNCTIONAL PROPERTIES OF LIPOPROTEIN FAMILIES

It has been demonstrated previously that apolipoprotein B (apoB)-containing lipoproteins consist of four major lipoprotein families: those containing only apoB (LpB), those containing apoB and apoC's (LpB:C's), those containing apoB and apoE (LpB:E), and those containing all three of these apolipoproteins (LpB:C's:E) (Alaupovic 1991). All these lipoproteins are distributed throughout the entire density spectrum. Although the major part of LpB occurs in LDL, this lipoprotein particle has also been detected in very low density lipoproteins (VLDL) and intermediate-density lipoproteins (IDL). LpB:C's and LpB:C's:E represent the major components of VLDL and IDL, but may also be present in significant amounts in LDL. LpB appears to be cholesteryl ester-rich, while the complex particles seem to be enriched in triglycerides. In the latter, the apoC and apoE content decreases with increasing density. The binding properties of these lipoproteins for the LDL receptor appear to be very much dependent on the apolipoprotein composition (Agnani *et al* 1991). ApoE with phenotypes E3 and E4 increases the affinity of the particle for the LDL receptor, but reduces the apparent number of binding sites. In contrast, LpB:E isolated from subjects with the E2/E2 phenotype does not bind to the receptor, indicating that LpB:E isolated from subjects with the E3 and/or E4 phenotypes binds to the receptor through apoE and not apoB. These results suggest that apoE may mask the receptor binding site of apoB. Also, LpB:C-III, free of apoE, does not bind to the receptor and addition of apoC's, particularly apoC-III, to triglyceride-rich LpB reduces the affinity of the particle for the LDL receptor. Recent work indicating that C apolipoproteins are located near residue 3249 of apolipoprotein B100 on VLDL suggests that apoC-III may impair binding, probably by the same mechanism we have hypothesized for apoE (Yang *et al* 1993).

It is now well established that apoA-I-containing lipoproteins exist as two major families, those containing apoA-I and apoA-II (LpA-I:A-II) and those containing apoA-I but free of apoA-II (LpA-I) (Fruchart *et al* 1993). However, small amounts of LpA-II particles, i.e. those containing apoA-II but free of apoA-I, may be detected in most normolipidemic subjects. This minor form may become predominant in some rare diseases such as apoA-I deficiency. Our understanding with respect to the metabolism of apoA-I-containing lipoprotein families is limited. However, Brewer and Rader (1991) have recently shown that both families are synthesized by the liver, but that the intestine is the major site of synthesis of the LpA-I family. Metabolic studies utilizing radiolabeled lipoprotein particles suggest that there is a kinetic difference between LpA-I and LpA-I:A-II families and support the concept that there may be important functional differences between the lipoprotein particles present within HDL. In this regard, the finding that proteins stimulating reverse cholesterol transport (LCAT, lectin-cholesterol acyltransferase; CETP, cholesteryl ester-transfer protein) are mainly present in the LpA-I and not in the LpA-I:A-II family is of considerable significance. Cholesterol efflux mediated by apoA-I-containing particles has been studied in different cells. Long-term exposure to the LpA-I family promoted cholesterol efflux, whereas little or no efflux was observed in the presence of the LpA-I:A-II family. The fact that the LpA-I:A-II family can inhibit this LpA-I-promoted cholesterol efflux strongly supports the role of apoA-II as an antagonist in the production of cholesterol efflux (Fruchart *et al* 1993). These results, which emphasize that LpA-I and LpA-I:A-II families behave as distinct entities, have been confirmed in other studies showing that they differ in clinical significance (Fruchart *et al* 1993). Recent studies from transgenic mice more clearly demonstrate that protein composition determines the antiatherogenic properties of HDL. Rubin *et al* (1991) have reported that transgenic mice expressing large amounts of human plasma apoA-I and with high HDL levels were significantly protected from the development of fatty streak lesions, whereas despite similar HDL cholesterol concentrations, the area of atherogenic lesions in human apoA-I plus apoA-II transgenic mice was 15-fold greater than in the apoA-I animals (Schultz *et al* 1993). Also, increased expression of mouse apoA-II in mice appeared to promote rather than retard aortic fatty streak development (Warden *et al* 1993).

MEASUREMENT OF LIPOPROTEIN FAMILIES

Three different immunological procedures have been developed to quantify lipoprotein particles: sequential immunoprecipitation, immunoenzymometric assay, and differential electroimmunoassay. The first is time consuming and requires a larger amount of specific antibodies. Nevertheless, it is the original procedure used to isolate the lipoprotein families.

Immunoenzymometric assay is based on a sandwich ELISA test and is performed with microtiter plates as a solid-phase antibody and enzyme-labeled antibodies as conjugate. It is thus possible to measure lipoprotein particles that contain at least two different apolipoproteins (for example, the LpE:B family) by using two antibodies with different specificities (anti-apoE as the first antibody and anti-apoB conjugated with enzyme as the second antibody, in the same example). The LpC-III:B or LpA-I:A-II family may be measured using the same principle.

To determine LpA-I directly, a simpler procedure using differential electroimmunoassay has been developed. By using a large excess of anti-apoA-II, LpA-I:A-II particles are retained in a first peak and LpA-I migrates as a second peak. This second peak is measured to estimate LpA-I.

LIPOPROTEIN FAMILIES AND ATHEROSCLEROSIS

Using these different methodologies, we have evaluated the clinical significance of apoA-I- and apoB-containing lipoprotein families.

ApoB-containing Lipoprotein Families

Using sequential immunoprecipitation, it has recently been shown that the major lipoprotein families (LpB, LpB:C:E, LpB:E, and LpB:C) are present in both normolipidemic and hyperlipoproteinemic subjects, despite several quantitative differences between groups. LpB particles are the main lipoprotein family in normal and hypercholesterolemic subjects, whereas LpB:C and LpB:C:E are the major lipoprotein families occurring in hypertriglyceridemic patients. Hypercholesterolemia leads to a 3- to 4-fold higher concentration of LpB, compared to normolipidemic or hypertriglyceridemic subjects, whereas patients with various types of hypertriglyceridemia have significantly higher levels of LpB:C:E and LpB:C. In some cases, an increase in LpB:E may be the most striking abnormality. This has been observed in type III hyperlipoproteinemia (Lussier-Cacan *et al* 1989). However, hypercholesterolemic patients also have significantly increased levels of LpB:E particles present, mainly in LDL_2. From these observations, it has been suggested that LpB particles may be the most atherogenic of the apoB-containing lipoproteins. However, a few studies indicate that complex lipoprotein particles LpB:C, LpB:E, and LpB:C:E may approach or even surpass the atherogenicity of LpB. This was the conclusion of a recent study in which 47 males with angiographically documented coronary artery disease were analyzed for lipids, apolipoproteins, and lipoprotein particles. Of all the examined parameters, LpB:C and LpB:C:E showed the most significant correlation with severity of coronary disease (Koren *et al* 1989).

More recently, the clinical significance of these different apoB-containing particles has been investigated in a retrospective epidemiological study (ECTIM Study) (Parra *et al* 1992). This study was performed in four populations at different risk for myocardial infarction. Male patients who had suffered an infarct and control subjects were recruited at three centers in France (Strasbourg, Toulouse, Lille) and a center in Northern Ireland (Belfast). The mortality rate for myocardial infarction was three to four times higher in Belfast than in France. The LpB:E family and, to a lesser extent, the LpB:CIII family were significantly increased in the population with the highest mortality rate. Similar results have been confirmed elsewhere in men with angiographically diagnosed coronary artery disease (Genest *et al* 1991).

ApoA-I-containing Lipoprotein Families

It has been shown that women have slightly higher concentrations of LpA-I and lower concentrations of LpA-I:A-II than men. In women, 35–45% of total apoA-I occurs in LpA-I and 55–66% in LpA-I:A-II. The corresponding data for men are 26–42% of the total apoA-I in LpA-I and 58–74% in LpA-I:A-II. From clinical studies, it seems obvious that LpA-I is a better marker and predictive factor than LpA-I:A-II in evaluating the risk of atherosclerosis. Puchois *et al* (1987) have shown that the concentration of LpA-I was lower in normolipidemic patients with angiographically proven coronary artery disease, whereas LpA-I:A-II was unchanged, compared to controls. Results from the ECTIM Study indicate that LpA-I is lower in Belfast (i.e., in the population with the highest mortality rate for myocardial infarction) than in France, while apoA-I does not differ between the populations. Moreover, within each population, patients with cardiovascular disease have lower concentrations of LpA-I than controls (Parra *et al* 1992).

Recently, it has also been observed that the level of LpA-I (but not LpA-I:A-II) in children whose parents suffer from a premature form of CHD is lower than that in a control group with no family history of CHD (Amouyel *et al* 1993).

Assuming that octogenarians, who have survived periods during which the incidence of CHD was very high, should have several protective factors, we have compared octogenarians and younger control subjects (30-50 years of age) with regard to levels of apoA-I-containing particles: LpA-I is significantly elevated and LpA-I:A-II clearly lowered in octogenarians (Luc *et al* 1991).

Brewer *et al* (1990) have recently investigated LpA-I and LpA-I:A-II in a kindred with hyperalphalipoproteinemia and a decreased risk of coronary artery disease. The selective increase in LpA-I in a 60-year-old putative homozygote proband with a family history of longevity supports the concept that these particles may represent the "antiatherogenic" fraction of HDL.

These results, taken as a whole, strongly suggest that LpA-I may represent a protective factor against atherosclerosis and confirm the potential beneficial effect of this particle that has already been suggested by basic studies.

SUMMARY

The separation of lipoproteins based on apolipoprotein composition has improved our understanding of the physiological functions of the discrete lipoprotein families. The introduction of new immunological methods permitting the separation of various lipoproteins particles has revealed the existence of subpopulations with different metabolic functions and clinical significance.

The data presented here suggest that the common forms of dyslipoproteinemia encountered in patients with coronary artery disease represent a broad spectrum of overlapping disorders characterized by increased plasma levels of apoB-containing particles (LpB, LpB:E, etc.) and/or by decreased plasma levels of LpA-I.

The quantification of these particles allows greater accuracy in predicting the risk of developing premature atherosclerosis. This approach may also provide a new basis for the classification of dyslipoproteinemic states and the study of the effects of diet and hypolipemic drugs.

REFERENCES

Agnani G, Bard JM, Candelier L, Delattre S, Fruchart JC, Clavey V 1991 Interaction of LpB, LpB:E, LpB:C-III and LpB:C-III:E lipoproteins with the low density lipoprotein receptor on HeLa cells. Arteriosclerosis 11: 1021–1029

Alaupovic P 1991 Apolipoprotein composition as the basis for classifying plasma lipoproteins: Characterization of apo A- and apo B-containing lipoprotein families. *In*: Lee DM (Ed) Progress in lipid research, Pergamon Press, New York, Vol 30, No 2/3, pp 105–138

Amouyel P, Isorez D, Bard JM, Goldman M, Zylberberg G, Fruchart JC 1993 Parental history of early myocardial infarction is associated with decreased levels of lipoparticle A-I adolescents: Arterioscler Thromb 13: 1640–1644

Brewer HB, Rader DJ 1991 Structure, function and metabolism. *In*: Lee DM (Ed) Progress in lipid research, Pergamon Press, New York, Vol 30, No 2/3, pp 139–144

Brewer HB, Rader D, Fojo S, Hoeg JM 1990 Frontiers in the analysis of HDL structure, function, and metabolism. *In*: Carlson LA (Ed) Disorders of HDL, Proceedings of the International Symposium held at the

Karolinska Hospital, Stockholm 7–8 June, Smith Gordon, London, pp 89–97

Fruchart JC, Ailhaud G, Bard JM 1993 Heterogeneity of high density lipoprotein particles. Circulation 87: 22–27

Genest JJ, Bard JM, Fruchart JC, Ordovas JM, Wilson PFW, Schaefer EJ 1991 Plasma apolipoprotein A-I, A-II, B, E and C-III containing particles in men with premature coronary artery disease. Atherosclerosis 90: 149–157

Koren E, Wilson P, Corder C, Alaupovic P 1989 Lipoprotein particles in patients with coronary artery disease. FASEB J, Abst No 5759, 3: A1218

Luc G, Bard JM, Lussier-Cacan S *et al* 1991 High density lipoprotein particles in octogenarians. Metabolism 40: 1238–1243

Lussier-Cacan S, Bard J-M, Boufet L *et al* 1989 Lipoprotein composition changes induced by fenofibrate in dysbetalipoproteinemia type III. Atherosclerosis 78: 167–182

Parra HJ, Arveiler D, Evans AE *et al* 1992 A case control study of lipoprotein particles in two populations at contrasting risk for coronary heart disease: The ECTIM Study. Arterioscler Thromb 12: 701–707

Puchois P, Kandoussi A, Fievet P *et al* 1987 Apolipoprotein A-I containing lipoproteins in coronary artery disease. Atherosclerosis 68: 35–40

Rubin EM, Krauss RM, Spangler EA, Verstuyft JG, Clift SM 1991 Inhibition of early atherogenesis in transgenic mice by human apolipoprotein A-I. Nature 353: 262–267

Schultz JR, Verstuyft JG, Gong EL, Nichols AV, Rubin EM 1993 Protein composition determines the anti-atherogenic properties of HDL in transgenic mice. Nature 365: 782–784

Warden CH, Hedrick CC, Qiao JH, Castellani LW, Lusis AJ 1993 Atherosclerosis in transgenic mice overexpressing apolipoprotein A-II. Science 261: 469–472

Yang CY, Gu ZW, Valentinova N *et al* 1993 Human very low density lipoprotein structure: Interaction of the C apolipoproteins with apolipoprotein B-100. J Lipid Res 34: 1311–1321

Multiple Risk Factors in Cardiovascular Disease, ed. by A. Yamamoto, Churchill Livingstone Japan, Tokyo, pp. 137–142 (1994)

A NEW APPRAISAL OF TRIGLYCERIDE

Antonio M. GOTTO, Jr

*Department of Medicine, Baylor College of Medicine**

Key words: triglyceride, coronary heart disease, atherosclerosis, risk factors, hypertriglyceridemia

There is a resurgence of interest in serum triglyceride level as a predictor of coronary heart disease (CHD). Although the status of triglyceride as an independent CHD risk factor remains controversial, mounting evidence from observational and clinical studies suggests its importance as part of a combination of risk factors that, considered together, may refine CHD risk assessment. Advances in lipoprotein metabolism research provide better understanding of the interaction between triglyceride and the other lipids and underscore the need to evaluate a complete lipid profile, not only for risk assessment but also to make treatment decisions.

LIPID METABOLISM

Triglyceride is transported through the bloodstream packaged in lipoproteins, which are composed of a core of triglyceride and cholesteryl ester, in various proportions, surrounded by a surface monolayer of phospholipids, unesterified cholesterol, and apolipoproteins. These proteins enable the lipoprotein to interact with enzymes and to bind to cell membrane receptors and so determine the lipoprotein's metabolic fate.

Of the triglyceride-rich lipoproteins, chylomicrons are the primary lipoprotein of exogenous lipid transport, and very-low-density lipoprotein (VLDL) particles, composed mostly of triglyceride synthesized in the liver, begin the endogenous lipid cascade. During lipolysis, triglyceride is hydrolyzed from the chylomicron and VLDL cores through the action of lipoprotein lipase, and the excess surface phospholipids are transferred to high-density lipoprotein (HDL) particles. The chylomicron remnants are then removed from the circulation through receptor-mediated uptake by hepatocytes, as are some of the VLDL remnants, termed intermediate-density lipoprotein (IDL) particles. Other IDL particles remain in the plasma, where more of their triglyceride is hydrolyzed through the action of hepatic lipase until low-density lipoprotein (LDL) particles are formed. LDL is the main supplier of cholesterol to cells.

HDL is secreted by the liver, intestine, and macrophages as discoidal precursor particles composed of apolipoproteins and phospholipids, primarily lecithin. These nascent HDL particles acquire unesterified cholesterol from cell membranes during cell

* 6550 Fannin, M.S. SM-1423, Houston, TX 77030, USA.

renewal or death, in addition to the excess phospholipids acquired from the hydrolysis of triglyceride-rich lipoproteins. The enzyme lecithin-cholesterol acyltransferase (LCAT) then acts upon the lecithin and unesterified cholesterol in HDL to form a core of cholesteryl ester and to transform the disks into mature, spherical HDL. Mature HDL exists in two major subclasses: smaller HDL_3, whose levels do not vary much among individuals, and larger HDL_2, formed through the action of LCAT on HDL_3. HDL_2 has a greater cholesterol-carrying capacity that enables HDL to return cholesterol from peripheral tissues to the liver in a process termed reverse cholesterol transport. Most of the interindividual variation in HDL levels is due to different levels of HDL_2.

Since HDL is formed in part from products of the catabolism of the triglyceride-rich lipoproteins, the effectiveness of this catabolism and consequent availability of phospholipids and cholesterol influence HDL levels. Rapid lipolysis of chylomicrons and VLDL is reflected by high HDL_2 levels, whereas delayed lipolysis favors HDL_3 formation at the expense of the larger HDL_2, thus compromising the reverse cholesterol transport process.

Reverse cholesterol transport is also reduced by the conversion of HDL_2 back to HDL_3 through the action of cholesteryl ester transfer protein (CETP), which is more active in the presence of elevated plasma triglyceride levels. CETP allows triglyceride from chylomicrons and VLDL to be transferred to HDL in exchange for cholesteryl ester. The acquired triglyceride is then hydrolyzed from HDL by hepatic lipase, and these smaller, denser HDL particles are removed more quickly from the circulation, so that HDL levels are decreased.

CETP permits a similar exchange between the triglyceride-rich lipoproteins and LDL. As cholesteryl ester is removed from LDL, the accumulated triglyceride becomes a substrate for further lipolysis by hepatic lipase, and small, dense LDL results. These small, dense LDL particles, which are often characteristic of hypertriglyceridemia, are associated with an increased risk for myocardial infarction and may be more atherogenic than normal LDL.

TRIGLYCERIDE AND CHD RISK

When triglyceride levels are elevated, the action of CETP causes the accumulation of cholesteryl ester in chylomicrons and VLDL particles, which increases their atherogenic potential by promoting cholesteryl ester uptake by macrophages. Elevated triglyceride levels have also been associated with alterations in coagulation factor levels that may promote thrombosis or inhibit fibrinolysis, and as discussed, triglyceride can influence atherogenesis indirectly by affecting the structure of HDL and LDL.

In most case-control studies and many prospective studies, a positive univariate association has been established between serum triglyceride level and CHD incidence (Austin 1991). However, upon multivariate analysis controlling for other risk factors such as blood pressure, physical activity, and obesity, this association tends to diminish and may disappear when HDL cholesterol, coagulation factors, or indicators of abnormal glucose metabolism are added. Because of the strong inverse relation between HDL and triglyceride-rich lipoprotein levels, the association between triglyceride and CHD risk may be underestimated when HDL is included in the statistical model. Also, the variability of triglyceride values both within and between individuals may cause misclassification of subjects with respect to their triglyceride level and suggests that triglyceride is less accurately measured than other lipids. In addition, different triglyceride-rich lipoproteins may vary in their atherogenicity: large, buoyant VLDL particles, which are associated with a low-fat vegetarian diet, and chylomicrons do not appear to confer atherosclerotic risk, whereas small, dense VLDL (β-VLDL) particles and chylomicron remnants are potentially atherogenic.

Although the association of triglyceride with CHD is inconsistent, serum triglyceride levels may have predictive value for CHD incidence if used in conjunction with other lipid levels. When triglyceride levels are evaluated in the context of the rest of the lipid profile, a more refined assessment of CHD risk can be made.

The joint effects of triglyceride, LDL cholesterol, and HDL cholesterol levels on CHD risk were studied in the Helsinki Heart Study (Manninen *et al* 1992), a 5-year, placebo-controlled, double-blind clinical trial conducted in 4,081 dyslipidemic, middle-aged men to test the effect of gemfibrozil-induced decreases in LDL cholesterol level and increases in HDL cholesterol level on CHD risk. While the LDL cholesterol:HDL cholesterol ratio was found to be the best single predictor of cardiac events, defined as fatal and nonfatal myocardial infarction and cardiac death, serum triglyceride levels of more than 2.3 mmol/L combined with LDL cholesterol:HDL cholesterol ratios of more than 5 defined a high-risk subgroup whose relative risk was 3.8 compared with subjects with triglyceride levels of 2.3 mmol/L or less and LDL cholesterol:HDL cholesterol ratios of 5 or less. The high-risk subgroup also benefited most from gemfibrozil treatment, as demonstrated by a 71% lower incidence of cardiac events in that treatment group than in the corresponding placebo group. Serum triglyceride level was found to be a strong indicator of CHD risk, and its interdependence with LDL cholesterol and HDL cholesterol suggests that the joint effects of triglyceride and lipoprotein cholesterol levels should be considered in the evaluation of CHD risk.

A comparable high-risk subgroup was identified among 4,576 men, aged 40–60 years, as part of the Prospective Cardiovascular Münster (PROCAM) study (Assmann & Schulte 1992). Triglyceride levels were 2.3 mmol/L or higher in 39.3% of the 122 subjects who suffered myocardial infarction or fatal CHD during a 4-year period and in 21.2% of the 4,352 surviving subjects who had not had myocardial infarction or stroke. Although univariate analysis showed a significant association between triglyceride level and CHD incidence, this relation disappeared after adjustment for total cholesterol or HDL cholesterol. However, when subjects were stratified by total cholesterol, LDL cholesterol, or HDL cholesterol, triglyceride levels of 2.3 mmol/L or greater were associated with a much higher incidence of CHD than were lower triglyceride levels. As in the Helsinki Heart Study, the group at highest risk for CHD was characterized by a combination of triglyceride levels of 2.3 mmol/L or greater and LDL cholesterol: HDL cholesterol ratios of 5 or more. This subgroup, which represented only 3.7% of subjects, accounted for almost 25% of all CHD events. Because this high-risk subgroup would not have been detected by evaluations of LDL cholesterol alone, this study suggests the advisability of obtaining a full lipid profile, including triglyceride level, before evaluating CHD risk or planning treatment.

In the Framingham Heart Study, which began in 1948 with a cohort of 5,127 men and women free from overt disease, stratification of triglyceride level by HDL cholesterol level was again predictive of CHD incidence (Castelli 1992). Men with triglyceride levels higher than 1.57 mmol/L and HDL cholesterol levels lower than 1.03 mmol/L had the highest incidence of CHD, almost twice that of any other group, during a 14-year period. Although the subgroup with low triglyceride and low HDL cholesterol levels also had a high rate of disease, the infrequency of this combination yielded fewer cases. Among women as well, the subgroup with high triglyceride and low HDL cholesterol levels produced almost twice as many cases as any other subgroup; in women, unlike in men, both an impact of the triglyceride tertile on CHD risk and a gradient of risk on the tertile of HDL cholesterol were found. This study suggests that the subgroup characterized by combined high triglyceride and low HDL cholesterol levels will produce a disproportionately large share of CHD cases because of the frequency of this combination in the general population. Since this subgroup may not have particularly high total cholesterol or LDL cholesterol levels, risk assessment that evaluates only these lipid concentrations may not identify individuals at the highest risk for CHD.

New evidence has found triglyceride to be an independent CHD risk factor even when HDL is included in the analysis. Recent meta-analysis of 16 population-based, prospective studies (Hokanson & Austin 1993), 12 conducted in a total of 33,214 men and 4 conducted in a total of 5,836 women, with follow-up intervals ranging from 3 to 14.5 years, showed that triglyceride is a risk factor for CHD in both men and women, independent of the effect of HDL cholesterol. Also, logistic regression analyses performed on 2-year data from the Cholesterol-Lowering Atherosclerosis Study (CLAS) (Miller *et al* 1993), a randomized, placebo-controlled trial of the effects of colestipol-plus-niacin therapy on angiographically defined CHD in 162 men with previous coronary bypass surgery, found that a higher baseline plasma triglyceride level predicts greater benefit of therapy on angiographic global change scores. This benefit was associated with greater triglyceride lowering but was not due to larger reductions in LDL or to greater increases in HDL.

TREATMENT OF HYPERTRIGLYCERIDEMIA

The importance of triglyceride in assessing CHD risk has been recognized in several major national and international treatment guidelines and recommendations. The European Atherosclerosis Society includes triglyceride among its CHD risk factors (International Task Force 1992), citing the concurrence of high triglyceride levels and low HDL cholesterol levels as predictive of CHD. For moderate hypertriglyceridemia, defined as triglyceride levels of 2.3–4.6 mmol/L, and for severe hypertriglyceridemia, defined as triglyceride levels greater than 4.6 mmol/L, treatment is to be a combination of correcting the underlying causes, weight control, lipid-lowering diet, and regular physical exercise. If response to hygienic therapy is inadequate or if a high overall risk profile is present, the recommended lipid-lowering agents are fibric-acid derivatives, nicotinic acid, and marine oils rich in omega-3 polyunsaturated fatty acids.

The U.S. National Cholesterol Education Program's second Adult Treatment Panel classifies triglyceride levels of 2.3–4.5 mmol/L as borderline-high, 4.5–11.3 mmol/L as high, and greater than 11.3 mmol/L as very high (1993). For all patients with elevated triglyceride levels, hygienic therapy is recommended and should comprise weight reduction if overweight, restriction of alcohol intake, and increased physical activity. Drug therapy may be indicated when elevated triglyceride levels are associated with recognized atherogenic dyslipidemias. In patients with very high triglyceride levels, drug therapy is generally indicated to prevent acute pancreatitis.

The International Committee for the Evaluation of Hypertriglyceridemia as a Vascular Risk Factor recommends complementing emphasis on LDL as the primary atherogenic lipoprotein with increased attention to the atherogenic potential of the triglyceride-rich lipoproteins (1991). Triglyceride levels greater than 2.3 mmol/L are defined as elevated; triglyceride levels between 2.3 and 4.5 mmol/L are defined as moderately elevated, and information on LDL cholesterol and HDL cholesterol concentrations is required for proper classification of the lipid abnormality. Triglyceride levels greater than 11.2 mmol/L increase the risk for pancreatitis. Recommended stepwise treatment of hypertriglyceridemia comprises identification of the cause of the triglyceride elevation, identification of the individual's overall risk pattern, treatment according to this overall risk pattern, diet as first-line treatment, and consideration of drug therapy if diet is ineffective, although this last step is admitted to be controversial.

The 1992 NIH Consensus Development Panel on Triglyceride, High-Density Lipoprotein, and Coronary Heart Disease recommends measuring triglyceride levels to assess the risk for further disease in individuals with established CHD; to refine CHD risk assessment in individuals with elevated total cholesterol, two or more CHD risk factors, or disorders associated with elevated triglycerides and increased CHD risk, such as diabetes mellitus or hypertension; to determine the presence of familial hyperlipidemic disorders and the likelihood of recurrent pancreatitis; and to assess the response to triglyceride-lowering therapy (1993). The panel recommends that the primary emphasis of treatment be diet and weight control, exercise, and smoking cessation. Although drug therapy is relegated to a secondary role, the triglyceride-lowering drugs recommended if non-pharmacological therapy fails are nicotinic acid and fibric-acid derivatives. For distinct hypertriglyceridemia, defined as triglyceride levels greater than 5.65 mmol/L, initial treatment is to be hygienic, followed by drug therapy if necessary to reduce the risk for pancreatitis; in patients with a history of pancreatitis, drug therapy in conjunction with hygienic treatment is considered the initial therapy. In patients with desirable LDL cholesterol levels, borderline hypertriglyceridemia, defined as triglyceride levels of 2.28–5.65 mmol/L, is to be treated with non-pharmacological therapy, although drug therapy should be considered if hygienic measures fail and CHD or a strong CHD risk profile is present.

SUMMARY

The role of serum triglyceride level in CHD risk assessment has become the subject of increased attention. Although a positive association between triglyceride level and CHD incidence has been established in univariate analysis of data from case-control and prospective studies, this association tends to weaken or disappear upon adjustment for other factors, including HDL. However, HDL levels may be largely determined by the effectiveness of the catabolism of triglyceride-rich lipoproteins and by the level of triglyceride in the circulation. Elevated triglyceride levels also affect the structure of HDL and LDL, resulting in smaller, denser particles, which, in the case of HDL, compromise reverse cholesterol transport, and in the case of LDL, are associated with an increased risk for myocardial infarction and may be more atherogenic than normal LDL. In the presence of elevated triglyceride levels, chylomicrons and VLDL accumulate cholesteryl ester and so become more atherogenic themselves, since they promote the uptake of cholesteryl ester by macrophages.

The varying atherogenicity of the different triglyceride-rich lipoproteins may also account for the inconsistent association between triglyceride and CHD incidence, as may the variability of triglyceride levels both within and between individuals. Despite the inconsistency, however, evaluating serum triglyceride levels in the context of other lipid levels may help to refine CHD risk assessment. Several major studies have identified a high-risk subgroup defined by elevated triglyceride levels combined with high LDL cholesterol : HDL cholesterol ratios or low HDL levels. Recognition of triglyceride as an important variable in assessing CHD risk has led to recommendations for the hygienic treatment and, if necessary, drug treatment of hypertriglyceridemia.

REFERENCES

Assmann G, Schulte H 1992 Role of triglycerides in coronary artery disease: Lessons from the Prospective Cardiovascular Münster study. Am J Cardiol 70: 10H–13H

Austin MA 1991 Plasma triglyceride and coronary heart disease. Arterioscler Thromb 11: 2–14

Castelli WP 1992 Epidemiology of triglycerides: A view from Framingham. Am J Cardiol 70: 3H–9H

Expert Panel on Detection, Evaluation, and Treatment of High Blood Cholesterol in Adults 1993 Summary of the second report of the National Cholesterol Education Program (NCEP) Expert Panel on Detection, Evaluation, and Treatment of High Blood Cholesterol in Adults (Adult Treatment Panel II). JAMA 269: 3015–3023

Hokanson JE, Austin MA 1993 Triglyceride is a risk factor for coronary disease in men and women: A meta-analysis of population-based prospective studies (abstract 2748). Circulation 88: I-510

International Committee for the Evaluation of Hypertriglyceridemia as a Vascular Risk Factor 1991 The hypertriglyceridemias: Risk and management. Am J Cardiol 68 (suppl): 1A–42A

International Task Force for the Prevention of Coronary Heart Disease 1992 Prevention of coronary heart disease: Scientific background and new clinical guidelines: Recommendations of the European Atherosclerosis Society. Nutr Metab Cardiovasc Dis 2: 113–156

Manninen V, Tenkanen L, Koskinen P *et al* 1992 Joint effects of serum triglyceride and LDL cholesterol and HDL cholesterol concentrations on coronary heart disease risk in the Helsinki Heart Study: Implications for treatment. Circulation 85: 37–45

Miller BD, Krauss RM, Cashin-Hemphill L, Blankenhorn DH 1993 Baseline triglyceride levels predict angiographic benefit of colestipol plus niacin therapy in the Cholesterol-Lowering Atherosclerosis Study (CLAS) (abstract 1946). Circulation 88: I-363

NIH Consensus Panel on Triglyceride, High-Density Lipoprotein, and Coronary Heart Disease 1993 Triglyceride, high-density lipoprotein, and coronary heart disease. JAMA 269: 505–510

Multiple Risk Factors in Cardiovascular Disease, ed. by A. Yamamoto, Churchill Livingstone Japan, Tokyo, pp. 143–148 (1994)

HYPERAPOB: AN UPDATE

Allan D. SNIDERMAN and Katherine CIANFLONE

*McGill Unit for the Prevention of Cardiovascular Disease, McGill University**

Key words: familial combined hyperlipidemia, HyperapoB, apoB

HyperapoB is that group of metabolic disorders which produce an elevated number of low-density lipoproteins (LDL) particles in plasma due to increased secretion of B100 lipoprotein particles by the liver (Teng *et al* 1986). Patients with HyperapoB are indistinguishable from those with familial combined hyperlipidemia (FCH) (Grundy *et al* 1987), but we believe the term HyperapoB is preferable to FCH for the following reasons. First, combined hyperlipidemia is now used both to mean that some individuals within a family are hypertriglyceridemic while others are hypercholesterolemic (Goldstein *et al* 1973) (the original sense) applying therefore to all affected members within the family, no matter their lipoprotein phenotype, but also, and quite differently, to mean that particular individuals are both hypertriglyceridemic and hypercholesterolemic (the sense which has been added with time). Second, depending on the diagnostic cut-off points which differ considerably depending on which lipid guidelines are being applied, a variable fraction of patients with HyperapoB or FCH may be normolipidemic but still have an elevated number of plasma LDL particles and therefore still be at high individual risk of premature vascular disease. If only lipids are examined, their increased risk will be overlooked. A striking extension of this view has recently been provided by Genest *et al* (1993) who showed that individuals with familial hypoalphalipoproteinemia and coronary disease had elevated apolipoprotein B (apoB) as well. If apoB had not been measured, there would have been no evidence of this abnormality in LDL which almost certainly led to their clinical disease. Third, if only lipid cut-off points are used, hypertriglyceridemic patients with FCH cannot be distinguished from hypertriglyceridemic patients with familial hypertriglyceridemia (Brunzell *et al* 1983), a distinction that should be possible given that the former is associated with increased coronary risk whereas the latter is not (Brunzell *et al* 1976). Fourth, the diagnosis of FCH cannot be made unless the family is studied. Doctors in practice are rarely able to do so, and even when they can, the family must be sufficiently large and its members sufficiently old for a diagnosis of FCH to be possible. On the other hand, HyperapoB is a diagnosis made in an individual which can be applied in a family, if and when that is necessary and appropriate.

* 687 Pine Avenue West, Montreal, Quebec H3A 1A1, Canada.

Since doctors must make decisions with the individuals in front of them, what use is a diagnostic construct that demands the rest of the family be there too and be large enough as well as to be informative. Fifth, FCH is only familial and overproduction of hepatic apoB particles can be acquired such as occurs in omental obesity (Anderson *et al* 1988) and with steroid administration (Ettinger & Hazzard 1988). Once again, measurement of apoB allows the doctor to deal effectively with the individual patient. Sixth, the term FCH does not imply anything about pathophysiology or therapy whereas HyperapoB is clear on both. Lowering the LDL particle number is the primary objective of therapy, an approach which is now solidly established as being of clinical benefit (Sniderman & Ghezzo 1994; Law *et al* 1994). Seventh and finally — measurement of apoB has now been standardized (Marcovina *et al* 1994) whereas that of lipoprotein lipids and triglycerides has not. For these reasons, therefore, we prefer the term HyperapoB to FCH.

PATHOPHYSIOLOGY OF HYPERAPOB

1. Mechanisms Leading to Increased Numbers of Smaller Denser LDL Particles in Plasma

The pathophysiology of HyperapoB is complex to the extent that the consequences are far removed from the metabolic causes of the syndrome. Our examination of this long-linked chain of events will begin, therefore, with the consequences of the increased secretion of hepatic apoB100 lipoprotein particles by the liver. In man, most very low-density lipoprotein (VLDL) particles are converted to LDL particles. Unfortunately, the LDL pathway, although specific with high affinity binding, has a limited capacity to remove LDL particles from plasma. Therefore, if production of the LDL particles increases sufficiently, the capacity of the LDL pathway to remove them is exceeded and the LDL particle number in plasma rises. Overproduction has thus led to an increased number of LDL particles in spite of the fact that the LDL pathway is entirely normal in function.

The next feature to account for in HyperapoB is the increased number of dense LDL. There are two possibilities, with some evidence for each. The most straightforward is that the liver secretes increased numbers of these smaller denser particles, a hypothesis supported by some data from turnover studies of radiolabelled VLDL and LDL (Teng *et al* 1986). The alternate — and often likely to be the more important explanation — is that the smaller denser LDL particles are generated by exaggeration of the cholesterol ester-triglyceride exchanges that occur normally in plasma (Tall 1986).

These work as follows: core lipid can, and does, exchange amongst the plasma lipoproteins by virtue of the action of a plasma protein known as cholesterol ester transfer protein (CETP). In the presence of CETP, a molecule of either cholesterol ester or triglyceride in one plasma lipoprotein is exchanged for a molecule of either one of these in another plasma lipoprotein. If like exchanges with like, nothing of consequence occurs. However, if cholesterol ester exchanges with triglyceride then changes of significance do follow. The lipoprotein particle which has received triglyceride in exchange for cholesterol ester remains almost the same with respect to size and density. However, if the triglyceride is then hydrolyzed, the mass of core lipid is reduced and the particle is therefore smaller. Because lipid is less dense than protein, if the mass of protein remains the same, since there is now less lipid, the particle is now denser as well as smaller.

Cholesterol ester-triglyceride exchanges are most likely to occur when the lipoproteins with predominantly cholesterol ester in their core, LDL and HDL, contact others with predominantly triglyceride in theirs, VLDL and chylomicrons. Each B100 lipoprotein particle secreted by the liver contains exactly one molecule of apoB100 which remains with the particle until it is irreversibly removed from plasma. The total number of lipoprotein particles of hepatic origin in plasma at any time is given by the sum of all the VLDL, IDL, and LDL particles and is equal to the total apoB. Furthermore, although most LDL particles arise from VLDL particles from which most of the triglycerides and all the apoproteins except apoB have been removed, because their plasma half-lives are so different, there are at least nine times more LDL than VLDL particles present at any time (Durrington *et al* 1978; Sniderman *et al* 1991). Thus, the total plasma apoB, even in hypertriglyceridemic patients, is determined for all practical purposes by the LDL apoB.

Even in normals, LDL particles differ in size and density, some being larger with more cholesterol within their core, others smaller and denser with less cholesterol within (Krauss & Burke 1982). When VLDL particles are overproduced, these differences are exaggerated resulting in increased numbers of smaller denser LDL particles (Teng *et al* 1983). The LDL particles become smaller and denser because the extent of cholesterol ester-triglyceride exchange depends on the rate of secretion of VLDL particles, the number of LDL particles, only in a limiting case on the amount of CETP, and finally — and probably quite importantly — the ambient plasma fatty acid concentration, since higher levels produce a greatly accelerated exchange. All these conditions are met in HyperapoB including an elevated plasma fatty acid concentration, particularly in the postprandial period, and so most often not only is LDL particle number increased in this disorder but many or most of the LDL particles are smaller and denser than normal. Clinically, based on the relationships between core cholesterol and apoB outlined above, mean LDL particle size can be estimated by the ratio of LDL cholesterol to LDL apoB. Indeed, even the ratio of LDL cholesterol to total plasma apoB will serve this purpose almost as well.

Even though these smaller LDL particles contain less cholesterol than normal, they are, it now appears, particle for particle, more atherogenic than LDL particles of normal size and composition. That is they penetrate the arterial wall more easily (Zilversmit & Nordestguard 1989), oxidize more easily (DeGraaf *et al* 1993), bind to the glycosaminoglycans more easily (Hurt-Camejo *et al* 1990) and stimulate more profoundly the production of thromboxane A2 by endothelial cells (Weisser *et al* 1993). The elevated LDL particle number and their increased atherogenicity undoubtedly explain largely why these patients with HyperapoB are at such increased risk of premature vascular disease. However to the extent that VLDL contribute to this risk, and more particularly to the extent that IDL do, both of these are also present in increased numbers.

2. Regulation of Hepatic B100 Lipoproteins

Only a few years ago, little was known about what controlled the rate at which hepatic B100 lipoproteins were secreted and now suddenly the major details seem clear. In the first instance, it is clear that the rate of secretion of these particles is determined principally by the mass of sterol and fatty acids delivered to the liver. Increase either- or both- and B100 secretion rises markedly (Sniderman & Cianflone 1993). Second, in these instances, the increased secretion rate is achieved by increased utilization of molecules of B100 which have been synthesized. That is to say, far more B100 molecules are synthesized on the rough endoplasmic reticulum than are finally secreted from the cell. Whether a molecule of B100 is eventually utilized for the purpose for which it was synthesized or whether it is hydrolyzed within minutes after its production seems to depend on the mass of core lipid present and being synthesized within the hepatocyte at that moment. That is, the utilization but not the synthesis of these enormous molecules is geared to the mass of lipid accumulating within the hepatocyte and which it is their function to remove.

This relation seems straightforward given the necessity to coordinate the two processes, synthesis of the essential structural molecule of the package, apoB100, and ensuring that unwanted masses of core lipid do not accumulate within the liver. That is, the packaging to remove lipid is being synthesized at a steady and usually excessive rate. Changing the proportion of these molecules which are destroyed allows instant and easy response to changes in lipid mass within the hepatocyte.

Two critical features of the handling of fatty acids by the liver are often overlooked. First, there is for all practical purposes no barrier to their entry into this organ. Heimberg and his colleagues (1969) showed definitively that the fractional extraction of fatty acids from plasma does not even begin to diminish until concentrations much above those seen in life are achieved. Second, although the uptake of fatty acids is unlimited, the liver is quite limited in the use it can make of them (Fukuda & Ontko 1984). That is to say, the capacity to oxidize them is not great and only relatively small amounts are needed for incorporation into other molecules which are being synthesized. What then happens to the rest? The answer is that they are re-exported once they have been reformed into triglycerides. If they were not virtually all immediately re-exported, hepatocytes would soon be swollen by triglycerides derived from the plasma fatty acids.

What then is the purpose of this apparently futile exercise- fatty acids taken up one moment without limit and then almost immediately resecreted?. The answer, we suggest, lies in the need to regulate the plasma fatty acid concentration. Adipocytes are the only tissue in the body able to store energy in significant quantities and, as many of us have discovered to our sorrow, their capacity to do so is limitless. When required, energy in the form of fatty acids is liberated from adipocytes. However, the number released are not carefully regulated by the need, for the need is not known until the task is complete. To ensure our muscles do not suffer a shortage of energy, release exceeds need. However, that creates a potential risk given the cytotoxicity of fatty acids. Therefore, to prevent the plasma concentration of fatty acids from rising to dangerous levels, the liver acts as a buffer, soaking up excessive fatty acids quickly, but then releasing them in the form of VLDL triglycerides in a slower less dangerous fashion. Back they go to myocytes to be oxidized or to adipocytes to be stored again, on call if needed. Thus, adipose tissue and the liver play complex and interlocking roles in energy storage and release.

3. *Mechanisms Leading to Increased Secretion of Hepatic B100 Particles*

a) Increased delivery of fatty acids to the liver
Normally, most of the chylomicron triglycerides should be stored in adipocytes or utilized immediately by myocytes. Very little, it is thought, should go directly to the liver. Increased release of fatty acids from adipocytes (Rebuffé-Scrive *et al* 1989), particularly omental adipocytes, delivered to the liver via the portal circulation has been thought to be responsible for the HyperapoB type dyslipidemia seen with omental obesity (Després *et al* 1990). The more common cause, we believe, is limitation in adipocyte triglyceride synthetic capacity (Maslowska *et al* 1993). Only recently has it been recognized that the rate at which adipocytes can synthesize triglycerides depends upon the activity of the Adipsin-acylation stimulating protein (ASP) pathway (Baldo *et al* 1993). Although space does not permit this pathway to be described in detail here, in essence, the human adipocyte can synthesize and secrete, factor B, adipsin and the third component of complement (C3). These are the components of the alternate complement pathway and they interact to produce ASP. ASP is identical to C3a, a fragment of C3. Carboxypeptidases present in plasma rapidly convert C3a to C3adesarg. Both forms of ASP, C3a and C3adesarg, however, are bioactive with regard to triglyceride synthesis. Adipocytes from patients with HyperapoB synthesize triglyceride less rapidly than do adipocytes from normals (Teng *et al* 1988), and skin fibroblasts cultured from patients with HyperapoB also synthesize triglycerides less rapidly than do fibroblasts from normals or

patients with other dyslipoproteinemias (Clanflone *et al* 1990). The defect appears to be a diminished response to ASP, apparently due to a defective or diminished number of cell membrane receptors for ASP (Clanflone *et al* 1990).

The functional consequences of such a diminished response are now easy to trace. First, lipoprotein lipase activity (LPL) is inhibited by the fatty acids which accumulate in the microcirculation because they are not being cleared by the adipocytes. The LPL is then detached from the endothelial surface and so also is the chylomicron particle which it was binding to that surface. This remnant with more triglyceride than normal is swept away to the liver where it is rapidly taken up. The consequence of the reduced adipocyte triglyceride synthetic rate is a diversion of fatty acids and triglyceride-enriched chylomicron remnants to the liver, the consequence of this being an increased secretion of B100 particles by this organ.

Omental adipocytes synthesize triglycerides less rapidly than subcutaneous adipocytes (Maślowska *et al* 1993) and so incomplete hydrolysis of triglyceride-rich lipoproteins is more likely to occur here than under the skin. This, rather than excessive hydrolysis, is the likely explanation for the HyperapoB type dyslipoproteinemia encountered so often in patients with omental obesity.

b) Increased delivery of sterol to the liver or abnormal sterol metabolism

In vitro studies have established that increased delivery of cholesterol to HepG2 cells results in increased secretion of B100 particles (Sniderman & Cianflone 1993). As in the case of fatty acids, post-translational mechanisms appear responsible. Again, as in the case of fatty acids, there is evidence that alteration in the mass of cholesterol ester is the key to altering the proportion of B100 particles that are secreted as opposed to hydrolyzed. Clinically, this is the likely mechanism responsible for the abnormal secretion of B100 particles in patients with nephrotic syndrome and with heterozygous and homozygous familial hypercholesterolemia. That is, even though the LDL pathway is normal in the first instance but not in the second, in both disorders, delivery of cholesterol to the liver is increased and this is almost certainly the basis for the increase in B100 secretion rates and the altered composition of the particles which are secreted.

In summary, much is now known about the mechanism responsible for the overproduction of B100 particles in patients with HyperapoB. Given the evidence — of angiographic benefit (Law *et al* 1994) and, in particular, the recent evidence of clinical benefit from the angiographic trials in which LDL particles were markedly lowered (Sniderman & Ghezzo in press 1994) — the challenge is to convert these concepts into routine clinical application.

REFERENCES

Anderson AJ, Sobocrinski KA, Freedman DS *et al* 1988 Body fat distribution, plasma lipids, and lipoproteins. Arteriosclerosis 8: 88–94

Baldo A, Sniderman AD, St-Luce S *et al* 1993 The adipsin-acylation stimulating protein system and regulation of intracellular triglyceride synthesis. J Clin Invest 92: 1543–1558

Brunzell JD, Schrott HG, Motulsky AG, Bierman EL 1976 Myocardial infarction in the familial forms of hypertriglyceridemia. Metabolism 25: 313–320

Brunzell JD, Albers JJ, Chait A *et al* 1983 Plasma lipoproteins in familial combined hyperlipidemia and monogenic familial hypertriglyceridemia. J Lipid Res 24: 147–155

Cianflone K, Maslowska M, Sniderman AD 1990 Impaired response of fibroblasts in patients with hyperapobetalipoproteinemia to Acylation Stimulating Proteins. J Clin Invest 85: 722–730

DeGraaf J, Hendricks JCM, Demacker PWM, Stalenhalf AFH 1993 Identification of multiple dense LDL subfractions with enhanced susceptibility to *in vitro* oxidation among hypertriglyceridemic subjects. Arterioscler Thromb 13: 712–719

Desprès JP, Moorjani S, Lupien P, Tremblay A, Nadeau A, Bouchard C 1990 Regional differences of body fat, plasma lipoproteins and cardiovascular disease. Arteriosclerosis 10: 497–511

Durrington PN, Bolton CH, Hartog M 1978 Serum and lipoprotein apolipoprotein B levels in normal subjects and patients with hyperlipoproteinemia. Clin Chim Acta 82: 151–160

Ettinger WH Jr., Hazzard WR 1988 Elevated apolipoprotein-B levels in corticosteroid treated patients with systemic lupus erythematosus. J Clin Endocrinol Metab 67: 425–428

Fukuda N, Ontko J 1984 Interactions between fatty acid synthesis, oxidation, and esterification in the production of triglyceride-rich lipoproteins by the liver. J Lipid Res 25: 831–842

Genest J Jr, Bard JM, Fruchart JC *et al* 1993. Familial hypoalphalipoproteinemia in premature coronary artery disease. Arterioscler Thromb 13: 1728–1737

Goldstein JL, Schrott HG, Hazzard WR, Bierman EL, Motulsky AG 1973 Hyperlipidemia in coronary heart disease. Il: Genetic analysis of lipid levels in 176 families and delineation of a new inherited disorder, combined hyperlipidaemia J Clin Invest 52: 1544–1568

Grundy SM, Chait A, Brunzell JD 1987 Familial Combined Hyperlipidemia Workshop. Arteriosclerosis 7: 203–207

Heimburg M, Weinstein I, Kohout M 1969 The effects of glucagon, dibutyryl cyclic adenosine 3′5' monophosphate and concentration of free fatty acid on hepatic lipid metabolism. J Biol Chem 244: 5131–5139

Hurt-Camejo E, Camejo G, Rosengren B, Lopez F, Wikland O, Bonders G 1990 Differential uptake of proteoglycan-selected subfractions of low density lipoprotein by human macrophages. J Lipid Res 31: 1387–1398

Krauss RM, Burke JD 1982 Identification of multiple subclasses of plasma low density lipoproteins in normal humans. J Lipid Res 23: 97–104

Law MR, Wald NG, Thompson SG 1994 By how much and how quickly does reduction in serum cholesterol lower risk of ischemic heart disease. BMJ 308: 367–372

Marcovina SM, Albers JJ, Kennedy H, Mei JU, Henderson LO, Hannon WH 1994 International Federation of Clinical Chemistry Standardization Project for measurements of apolipoproteins A-1 and B. Comparability of apolipoprotein B values by use of international reference material. Clin Chem 40: 586–592

Maslowska MH, Sniderman AD, MacLean LD, Cianflone K 1993 Regional differences in triacylglycerol synthesis in adipose tissue. J Lipid Res 34: 219–228

Rebuffé-Scrive M, Andersson B, Olbe L, Bjorntorp P 1989 Metabolism of adipose tissue in intraabdominal depots of nonobese men and women. Metabolism 38: 453–458

Sniderman A, Cianflone K 1993 Substrate delivery as a determinant of hepatic apoB secretion. Arterioscler Thromb 13: 629–636

Sniderman AD, Ghezzo R 1994 A meta-analysis of the clinical outcomes of the recent quantitative angiographic trials to lower plasma LDL in patients with coronary artery disease. Can J Cardiol 10 (suppl B):10B–16B

Sniderman AD, Vu H, Cianflone K 1991 The effect of moderate hypertriglyceridemia on the relation of plasma total and LDL apoB levels. Atherosclerosis 89: 109–116

Tall AR 1986 Plasma lipid transfer proteins. J Lipid Res 27: 361–366

Teng B, Thompson GR, Sniderman AD, Forte TM, Krauss RM, Kwiterovich PO Jr 1983 Composition and distribution of low-density lipoprotein fractions in hyperapobetalipoproteinemia, normolipidemia and familial hypercholesterolemia. Proc Natl Acad Sci. USA 80: 6662–6666

Teng B, Sniderman AD, Soutar AK, Thompson GR 1986 Metabolic basis of hyperapobetalipoproteinemia: Turnover of apolipoprotein B in low density lipoprotein and its precursors and subfractions compared with normal and familial hyper-cholesterolemia. J Clin Invest 77: 663–672

Teng B, Forse A, Rodriguez MA, Sniderman AD 1988 Adipose tissue glyceride synthesis inpatients with hyperapobetalipoproteine-mia. Can J Pharmacol Physiol 66: 239–242

Weisser B, Locher R, DeGraaf J, Moser R, Sachinides A, Vetter W 1993 Low density lipoprotein subfractions increase thrombox-ane formation in endothelial cells. Biochem Biophys Res Commun 192: 1245–1250

Zilversmit DB, Nordestguard BG 1989 Compar-ison of arterial intimal clearances of LDL from diabetic and non-diabetic cholesterol-fed rabbits. Arteriosclerosis 9: 176–183

Multiple Risk Factors in Cardiovascular Disease, ed. by A. Yamamoto, Churchill Livingstone Japan, Tokyo, pp. 149–153 (1994)

LIPOPROTEIN(a) PHENOTYPES IN HEALTHY JAPANESE SUBJECTS AND IN PATIENTS WITH CORONARY ARTERY DISEASE

Akio Noma

*Department of Laboratory Medicine, Gifu University School of Medicine**

Key words: lipoprotein (a), phenotype, frequency distribution, Japanese, coronary artery disease

Lipoprotein (a) (Lp(a)) was first detected in human plasma by Berg and is believed to be inherited as an autosomal dominant trait. A great deal of clinical interest was generated by quantitative studies that demonstrated a strong association between high Lp(a) concentrations and both cardiovascular and cerebrovascular diseases. Lp(a) exhibits a density heterogeneity within and between individuals, as well as a size heterogeneity of apolipoprotein(a) (apo(a)), the Lp(a) specific glycoprotein.

The cDNA sequence of apo(a) has revealed a high degree of homology with plasminogen (McLean *et al* 1987). Apo(a) contains the signal domains, lacks the tail and kringle 1 through 3, but includes a variable number of kringle 4-like domains, a single copy of a kringle 5-like domain and the serine protease domain of plasminogen. The differences in size of apo(a) isoforms are due to allelic differences in the number of kringle 4-like units.

Although the frequency distribution of Lp(a) phenotypes and the relationships between these phenotypes and plasma concentrations have been studied in Caucasian and other populations, no similar work has been carried out in a Japanese population. The present study was designed to fill this gap with our investigation of Lp(a) concentrations and phenotype frequencies in healthy Japanese and also to study the relationships between the severity of coronary artery disease (CAD) and cholesterol and Lp(a) plasma concentrations with respect to Lp(a) phenotypes.

FREQUENCY DISTRIBUTION OF SERUM LP(A) CONCENTRATIONS AND PHENOTYPES

The frequency distribution for serum Lp(a) concentrations in healthy Japanese ($n = 500$; 272 males, 33 ± 12 years, 218 females, 29 ± 13 years) was highly skewed, as has been observed in previous studies, with a mean ± SD of 14.6 ± 13.6 mg/dl and a median of 11.0 mg/dl. The distribution, together with mean and median values, was in good agreement with that in Tyrolean subjects, whereas it is significantly different from those for Asian and African populations, i.e., Chinese, Indian and Malaysians, and Sudanese, reported by Sandholzer *et al* and Helmhold *et al* (Abe & Noma 1992).

* 40 Tsukasa-machi, Gifu 500, Japan.

When the observed phenotype frequencies in healthy subjects were compared with those expected assuming a Hardy-Weinberg equilibrium, there was no significant deviation of observed from expected frequencies. The estimated frequency of apo(a) alleles in the healthy Japanese population also was not significantly difference from that in Tyroleans, whereas it is significantly different from those of the above-mentioned Asian and African populations, reported by Sandholzer *et al*. The present results on the Lp(a) phenotype, however, cannot be compared directly with those of Helmhold *et al*, because they observed higher numbers of apo(a) polymorphs using a gel system with a lower acrylamide concentration.

These results are ethnologically very interesting, because it has been accepted that the ancient Japanese came from China. The results also suggest the possibility that natural selection has occurred since that time due to changes in environmental conditions.

RELATIONSHIP BETWEEN Lp(a) PHENOTYPES AND PLASMA CONCENTRATIONS

It is well known that there is an inverse relationship between the apparent molecular weights of apo(a) isoforms and plasma Lp(a) concentrations.

In the present study, a new system has been employed to determine the Lp(a) phenotypes (Abe *et al* 1993). Electrophoresis was routinely performed using an sodium dodecyle sulfate (SDS)-4% polyacrylamide slab gel and a discontinuous buffer system. After electrophoresis, transferring and immunoblotting with a double-antibody procedure, the R_f values of apo(a) isoform bands were measured using a computerized micro scale and Lp(a) phenotypes were categorized automatically based on their R_f values. Lp(a) phenotypes were designated F, B, Sl, S2, S3, and S4, and the respective double-band phenotypes, compared with the mobility of apo B-100 as a marker, according to Utermann (Utermann *et al* 1987). As shown in Fig. 1, a positive correlation was found between serum Lp(a) concentrations and R_f values, estimated as described above, in the single-band phenotypes ($n = 111$, $r = 0.675$, $p < 0.001$). These results also indicated that serum Lp(a) concentrations are inversely related to the apparent molecular weight of apo(a). Phenotypes B, Sl and S2 are associated with high levels and phenotypes S3 and S4 with low levels of Lp(a). There is, however, considerable overlap between the Lp(a) concentrations of the different phenotypes and it is impossible to predict Lp(a) concentrations from Lp(a) phenotypes, or vice versa. The apo(a) size variation has been estimated to be responsible for ~40% of the variation in plasma Lp(a) concentrations. Lp(a) concentrations also vary substantially within each apo(a) isoform class, indicating that factors other than apo(a) phenotype affect Lp(a) levels.

Lp(a) CONCENTRATIONS AND THEIR DISTRIBUTION IN CAD PATIENTS

The frequency distribution of serum Lp(a) levels in the CAD patients ($n = 470$; 402 males, 50 ± 9 years, 68 females, 54 ± 7 years) was also highly skewed, with a mean ± SD of 23.5 ± 23.3 mg/dl and a median value of 16.4 mg/dl. The Lp(a) distribution in the CAD patients was markedly shifted to higher values.

Furthermore, serum Lp(a) concentrations were significantly increased in proportion to the number of diseased vessels in the CAD patients. In addition, serum cholesterol and HDL-cholesterol levels were also significantly different in the CAD patients compared with those in the healthy group, whereas no change was observed in the subgroups divided according to the number of diseased vessels.

In order to confirm these results, the relationships between severity of CAD and either Lp(a) or cholesterol levels were investigated, using 769 CAD patients with known Lp(a) and cholesterol levels and a known number of diseased vessels. We de-

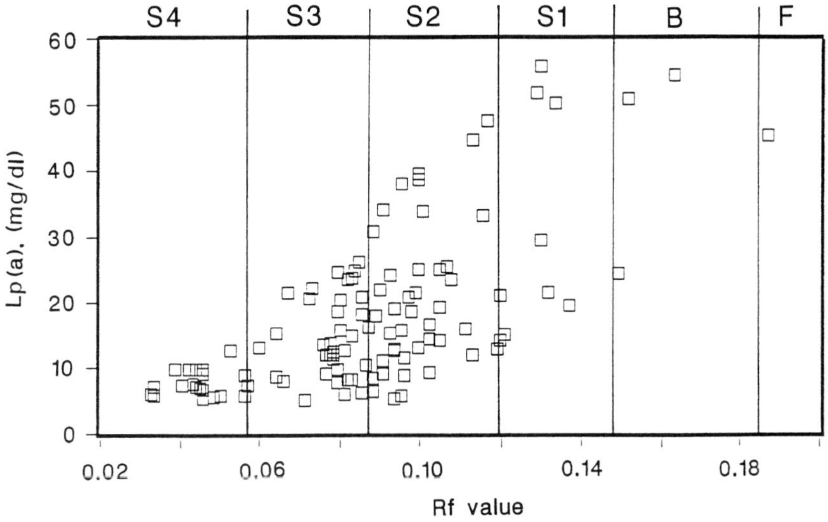

Fig. 1. Relationships between serum Lp(a) levels and *R*f values of apo(a) isoforms on SDS-PAGE. $n = 111$; $r = 0.675$. (Reprinted from Clin. Clin. Acta 219, p. 153)

fined hypercholesterolemia as a plasma cholesterol level above 220 mg/dl and hyperLp(a)emia as a plasma Lp(a) level above 30 mg/dl. There was no significant difference in the frequencies of the number of diseased vessels in hyper- and normo-cholesterolemia, whereas there was a significant difference between hyper- and normo-Lp(a)emia ($\chi^2 = 16.0$, $p < 0.01$). Furthermore, the frequencies of hyperLp(a)emia increased with the number of diseased vessels.

FREQUENCIES OF Lp(a) PHENOTYPES AND ALLELES IN CAD PATIENTS

Since Lp(a) levels are elevated 1.5- to 2-fold in sera from patients with CAD, it is possible to suppose that the elevation may be due to a high frequency of those Lp(a) phenotypes associated with high Lp(a) concentrations. The frequency of double-band phenotypes was significantly higher in the CAD patients than in the healthy subjects and was proportional to the number of diseased vessels in the CAD patients. Although the possibility cannot be ruled out that the detection of double-band phenotypes in the sera from CAD patients is due to their higher Lp(a) levels, no difference in Lp(a) phenotypes was observed when SDS-PAGE was carried out with sample volumes increased two-fold. Although the frequencies of these alleles in the CAD patients were calculated and shown to be significantly different ($\chi^2 = 13.3$, $p < 0.05$) from those in the healthy population, those in phenotypes were not statistically significant ($\chi^2 = 8.8$) when the null type was excluded, because the alleles of samples in the null-type cannot be assigned due to the sensitivity limit of the test (Abe *et al* 1992). Therefore, the differences in serum Lp(a) concentrations between the healthy and CAD groups cannot be explained by allele differences.

Lp(a) levels in each phenotype were compared in the healthy subjects and CAD patients. As shown in Table I, Lp(a) levels were significantly higher in the CAD patients than in healthy subjects in each common Lp(a) phenotype. These results agree with those from patients with familial hypercholesterolemia. The present results suggest that it is important to consider some post-translational or environmental modifications and other factors, e.g., other serum

TABLE I. Comparison of Serum Lp(a) Concentrations in Different Lp(a) Phenotypes between the Health and CAD Groups

Phenotype	Healthy subject				CAD patients			
	No	Mean	SD	Median	No	Mean	SD	Median
F	1				1	47.7		
B	4	42.3	6.7	45.1	1	85.5		
S1	14	22.0	18.0	18.5	4	38.0	31.4	31.5
S2	62	17.0	14.6	13.8	13	25.2	18.5	16.6
S3	133	12.5	8.4	10.9	106	18.5	13.8	14.7
S4	99	8.1	6.1	6.8	132	13.6	11.8	10.0
Null	38	2.6	2.2	1.7	10	3.9	4.4	1.9
F + S3	1	20.7			3	35.0	21.5	30.4
F + S4	0				3	25.5	4.3	23.3
B + S1	0				2	30.4		
B + S2	2	24.9			3	37.5	10.5	35.3
B + S3	2	34.7			16	34.6	29.8	21.4
B + S4	2	8.7			16	34.2	29.8	15.2
S1 + S2	10	43.9	28.2	39.5	4	38.7	25.4	31.1
S1 + S3	7	25.1	16.1	22.4	25	37.3	28.7	27.3
S1 + S4	2	27.8			9	34.4	40.9	20.3
S2 + S3	35	23.3	12.7	24.9	23	37.7	28.2	30.1
S2 + S4	26	19.7	12.0	16.9	33	28.9	34.1	13.1
S3 + S4	28	16.9	11.8	14.4	66	31.9	22.9	30.4
Total	465	14.6	13.6	11.0	470	23.5	23.3	16.4

(Redrown from Atherosclerosis 96, p. 5)

lipid and lipoprotein fractions, besides the genetic factor, as possible contributors to plasma Lp(a) levels.

SUMMARY

1. The frequency distribution of serum Lp(a) concentrations in healthy Japanese was highly skewed, with a mean ± SD of 14.6 ± 13.6 mg/dl and a median of 11.0 mg/dl.
2. Apo(a) isoforms were classified using their *Rf* values, determined using a computerized micro-scale, according to Utermann.
3. There was a strong inverse relationship between the apparent molecular weights of apo(a) isoforms and plasma Lp(a) concentrations.
4. The distribution of Lp(a) concentrations, mean and median values, and Lp(a) phenotypes and allele frequencies in healthy Japanese are in agreement with those for Europeans, whereas they are significantly different from other Asian populations.
5. Although the frequency of double-band phenotypes was significantly higher in the CAD group than in the healthy group, the frequencies of estimated Lp(a) alleles were not significantly different between these two groups.
6. Lp(a) levels in CAD patients were higher than in healthy subjects with the same phenotypes.

REFERENCES

Abe A, Noma A 1992 Studies on apolipoprotein(a) phenotypes. Part 1. Phenotype frequencies in a healthy Japanese population. Atherosclerosis 96: 1–8

Abe A, Noma A, Lee YJ, Yamaguchi H 1992 Studies on apolipoprotein(a) phenotypes.

Part 2. Phenotype frequencies and Lp(a) concentrations in different phenotypes in patients with angiographically defined coronary artery disease. Atherosclerosis 96: 9–15

Abe A, Noma A, Itakura H 1993 Lipoprotein(a) phenotyping using a computerized micro scale and phenotype frequencies in a healthy Japanese population. Clin Chim Acta 219: 149–157

McLean JW, Tomlinson JE, Kuang WJ *et al* 1987 cDNA sequence of human apolipoprotein(a) is homologous to plasminogen. Nature 330: 132–137

Utermann G, Menzel HJ, Kraft HG *et al* 1987 Lp(a) glycoprotein phenotypes. Inheritance and relation to Lp(a)-lipoprotein concentrations in plasma. J Clin Invest 80: 458–465

Multiple Risk Factors in Cardiovascular Disease, ed. by A. Yamamoto, Churchill Livingstone Japan, Tokyo, pp. 155–158 (1994)

SRC SIGNAL SEQUENCES IN APOPROTEIN B-100: DOES LDL OR LP(a) PLAY A ROLE IN SIGNAL TRANSDUCTION?

Juan GUEVARA, Jr.,*[1] James T. SPARROW,*[1] Natalia V. VALENTINOVA,*[1] Daniel DAVISON,*[2] and Joel D. MORRISETT*[1,3]

Division of Atherosclerosis and Lipoprotein Research, Departments of Medicine,[1] Cell Biology,*[2] and Biochemistry,*[3] Baylor College of Medicine*[1,2,3]*

Key words: apo B-100, apo(a), signaling, SH3, proline-rich

Apolipoprotein B-100 (apoB-100) and apoprotein (a) (apo(a)) are the two major apoprotein components of human lipoprotein (a) (Lp(a)). The primary structures of these extraordinarily large proteins have been elucidated (McLean *et al* 1987; Yang *et al* 1986). Two apo(a) kringle-like repeat sequences have been proposed to bind lysine and compete with plasminogen for fibrin(ogen) and thereby compromise fibrinolysis. In apoB-100, several functional regions such as heparin-binding sites, glycosylation sites, and the low-density lipoprotein (LDL) receptor-binding region have been identified (Yang *et al* 1986). A recently proposed hypothesis suggests that this massive apoprotein may also play a part in signal transduction (Voyno-Yasenetskaya *et al* 1993). In Lp(a), the association between apo(a) and apoB-100 probably involves a single disulfide bond between apo(a) Cys4057 and apoB-100 Cys3734, non-covalent interactions between amino acids flanking these respective residues and perhaps other interactions occurring at more remote sites.

In apo(a), the proline-rich, inter-kringle segments, such as AVAPPTVTPVPSLEAPSEQAPT between the LPaK2 repeats, exhibit similarities to the ten amino acid proline-rich segment of 3BP-1 that binds Ab1 *src* homology 3 (SH3). This observation has raised the question of whether there are non-covalent interactions between the proline-rich interkringle segments of apo(a) and the SH3-like regions that might be present in apoB-100. Accordingly, we have searched the sequence of apoB-100 for regions which exhibit similarities to the SH3 and/or SH2 domains common to signal transduction proteins (Ren *et al* 1993), these regulatory domains in signaling proteins can mediate enzymatic activity and participate in intracellular protein-protein interactions and bind to activated receptor tyrosine kinases (Koch *et al* 1991). SH3 domains are composed of 55 to 80 amino acids, while SH2 domains are made up of about 100 residues. Both types of domains are noncatalytic and may be part of, or associated with, a tyrosine kinase. Usually, but not always, SH2 domains are flanked by SH3 domains. In the signaling process, SH2 domains bind the phosphotyrosine of target proteins. The phosphotyrosine is part of a short amino acid motif that is also conserved in signal transduction mechanisms. SH2 and SH3 candidate sequences in apoB-100 are described in the present report.

*[1,2,3] 6565 Fannin Street, Houston TX 77030, USA.

LOCATION OF *SRC*-LIKE SEQUENCES IN apoB-100

A simple algorithm was used to search the sequence of apoB-100 for consensus motifs typical of SH3 (YDY, NT, YL) (Musacchio *et al* 1992) and SH2 (WYW, RES, THY) domains, as well as variations with conservative amino acid substitutions. Sixteen SH3-candidate regions were found in the apoB-100 sequence (Table I). The motif, YDF (and conservative variations thereof), is repeated in six of the SH3-like segments of the apoB-100 sequence. This motif is the most characteristic feature of SH3 domains and is a critical part of the receptor site that binds the proline-rich region of 3BP-1. In a separate study, we have obtained evidence which suggests that in Lp(a), apo(a) masks or alters the apoB-100 structure between residues 3341 and 3569 and hinders the binding of monoclonal antibodies specific for this

TABLE I. Location of SH3 and SH2-Candidate Regions of Apolipoprotein B-100

Sequence	Residue
10 20 30 40 50 60 70 80 90	
EEEMLENVSLVCPKDATRFKHLR**KYTYNYEAESSSGVPGTADSRSATRINCKVELEVPQLCSFILKTSQCTLKEV**YGF**NPEGKALLKKTKNSEEFAAAMS**	100
RYELKLAIPEGKQVFLYPEKDEPTYILNIKRGIISALLVPPETEEAKQVLFLDTVYGNCSTHFTVKTRKGNVATEISTERDLGQCDRFKPIRTGISPLAL	200
IKGMTRPLSTLISSSQSCQYTLDAKRKHVAEAICKEQH**LFLPFSYNNKYGMVAQVTQTLKLEDTPKINSRFFGEGTKKMGLAFESTKSTSPPKQAEAVLK**	300
TLQELKKLTISEQNIQRANLFNKLVTELRGLSDEAVTSLLPQLIEVSSPITLQALVQCGQPQCSTHILQWLKRVHANPLLIDVVTYLVALIPEPSAQQLR	400
EIFNMARDQRSRATLYALSHAVNNYHKTNPTGTQELLDIANYLMEQIQDDCTG**DEDYTYLILRVIGNMGQTMEQLTPELKSSILKCVQSTKPSLMIQKAA**	500
IQALRKMEPKDKDQEVLLQTFLDDASPGDKRLAAYLMLMRSPSQADINKIVQILPWEQNEQVKNFVASHIANILNSEELDIQDLKKLVKEALKESQLPTV	600
MDFRKFSRNYQLYKSVSLPSLDPASAKIEGNLIFDPNNYLPKESMLKTT**LTAFGFASADLIEIGLEGKGFEPTLEALFGKQGFFPDSVNKALYWVNGQVP**	700
DGVSKVLVD**HFGYTKDDKHEQDMVNGIMLSVEKLIKDLKSKEVPEARAYLRILGEELGFASLHDLQLLGK**LLLMGARTLQGIPQMIGEVIRKGSKNDFFL	800
HYIFMENAFELPTGAGLQLQISSSGVIAPGAKAGVKLEVANMQAELVAKPSVSVEFVTNMGIIIPDFARSGVQMNTNFFHESGLEAHVALKAGKLKFIIP	900
SPKRPVKLLSGGNTLHLVSTTKTEVIPPLIENRQSWSVCKQVFPGLNYCTSGAYSNASSTDSASYYPLTGDTRLELELRPTGEIEQYSVSATYELQREDR	1000
10 20 30 40 50 60 70 80 90	
ALVDTLKFVTQAEGAKQTEATMTFKYNRQSMTLSSEVQIPDFDVDLGTILRVNDESTEGKTSYRLTLDIQNKKITEVALMGHLSCDTKEERKIKGVISIP	1100
RLQAEARSEILAHWSPAKLLLQMDSSATAYGSTVSKRVAWHYDEEKIEFEWNTGTNVDTKKMTSNFPVDLSDYPKSLHMYANRLLDHRVPETDMTFRHVG	1200
SKLIVAMSSWLQKASGSLPYTQTLQDHLNSLKEFNLQNMGLPDFHIPENLFLKSDGRVKYTLNKNSLKIEIPLPFGGKSSRDLKMLETVRTPALHFKSVG	1300
FHLPSREFQVPTFTIPKLYQLQVPLLGVLDLSTNVYSNLYNWSASYSGGNTSTDHFSLRARYHMKADSVVDLLSYNVQGSGETTYDHKNTFTLSCDGSLR	1400
HKFLDSNIKFSHVEKLGNNPVSKGLLIFDASSSWGPQMSASVHLDSKKKQHLFVKEVKIDGQFRVSSFYAKGTYGLSCQRDPNTGRLNGESNLRFNSSYL	1500
QGTNQITGRYEDGTLSLTSTSDLQSGIIKNTASLKYENYELTLKSDTNGKYKNFATSNKMDMTFSKQNALLRSEYQADYESLRFFSLLSGSLNSHGLELN	1600
ADILGTDKINSGAHKATLRIGQDGISTSATTNLKCSLLVLENELNAELGLSGASMKLTTNGRFREHNAKFSLDGKAALTELSLGSAYQAMILGVDSKNIF	1700
NFKVSQEGLKLSNDMMGSYAEMKFDHTNSLNIAGLSLDFSSKLDNIYSSDKFYKQTVNLQLQPYSLVTTLNSDLKYNALDLTNNGKLRLEPLKLHVAGNL	1800
KGAYQNNEIKHIYAISSAALSASYKADTVAKVQGVEFSHRLNTDIAGLASAIDMSTNYNSDSLHFSNVFRSVMAPFTMTIDAHTNGNGKLALWGEHTGQL	1900
YSKFLLKAEP**LAFTFSHDYKGSTSHHLVSRKSISAALEHKVSALLTPAEQTGTWKLKTQFNNNEYSQDLDAY**NTKDKIGVELTGRTLADLTLLDSPIKVP	2000
10 20 30 40 50 60 70 80 90	
LLLSEPINIIDALEMRDAVEKPQEFTIVAFVKYDKNQDVHSINLPFFETLQEYFERNRQTIIVVVENVQRNLKHINIDQFVRKYRAALGKLPQQANDYLN	2100
SFNWERQVSHAKEKLTALTKKYRITENDIQIALDDAKINFNEKLSQLQTYMIQFDQYIKDSYDLHDLKIAIANIIDEIIEKLKSLDEHYHIRVNLVKTIH	2200
DLHLFIENIDFNKSGSSTASWIQNVDTKYQIRIQIQEKLQQLKRHIQNIDIQHLAGKLKQHIEAIDVRVLLDQLGTTISFERINDVLEHVKHFVINLIGD	2300
FEVAEKINAFRAKVHELIERYEVDQQIQVLMDKLVELTHQYKLKETIQKLSNVLQQVKIKDYFEKLVGFIDDAVKKLNELSFKTFIEDVNKFLDMLIKKL	2400
KSFDYHQFVDETNDKIREVTQRLNGEIQALELPQKAEALKLFLEETKATVAVYLESLQDTKITLIINWLQEALSSASLAHMKAKFRETLEDTR**DRMYDMD**	2500
IQQELQRYLSLVGQVYSTLVTYISDWWTLAAKNLTDFAEQYSIQDWAKRMKALVEQGFTVPEIKTILGTMPAFEVSLQALQKATFQTPDFIVPLTDLRIP	2600
SVQINFKDLKNIKIPSRFSTPEFTILNTFHIPSFTIDFVEMKVKIIRTIDQMQNSELQWPVPDIYLRDLKVEDIPLARITLPDFRLPEIAIPEFIIPTLN	2700
LNDFQVPDLHIPEFQLPHISHTIEVPTFGKLYSILKIQSPLFTLDANADIGNGTTSANEAGIAASITAKGESKLE**VLNFDFQANAQLSNPKINPLALKES**	2800
VKFSSKYLRTEHGSEMLFFGNAIEGKSNTVASLHTEKNTLELSNGVIVKINNQLTLDSNTKYFHKLNIPKLDFSSQADLRNEIKTLLKAGHIAWTSSGKG	2900
SWKWACPRFSDEGTHESQISFTIEGPLTSFGLSNKINSKHLRVNQNLVYESGSLNFSKLEIQSQVDSQHVGHSVLTAKGMALFGEGKAEFTGRHDAHLNG	3000
10 20 30 40 50 60 70 80 90	
KVIGTLKNSLFFSAQPFEITASTNNEGNLKVRFPLRLTGKIDFLNNYALFLSPSAQQASWQVSARFNQYKYNQNFSAGNNENIMEAHVGINGEANLDFLN	3100
IPLTIPEMRLPYTIITTPPLKDFSLWEKTGLKEFLKTTKQSFDLSVKAQYKKNKHRHSITNPLAVLCEFISQSIKSFDRHFEKNRNNALDFVTKSYNETK	3200
IKFDKYKAEKSHDELPRTFQIPGYTVPVVNVEVSPFTIEMSAFGYVFPKAVSMPSFSILGSDVRVPSYTLILPSLELPVLHVPRNLKLSLPHFKELCTIS	3300
HIFIPAMGN**ITYDFSFKSSVITLNTNAELFNQSDIVAHLLSSSSSVIDALQYKLEGTTRLTRKRGLKLATALSLSNKFV**EGSHNSTVSLTTKNMEVSVAK	3400
TTKAEIPILRMNFKQELNGNTKSKPTVSSSM**EFKYDFNSSMLYSTAKGAVDHKLSLESLTSYFSIESSTKGDVKGSVLSREYSGTIASEANTYLNSK**STR	3500
SSVKLQGTSKIDDIWNLEVKENFAGEATLQRIYSLWEHSTKNHLQLEGLFFTNGEHTSKATLELSPWQMSALVQVHASQPSSFHDFPDLGQEVALNANTK	3600
NQKIRWKNEVRIHSGSFQSQVELSNDQEKAHLDIAGSLEGHLRFLKNIILPVYD**KSLWDFLKLDVTTSIGRRQHLRVSTAFVYTKNPNGYSFSIPVKVLA**	3700
DKFITPGLKLNDLNSVLVMPTFHVPFTDLQVPSCKLDFREIQIYKKLRTSSFALNLPTLPEVKFPEVDVLTKYSQPEDSLIPFFEITVPESQLTVSQFTL	3800
PKSVSDGIAALDLNAVANKIADFELPTIIVPEQTIEIPSIKFSVPAGIVIPSFQALTARFEVDSPVYNATWSASLKNKADYVETVLDSTCSSTVQFLEYE	3900
LNVLGTHKIEDGTLASKTKGTLAHRDFSAEYEEDGKFEGLQEWEGKAHLNIKSPAFTDLHLRYQKDKKGISTSAASPAVGTVGMDMDEDDDFSKWNFYYS	4000
10 20 30 40 50 60 70 80 90	
PQSSPDKKLTIFKTELRVRESDEETQIKVNWEEEAASGLLTSLKDNVPKATG**VLYDYVNKYHWEHTGLTLREVSSKLRRNLQNNAEWVYQGAIRQIDDID**	4100
VRFQKAASGTTGTYQEWKDKAQNLYQELLTQEGQASFQGLKDNVFDGLVRVTQKFHMKVKHLIDSLIDFLN**FPRFQFPGKPGIYTREELCTMFIREVGTV**	4200
LSQVYSKVHNGSEILFSYFQDLVITLPFELRKHKLIDVISMYRELLKDLSKEAQEVFKAIQSLKTTEVLRNLQDLLQFIFQLIEDNIKQLKE**MKFTYLIN**	4300
YIQDEINTIFNDYIPYVFKLLKENLCLNLHKFNEFIQNELQEASQELQQIHQYIMALREEYFDPSIVGWTVKYYELEEKIVSLIKNLLVALKDFHSEYIV	4400
SASNFTSQLSSQVEQFLHRNIQEYLSILTDPDGKGKEKIAELSATAQEIIKSQAIATKKIISDYHQQFRYKLQDFSDQLSDYYEKFIAESKRLIDLSIQN	4500
YHTFLIYITELLKKLQSTTVMNPYMKLAPGELTIIL	

SH3 candidate segments are shown in **bold** with motifs characteristic of SH3 domains in **bold and underlined**; SH2 candidate segments are highligted with underline.

region. This part of the apoB-100 sequence includes I$_{3310}$T**YDF**SFKSSVITL**NT**NAELFN QSDIVAHLLSSSSSVIDALQYKLEGTTRLT RKRGLKLATALSLSNKF**V**E$_{3380}$ and S$_{3430}$ MEFK**YDF**NSSMLYSTAKGAVDHKLSLE**S** LTSYFSIESSTKGDVKGSVLSREYSGTIASE ANT**YL**NSKSTR$_{3500}$, which contain motifs common to SH3 domains. The putative LDL-receptor binding region of apoB-100 is located near the carboxyl-end of the former sequence. The binding of apoB-100 to the LDL-receptor is greatly reduced by the presence of the apo(a) molecule in Lp(a). It is possible that proline-rich, inter-kringle segments of apo(a) bind to these apoB-100 SH3-like regions by a mechanism similar to that used by the proline-rich segment of 3BP-1 which binds to the SH3 domain of a protein such as spectrin. Results from recent ligand binding experiments demonstrate that a synthetic peptide with the sequence of the proline-rich, inter-kringle segment of apo(a) (sequence shown above) binds specifically to LDL. This type of interaction provides a plausible explanation for the observed inhibition by free proline of recombinant apo(a) binding to LDL.

There are four SH2-like regions in the apoB-100 molecule. These are located in positions F$_{2046}$–L$_{2144}$, Y$_{2862}$–I$_{2961}$, F$_{3011}$–L$_{3110}$, and F$_{3997}$–I$_{4096}$. A comparison of these apoB-100 SH2-candidate regions with three known SH2 domains of signal transduction proteins is shown in Table II. The residues essential for binding to the phosphotyrosine-containing motif, arginine located near the amino-end and histidine located near the carboxyl-end of the region, are conserved in these SH2-candidate regions of apoB-100. The similarity between these sequences and those of well known SH2 domains in signaling proteins suggests that these regions impart to apoB-100, and hence to LDL, the capacity to bind intracellularly to the phosphotyrosine motif characteristic of membrane receptor tyrosine kinase proteins or perhaps to other phosphotyrosine moieties on extracellular protein.

SUMMARY

Close inspection of the human apoB-100 sequence reveals that regions which are similar to the SH3 and SH2 domains of signal

Table II. Comparison of Four ApoB-100 SH2-Candidate Sequences with Three Known SH2 Domain Sequences.

```
1. WYHG-------KL----D-R-TIAEER----LR--QAG-KSGSYLIRE-SDRRPGS-----FV-----------LS-FLS---QTN--VV-N-H----F-RII-A-
2. WFHG-------KLGAGRDGRH-IAE-RLLTEY-CIETGAPDGSFLVRE-SE----T-----FVGDY---------LS-FW--R-NG--KV--Q-HC-----RI-HSR
3. WYWG---------DISREE---V-NEK----LR--DT-A-DGTFLVRDAS-----T--KMH--GDY------T--LT--L--RKGGNNKLI---K----I--F-H-R
   FYYSPQSSPDKKL--------TIF--K--TELR------------VRE-SDEE--TQIKV----NW-EEEAASGLLTS-L--K---DN-VP---KAT-GVL-Y----
   YFH--------KLNI--------P--KL--DF-SSQ--A-D---L-RN--E------IK------------T-LL------K-AG--HIAW---TSSG--K--G-S
   FFSAQPFEITASTN---NEG-NL---KV----R-F----P-----LR-LT----G---KI----DFLNN---YAL--FLSP--SAQQ-ASWQV-SA----RF----
   FFETLQEYF----E--RN-RQTII---VV--V---E----N---VQRNL---------K-H-I-N-IDQ---------FV--RK--------Y-RAA--LGKLP---
=============================================================================================================
1. MCGD-Y---YI-GG-R----RFS--SLS-DL-IG---YY----------SHV--S-CL-----LKG-----------------E--KL----L-YPV
2. ---QD-A-----GTPKF----F----LT-D----NL-VFDSL-YDL-I-THY---QQV-P---LR-CNE-----F--------EM-RLSE-----PV
3. ---D--------G--KYG---FSD-PLT--F---N-SVVE-L-IN-----HY--------R-N----ESLAQ--Y-N-----P---KL-D--VKL--
   ---D-YVN-------KY---HW-E----H--T-G-LTL----R-E--VSSKL--------RRNL---QNNAEWVY-Q--GAI----R--Q--I----
   -----W---------KWACPRFSDEG-THE-S--QISF--TI--EGPLTS-FGLSNKINSKH-LRV-NQNL--VY-E-SGSL-NFSKL-E--I----
   ---NQY---------KY------NQ----NFSAGN--N-E--NI---MEAHVGI-N-GEA--NL---D------FLNIPLTIPEM-RL----P-Y--
   ---QQ-ANDYLN-S--F-N--W-E----RQ-----------------V-SHA----K-E-----KL--T-A----L-TKK----Y-RITENDIQIA-
```

Three known SH2 sequences are in rows 1–3. Conservation of several motifs were used as criteria in selection of these SH2-like sequences: WY, KL, VRE, and SHV or variations of these within certain limits. In the first instance, WY, the apoB-100 sequences start with FY, YF, and FF. The second motif, KL, which occurs throughout the SH2 sequence, is retained by two apoB-100 segments. The third motif, VRE, is one of the two essential characteristics of SH2 domains for binding to phosphotyrosine. The guanidinyl group of the arginine residue is believed to form a salt bridge with the orthophosphate of tyrosine. The imidazolium group of histidine stacks with the planar phenolic of the phosphotyrosine.

transduction proteins are contained by this large protein. The presence of proline-rich sequences between the kringle-like sequences of the apo(a) molecule and the association of apo(a) with apoB-100 in Lp(a) strongly suggest the existence of protein-protein interactions which may involve the SH3- and SH2-like region of the apoB-100 molecule. The association has been shown to occur extracellularly with recombinant apo (a) and LDL as well as *in vitro*. However, there is little evidence to suggest that this association occurs initially in the plasma compartment since free-apo(a) is not abundant in plasma. It is possible that LDL, through the "signal" domains of apoB-100, functions as an attenuator of signals such as are produced by cytokines or insulin. A second possibility may be that LDL and high-density lipoproteins (HDL) function as extracellular primary signals, acting more like a gross-level modulator than a micro-level signal such as a growth factor. Both apoB-100 and apoA-I have been reported to be phosphorylated and may be involved in a signaling mechanism. Whether these regions of apoB-100 are involved in this type of mechanism remains to be demonstrated.

REFERENCES

Koch CA, Anderson D, Moran MF, Ellis C, Pawson T 1991 SH2 and SH3 domains: elements that control interactions of cytoplasmic signaling proteins. Science 252: 668–674

McLean JW, Tomlinson JE, Kuang W-J, *et al* 1987 cDNA sequence of human apolipoprotein(a) is homologous to plasminogen. Nature 330: 132–137

Musacchio A, Noble M, Pauptit R, Wierenga R, Saraste M 1992 Crystal structure of a Src-homology 3 (SH3) domain. Nature 359: 851–855

Ren R, Mayer BJ, Cicchetti P, Baltimore D 1993 Identification of a ten-amino acid proline-rich SH3 binding site. Science 259: 1157–1161

Voyno-Yasenetskaya T, Dobbs LG, Erickson SK, Hamilton RL 1993 Low density lipoprotein- and high density lipoprotein-mediated signal transduction and exocytosis in alveolar type II cells. Proc Natl Acad Sci USA 90: 4256–4260

Yang C-Y, Chen S-H., Gianturco SH *et al* 1986 Sequence, structure, receptor-binding domains and internal repeats of human apolipoprotein B-100. Nature 323: 738–742

Multiple Risk Factors in Cardiovascular Disease, ed. by A. Yamamoto, Churchill Livingstone Japan, Tokyo, pp. 159–165 (1994)

HEREDITARY TRAITS AND INDIVIDUAL DIFFERENCES IN THE EXPRESSION OF HYPER- OR DYS-LIPOPROTEINEMIA

Akira YAMAMOTO, Taku YAMAMURA, Yasuko MIYAKE, Yasuyuki IKEDA, Atsuko TAKAGI, and Mariko HARADA-SHIBA

*Department of Etiology and Pathogenesis, National Cardiovascular Center Research Institute**

Key words: hyperlipoproteinemia, LDL receptor, apolipoprotein E, lipoprotein lipase deficiency, hepatic lipase deficiency

Hyperlipoproteinemia is classified into several types according to the presence of a definite metabolic defect and the clustering in special families. However, clinical manifestations vary from one individual to another, being influenced by other congenital factors interacting with each other. The appearance and extent of hyperlipoproteinemia is also strongly influenced by nutrition and some underlying diseases such as hypothyroidism, diabetes mellitus, etc. In this paper we would like to focus on the variety of the mutation of genes involved in lipoprotein metabolism and the interaction of various factors in the development of essential hyper- or dys-lipoproteinemia.

VARIETY OF MUTATIONS OF THE LDL RECEPTOR GENE IN FAMILIAL HYPERCHOLESTEROLEMIA AND ITS CLINICAL MANIFESTATIONS

Familial hypercholesterolemia (FH) is the most prominent and well defined herediatry trait associated with atherosclerosis. The average serum cholesterol of Japanese patients with heterozygous FH is 330–350 mg/dl. However, this level is markedly influenced by the number and extent of the functioning low density lipoproteins (LDL) receptors. The progression of atherosclerosis is much slower and ischemic heart disease appears later in those patients with a receptor-defective type of disease in which the cells can bind and degrade LDL at a rate of 20–40% of normal control, compared with the receptor-negative type, in which the cells cannot bind LDL at all (Yamamoto *et al* 1989).

Many kinds of mutation, nearly one hundred, have been identified worldwide (Hobbs *et al* 1990), and at least 18 in Japan (Fig. 1). All the mutations with a large deletion appear to be caused by Alu-Alu recombination, either in the same or reverse direction (Miyake *et al* 1992a). Kajinami *et al* (1988) detected a mutation, which showed a local distribution confined to the Tonami area. Four different point mutations have been identified in our laboratory (Fig. 1). Among them, one mutation is located at about the middle of the EGF-precursor homology domain and this mutation has been found in 3 non-blood related families. Another mutation at the splice-donor site of the intron 12, resulting in the absence of protein synthesis, was found in 5 out of 23 FH

* 5-7-1 Fujishiro-dai, Suita 565, Japan.

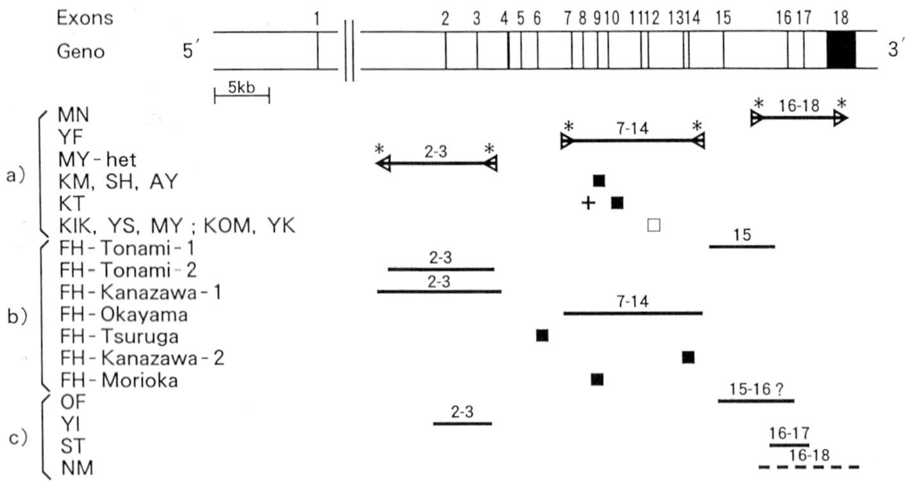

Fig. 1. Mutations of LDL-receptor gene in familial hypercholesterolemia in Japanese detected at a) National Cardiovascular Center, b) Kanazawa University, c) Tsukuba University.
—, deletion; *, deletion joint has been sequenced; ▷, Alu sequence with its orientation indicated by arrowhead; ■, missense mutation; □, splice sitemutation; +, insertion.

homozygotes from independent families. It was found in 15% of heterozygous FH patients and this type of mutation seems to be the most common among Japanese (Maruyama *et al* in preparation). Mutations in the region ranging from exon 15 to 18 also seem to be frequent in the Japanese population (Fig. 1).

A point mutation of apolipoprotein B (apoB), a ligand of the LDL-receptor, has been found in patients with severe hypercholesterolemia similar to FH (Tybjaerg-Hansen & Humphries 1992). Although this mutation of apoB (3500Arg to Gln) is reported to be common in Europeans, it has not yet been found among the Japanese.

APOLIPOPROTEIN E MUTATION AND DYSLIPOPROTEINEMIA

There are ten or more apoproteins associated with lipoprotein particles. Among them, apolipoprotein E (apoE) is peculiar in that it is synthesized in almost every tissue and functions as a mediator for reverse cholesterol transport. There are three major isoforms of apoE: apoE3 is thought to be the prototype or wild type, apoE4 is caused by the replacement of 112Cys by Arg, and E2 by the replacement of 158Arg by Cys. In the Japanese population, the gene frequency of apoE4, E3, and E2 was reported to be 0.090, 0.845, and 0.065, respectively (Yamamura *et al* 1990); the frequency of E3 being higher and that of E4 lower than in Western populations (Davignon *et al* 1988).

ApoE phenotypes strongly influence the LDL-cholesterol level in the general population. We have studied the difference in serum lipid levels in schoolchildren aged between 7 and 15 according to apoE phenotypes. Those children with apoE4/3 had higher LDL-cholesterol and those with E3/2 had lower LDL-cholesterol compared with those with E3/3 (E4/3, 176.4 ± 28.6; E3/3, 170.8 ± 27.8; E3/2, 155.3 ± 26.8 mg/dl). In addition, the lipoprotein (a) (Lp(a)) level of children with the apoE4 allele tended to be higher, and that of children with the apoE2 allele lower, compared with that of children with apoE3/3. Lp(a) is now thought to be a strong independent risk factor for atherosclerosis (Nomura *et al* 1993). Therefore, the combination of high LDL-cholesterol and high Lp(a) level seems to contribute to the development of atherosclerotic vascular diseases in people with the apoE4 allele.

A strong effect of apoE phenotypes on serum LDL-cholesterol was also observed in FH patients. Among the family members with a mutation caused by one base exchange G to C in exon 9, resulting in the substitution of Asp by His, those with apoE3/3 had a serum cholesterol ranging from 330 to 350 mg/dl, usually only seen in FH heterozygotes in Japan. In contrast, those family members with apoE3/2 had much lower cholesterol levels (230–250 mg/dl) (Miyake *et al* 1992b). The cholesterol-lowering effect of the E2 allele is almost equivalent to the effect of hypobetalipoproteinemia combined with FH.

In addition to the major isoforms, there are many mutations of the apoE molecule and a number of them are associated with dyslipoproteinemia. Homozygosity for apoE2 sometimes relates to Type III hyperlipoproteinemia, which is characterized by the presence of cholesterol-rich very low density lipoproteins (VLDL), or beta-VLDL. In some apoE mutants, with the mutation site in the receptor-binding domain (amino acid 140 150), Type III hyperlipoproteinemia appears even in heterozygotes (Rall & Mahley 1992). However such kinds of mutations are rare in Japan and only one case has been reported from Fukuoka (Moriyama *et al* 1992).

There are two relatively common mutations of apoE in the Japanese , E5 and E7, the frequency of which is about 0.5 to 1.0% in the form of heterozygosity with E3 (Yamamura *et al* 1990). ApoE5 seems to cause hyperlipoproteinemia through a mechanism similar to E4. ApoE7 could be related to dyslipoproteinemia and atherosclerosis due to its low affinity for cell surface receptors and high affinity for heparin (Yamamura *et al* 1990). The association between apoE5 or E7 and atherosclerosis appears to be not so strong as the mutations peculiar to European populations and it is not clear if it is due to the hereditary trait itself or to a difference in dietary conditions.

HYPERLIPOPROTEINEMIA ASSOCIATED WITH A DEFICIENCY IN LIPOLYTIC ENZYMES

Lipoprotein Lipase Deficiency and Type IV Hyperlipoproteinemia

Recently, the significance of triglyceride as a risk factor in cardiovascular diseases has been widely discussed. There are two major causes leading to hypertriglyceridemia: an increase in synthesis and a decrease in the catabolism of triglyceride-rich lipoproteins. It has well been documented that the homozygosity for lipoprotein lipase (LpL) deficiency manifests itself in severe hyper-

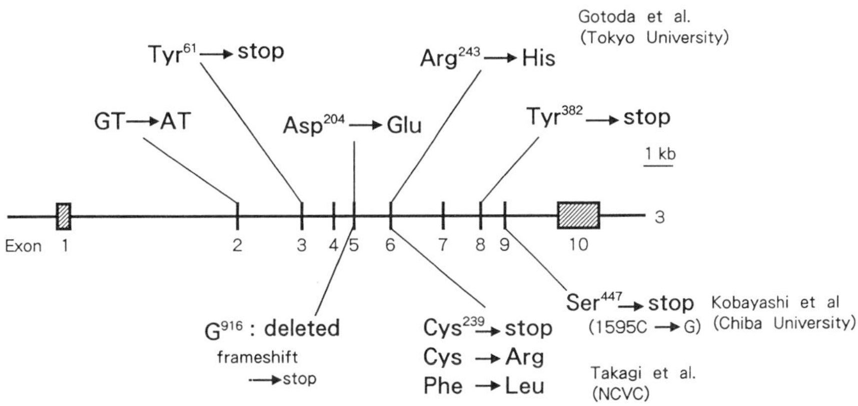

Fig. 2. Lipoprotein lipase gene mutation identified in Japan.

triglyceridemia characterized by the accumulation of chylomicrons, i.e. Type I hyperlipoproteinemia. This type of hyperlipidemia is frequently associated with pancreatitis. There is a wide variety of mutations of the LpL gene, at least 10 have been characterized in Japan (Fig. 2). One mutation, named LpL arita was found to be widely distributed in the western part of Japan (Takagi et *al* 1992). The abnormality can be detected by DNA fragment analysis with the Alu I restriction site.

In contrast to the homozygote, which is associated with severe clinical manifestations, the clinical significance of the heterozygosity for LpL deficiency has not yet been established. We studied the relationship between hypertriglyceridemia and LpL deficiency using a newly developed assay system with monospecific antibodies for the two lipolytic enzymes in postheparin plasma (PHP), LpL and hepatic triglyceride lipase (HTGL) (Ikeda *et al* 1990). Deficiency in LpL is frequently found in essential Type IV and V hyperlipoproteinemias, in about 1/3 of patients with Type IV and 3/4 of those with Type V. Analysis of genes using samples of peripheral mononuclear cells revealed a defect in the genomic DNA in nine cases (5 LpL arita and 4 others), out of a total of 22 samples. We suggest that almost all the cases with essential Type IV and V hyperlipoproteinemias exhibiting a significant reduction of LpL mass (40 percentile of the normal control) in PHP is the result of an abnormality in the LpL gene. Suppose that the frequency of essential Type IV hyperlipoproteinemia with triglyceride levels exceeding 250 mg/dl and without glucose intolerance is 1% and approximately 20% of such a population has a defect in the LpL gene, the frequency of the LpL gene abnormality would be about 1 in 500 of the population (Ikeda *et al* 1994b).

Not all the heterozygotes of LpL deficiency develop hypertriglyceridemia in the fasting state. Multivariate analysis of the medical background of our patients showed that obesity and alcohol are the major factors involved in the expression of hypertriglyceridemia (Table I). It is also noteworthy that ΣIRI also contributes to the expression of hypertriglyceridemia, in spite of the fact that we excluded patients with diabetes mellitus or glucose intolerance from the present study.

Hepatic Triglyceride Lipase Deficiency and Triglyceride-Rich LDL

Another aspect of the lipolytic enzyme-related dyslipoproteinemia is HTGL deficiency. A reduction of this enzyme is generally observed in hypothyroidism, but very low levels of this enzyme attributable to the hereditary trait have also been reported by several laboratories including our own. We compared the laboratory data obtained from two male patients with HTGL deficiency and the data from patients with ordinary Type IV hyperlipoproteinemia with triglyceride levels comparable with those patients having HTGL deficiency.

TABLE I. Multiple Regression Analysis of Factors Affecting Serum Triglyceride in Hypertriglyceridemic (n = 31) and Normolipidemic (n = 36) Subjects

Variables					
Dependent	Independent	b	p value	r	contribution (%)
log (TG)	log (LPL mass)	−0.51	0.0001	−0.57	29.07
	apo C-II/C-III	−0.04	ns	−0.12	0.48
	ΣIRI	0.33	0.0002	0.53	17.49
	alcohol intake	0.26	0.0014	0.39	10.14
	age	0.31	0.0004	0.30	9.30
	R2	0.66	0.0001		66.00

TG, serum triglyceride concentration; LPL, lipoprotein lipase in postheparin plasma.

Lipid analysis of the lipoprotein fractions obtained by ultracentrifugation revealed increases in VLDL and intermediate density lipoproteins (IDL) and, most importantly, the presence of triglyceride-rich LDL with apoB as the only apolipoprotein. The increase in IDL was found in both HTGL deficiency and Type IV hyperlipoproteinemia patients and there was no significant difference in the lipoprotein lipid composition of IDL between these two groups. In contrast, the triglyceride content of LDL was significantly increased and the ratio of triglyceride to apoB was significantly elevated in HTGL-deficiency, but not in Type IV hyperlipoproteinemia compared with normal controls:

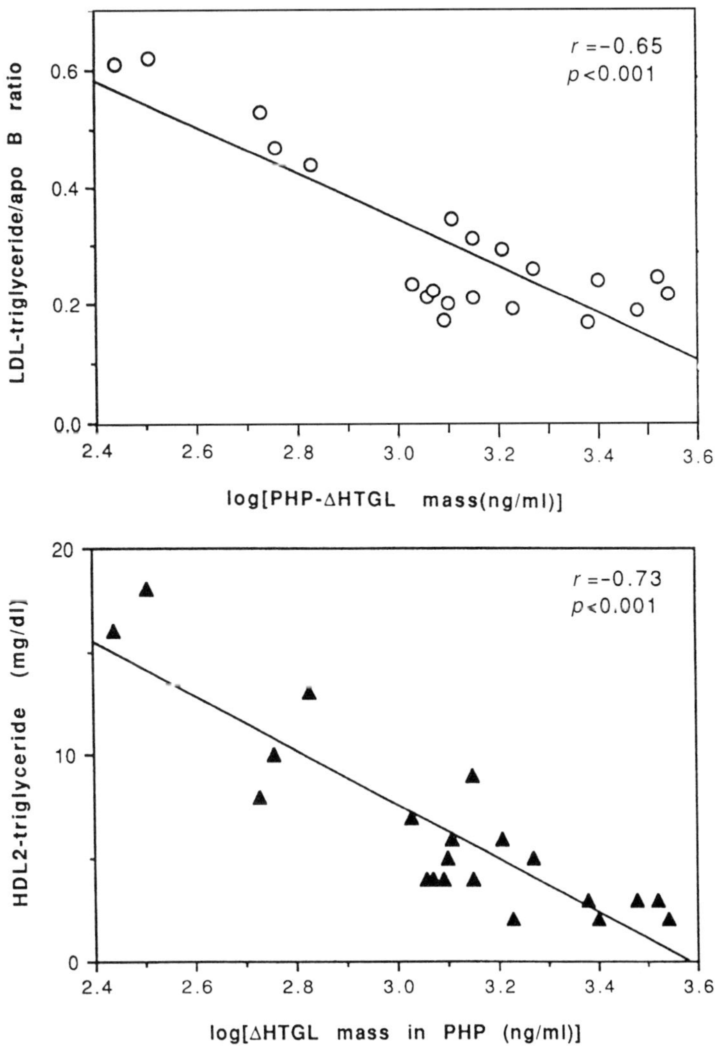

Fig. 3. Correlation between triglyceride/apoB ratio in LDL fraction and hepatic triglyceride lipase (HTGL) in postheparin plasma (PHP) (top) and between triglyceride in HDL_2 fraction and HTGL in PHP (bottom).
Data were obtained from 15 healthy male volunteers, 4 patients (males) with Type IV hyperlipoproteinemia, and 2 male patients with hepatic triglyceride lipase deficiency.

triglyceride/apoB : 0.6, 0.3, 0.3, respectively for the three groups (Tsutsumi *et al* in preparation). There was a significant correlation between the ratio of LDL-triglyceride to apoB and HTGL mass in PHP and also between high density lipoprotein (HDL_2) triglyceride and HTGL mass in PHP (Fig. 3). In an extreme case of HTGL deficiency, the blood serum looked clear in spite of the presence of hypertriglyceridemia, which normally produces a turbid serum in the case of ordinary Type IV hypertriglyceridemia (Ikeda *et al* 1994a).

Two cases of HTGL deficiency have been reported, one from Carlson's group (1986) in Scandinavia and another from Little's group in Canada (Hegele *et al* 1993). From the reports of these authors and our own, we can speculate that the incidence of dyslipoproteinemia is increased in people predisposed to HTGL deficiency and these people become liable to atherosclerosis, when combined with some other factors, either nutritional or diabetic, which raise serum lipid levels. The situation seems to be similar to that observed in apoE2 homozygosity.

Cases where LpL and HTGL deficiency coexist have been reported (Yamamura *et al* 1979; Auwerx *et al* 1990). The proband of our family originally showed Type V hyperlipoproteinemia (Yamamura *et al* 1979). After restriction of fat, alcohol, and total calorie intake, electrophoresis of plasma lipoproteins showed a pattern characteristic of Type III hyperlipoproteinemia, although the VLDL cholesterol/triglyceride ratio was not as high as in the cases of apoE2 homozygosity. A type III-like pattern has also been found in another family (Auwerx *et al* 1990).

CONCLUSION

There is no doubt about the association of LDL and atherosclerosis. Familial hypercholesterolemia is a typical example of congenital hypercholesterolemia related to atherosclerosis. Cholesterol-rich VLDL also seems to be strongly related to atherosclerosis, as shown by the cases with Type III hyperlipoproteinemia. However, it is still not clear if moderate to mild hypertriglyceridemia is associated with atherosclerosis and the causes of common hyperlipidemias still remain to be identified in the light of the advanced gene technology. For a complete understanding of the relationship between hyperlipidemia and atherosclerosis and the effects of nutrition, it will be necessary to conduct a clinicoepidemiological study after classifying patients and family members according to their hereditary predisposition.

REFERENCES

Auwerx JH, Babirak SP, Hokamson JE *et al* 1990 Coexistence of abnormalities of hepatic lipase and lipoprotein lipase in a large family. Am J Human Genet 46: 470–477

Carlson LA, Holmquist L, Nilsson-Ehle P 1986 Deficiency of hepatic lipase activity in postheparin plasma in familial hyper-β-triglyceridemia. Acta Med Scand 219: 435–447

Davignon J, Gregg RE, Sing CF 1988 Apolipoprotein polymorphism and atherosclerosis. Arteriosclerosis 8: 1–21

Hegele RA, Little JA, Vezina C *et al* 1993 Hepatic lipase deficiency. Clinical, biochemical and molecular genetic characteristics. Arterioscler Thromb 13: 720–728

Hobbs HH, Russel DW, Brown MS, Goldstein JL 1990 The LDL receptor locus in familial hypercholesterolemia; mutational analysis of a membrane protein. Annu Rev Genet 24: 133–170

Ikeda Y, Takagi A, Ohkaru Y *et al 1990* A sandwich-enzyme immunoassay for the quantification of lipoprotein lipase and hepatic lipase in post heparin plasma using monoclonal antibodies to the corresponding enzymes. J Lipid Res 31: 1911–1924

Ikeda Y, Takagi A, Zenta T *et al* 1994a Physiological role of human hepatic triglyceride lipase (HTGL) : HTGL regulates the multiple lipoprotein metabolism of IDL, LDL, and HDL_2. This book, Section 4, p 181–185

Ikeda Y, Takagi A, Yamamoto A 1994b Elucidation of an underlying etiology of primary type IV hyperlipoproteinemia: heterozygous lipoprotein lipase deficiency as a causal genetic disorder. *In* Yamamoto A, Nakamura H, Nakai T (Eds) Current Advances in Triglyceride and Atherosclerosis, Churchill Livingstone, Osaka, pp 173–186

Kajinami K, Mabuchi H, Itoh H *et al* 1988 New variant of low density lipoprotein receptor gene. Arteriosclerosis 8: 187–192

Miyake Y, Tajima S, Funahashi T, Kigawa K, Yamamoto A 1992a Analysis of mutations of low density lipoprotein receptor in Japanese familial hypercholesterolemia. *In*: Yoshida TO, Wilson JM (Eds) Molecular approaches to the study and treatment of human diseases. Elsevier Science Publishers, Amsterdam, pp 31–35

Miyake Y, Tajima S, Funahashi T, Yamamura T, Yamamoto A 1992b A point mutation of low-density-lipoprotein receptor causing rapid degradation of the receptor. Eur J Biochem 210: 1–7

Moriyama K , Sasaki J, Matsunaga A *et al* 1992 Apolipoprotein E1 Lys146 — Glu with Type III hyperlipoproteinemia. Biochim Biophys Acta 1128: 58–64

Nomura S, Yamamura T, Yamamoto A *et al* 1993 The association between lipoprotein (a) and severity of coronary and cerebrovascular atherosclerosis, especially in non-hypercholesterolemic subjects. Cardiovasc Risk Factors 3: 336–343

Rall SC Jr, Mahley RW 1992 The role of apolipoprotein E genetic variants in lipoprotein disorders. J Intern Med 231: 653–659

Takagi A., Ikeda Y, Tsutsumi Z, Shoji T, Yamamoto A 1992 Molecular studies on primary lipoprotein lipase deficiency. One base deletion (G916) in exon 5 of the LPL gene causes no detectable LPL protein due to the absence of LPL mRNA transcript. J Clin Invest 89: 581–591

Tybjaerg-Hansen A. Humphries SE 1992 Familial defective apolipoprotein B-100. A single mutation that causes hypercholesterolemia and premature coronary artery disease (review). Atherosclerosis 96: 91–107

Yamamoto A, Kamiya T, Yamamura T *et al* 1989 Clinical features of familial hypercholesterolemia. Arteriosclerosis 9 (suppl I): 66–74

Yamamura T, Sudo H, Matsuzawa Y, Yamamoto A 1979 Familial hyperlipoproteinemia showing an interconversion between type III and V with a trait of xeroderma pigmentosum. Med J Osaka Univ 30: 5–14

Yamamura T, Tajima S, Miyake Y *et al* 1990 Hyperlipoproteinemia as a risk factor for ischemic heart disease. Jpn Circ J 54: 448–456

Multiple Risk Factors in Cardiovascular Disease, ed. by A. Yamamoto, Churchill Livingstone Japan, Tokyo, pp. 167–171 (1994)

RARE MUTATIONS IN THE *Apo*E GENE AND THEIR EFFECT ON CHYLOMICRON AND VLDL REMNANT METABOLISM IN FAMILIAL DYSBETALIPOPROTEINEMIC PATIENTS AND IN TRANSGENIC MICE

Louis M. HAVEKES,[*1] Bart van VLIJMEN,[*1] Rune FRANTS,[*2] and Marten HOFKER[*2]

[*1] *TNO-Institute of Prevention and Health Research, Gaubius Laboratory, and* [*2] *Department of Human Genetics*

Key words: apolipoprotein E, type III hyperlipoproteinemia, transgenic mice, lipoprotein metabolism, dominant inheritance

Apolipoprotein E (apoE) is a major constituent of chylomicron and very low-density lipoprotein (VLDL) remnants. It plays a major role in the clearance of these lipoproteins because it serves as a ligand for their recognition by hepatic lipoprotein receptors. Using isoelectric focusing (IEF), apoE can be separated into three commonly occurring isoforms: E2, E3, and E4.

Patients with familial dysbetalipoproteinemia (FD) show an increased plasma level of atherogenic chylomicron and VLDL remnants. The increased level of these lipoproteins leads to an enhanced risk of premature atherosclerosis and is thought to be due to both increased synthesis and decreased clearance.

FD WITH E2E2 PHENOTYPE

Most FD patients show homozygosity for the apoE2 variant. The major underlying metabolic defect in these patients is impaired clearance of the remnant particles due to defective binding of apoE2 to hepatic lipoprotein receptors.

In the general population, the frequency of E2E2 homozygosity is about 1%. However, only about 4% of all E2E2 homozygotes eventually develop FD, generally after the third decade of life in men and after menopause in women. This implies that FD is a recessively inherited multifactorial disease. In addition to E2E2 homozygosity, genetic and/or environmental factors are involved in the expression of this disease. It is commonly assumed that these additional factors are somehow related to the synthesis of chylomicrons and VLDL, and include such factors as nutrition, diabetes, obesity, and hormonal status (Mahley & Rall 1989). We addressed the question as to whether this multifactorial character was, in part, due to additional heterogeneity in the E*2 allele.

In order to investigate whether additional heterogeneity in the *apo*E gene is responsible for this reduced penetrance of FD, we evaluated the exact mutation in both E*2 alleles in 60 E2E2 homozygous FD patients. By employing polymerase chain reaction (PCR)-based restriction fragment length polymorphism (RFLP) analysis with restriction enzyme Hhal (Hixson & Vernier 1990). we were able to show that all FD patients were homozygous for the common E*2 (*arg*158 → *cys*) mutation. This indicates that factors not

[*1] P.O. Box 430, 2300 AK Leiden, The Netherlands
[*2] P.O. Box 9503, 2300 RA Leiden, The Netherlands

related to the E*2 allele determine the expression of FD in E2E2 homozygotes.

We measured the binding efficiency to the low-density lipoproteins (LDL) receptor of Hep G2 cells of the lipoprotein fraction with density $d < 1.019$ g/ml isolated from E2E2-homozygous FD patients before and after treatment with gemfibrozil. Treatment with gemfibrozil normalizes VLDL and intermediate-density lipoproteins (IDL) cholesterol levels in these patients. However, this normalization is not accompanied by improved binding of the $d < 1.019$ lipoprotein fraction to the LDL receptor. The absence of an effect of gemfibrozil treatment on the binding efficiency is also reflected by the absence of an effect of gemfibrozil treatment on the plasma level of apoE. We hypothesize that normal VLDL and IDL cholesterol levels in E2E2 homozygotes reflect a reduced production rate of VLDL particles rather than an improved binding efficiency of the $d < 1.019$ lipoprotein fraction to the LDL receptor.

FD WITH E3E2 PHENOTYPE

In addition to 60 FD patients with E2E2 homozygosity, we found 6 FD probands with the E3E2 phenotype. DNA sequence analyses revealed that all these probands carried the E2 (*lys*146 → *gln*) mutation described previously (Rall *et al* 1983). In addition, family analyses showed that almost all carriers of the E*2 (*lys*146 → *gln*) allele express FD, although with a variable degree of severity.

Thus, in contrast to the common E*2 (*arg*158 → *cys*) allele, the E*2 (*lys*146 → *gln*) allele is associated with a dominantly inherited form of FD with high penetrance (Smit *et al* 1990). The exact mechanism of the dominant behavior of the E2 (*lys*146 → *gln*) variant in the expression of FD is still subject to speculation. However, we obtained some evidence that the $d < 1.019$ lipoprotein fraction from carriers of the E*2 (*lys*146 → *gln*) allele is defective in lipolysis by bovine milk lipoprotein lipase. Since VLDL lipoproteins become more efficient in binding to the LDL receptor after treatment with lipoprotein lipase, this relative defect as a substrate for lipoprotein lipase could explain the relative defect of the E2 (*lys*146 → *gln*)-containing $d <$ 1.019 lipoprotein fraction in its receptor-mediated clearance. Although this variant was originally described by Rall *et al.* (1983) in two sibs, we suggest this variant to be a Dutch variant because of the number of probands found in the Dutch population. This hypothesis is further strengthened by the findings of Dr. Marais in Cape Town, South Africa. He described a patient with severe FD with heterozygosity for the E*2 (*lys*146 → *gln*) allele who originated from the Dutch-speaking part of the Belgian population, which is closely related genetically to the Dutch population. Genealogical studies are currently being performed to evaluate whether these FD patients carrying the E*2 (*lys*146 → *gln*) allele share a common ancestry.

FD WITH E3E3 PHENOTYPE

Six FD patients have been found with the E3E3 phenotype. These patients exhibit heterozygosity for the E*3-Leiden allele, which is characterized by a partial gene duplication of codons 120-126 (Wardell *et al* 1989; Van den Maagdenberg *et al* 1989). Family analyses have been carried out for five probands. Genealogical studies revealed that these five probands share a common ancestry in the second half of the 17th century (De Knijff *et al* 1991).

We collected blood from 128 family members, including 42 carriers of the E*3-Leiden allele. All carriers of the E*3-Leiden allele showed characteristics of FD, such as increased levels of cholesterol in the $d < 1.019$ lipoprotein fraction, increased ratios of cholesterol to triglyceride in this fraction, and strongly increased levels of plasma apoE. Although all carriers of the E*3-Leiden allele expressed FD, there was a variable degree of severity. Multiple linear regression analysis revealed that this variability in the expression of FD can be explained by age or body mass index. Gender did not show any significant additional influence on the expression of FD nor did it influence the age of onset of FD. This is in strong contrast with FD in E2E2 homozygosity.

Subdividing carriers of the E*3-Leiden allele according to the common, second *apo*E allele showed that the E*2 allele significantly enhanced the expression of FD, whereas the E*4 allele had the opposite effect. However, irrespective of the effect of the common, second *apo*E allele on the severity of FD, heterozygosity for the *apo*E*3-Leiden allele was absolutely associated with the expression of this disease. We conclude that, in carriers of the *apo*E*3-Leiden allele, FD is a dominantly inherited monofactorial disease, i.e., the presence of normally functioning apoE molecules in the plasma does not prevent the age- or body mass index-related expression of this disease.

By using quantitative Western blotting after IEF of samples with and without cysteamine treatment, we were able to measure the protein ratio of E3-Leiden to the common E variant. In complete plasma, the mean ratio of E3-Leiden to the common E variant was about 3 : 1. In the HDL fraction, this ratio was about 1:1, whereas the E3-Leiden isoform largely predominated in the VLDL-IDL fraction (mean ratio, 7 : 1). This large predominance of E3-Leiden in the VLDL-IDL fraction renders these lipoproteins "apparent homozygous" E3-Leiden particles and could therefore be the mechanism underlying the dominant behavior of E3-Leiden in the expression of FD.

SCREENING FOR NEW *APO*E VARIANTS

The use of a combination of IEF (Havekes *et al* 1987) and genotyping with allele-specific restriction enzymes such as HhaI (Hixon & Vernier 1990) permits screening for the presence of new mutations in the *apo*E gene. When the results of both methods are compared, typing discrepancies indicate the presence of new mutations in the *apo*E gene. However, for screening purposes, this combination of techniques is not 100% informative and is too laborious. In order to screen 120 hyperlipoproteinemic and normolipidemic individuals for the presence of new apoE variants, we introduced the technique of denaturing gradient gel electrophoresis (DGGE, Sheffield *et al* 1989). Using this technique, we were able to screen for the presence of mutations in predetermined parts of exon 4 of the *apo*E gene. Subsequently, we used the direct sequencing method to determine the exact nature of these four mutations: E2 (*val*236 → *glu*), E1 (*leu*252 → *glu*), E4 (*cys*112 → *arg*, *arg*274 → *his*), and E4 (*ser*296 → *arg*) (Van den Maagdenberg *et al* 1993b). Preliminary family analyses revealed no cosegregation of FD or any other type of hyperlipoproteinemia with any of these new variants. At present, we cannot rule out the possibility that mutations in the *apo*E gene can cause phenotypes different from FD. The DGGE method offers an efficient method for screening large numbers of individuals with regard to the occurrence of new mutations in predetermined parts of the *apo*E gene.

STUDIES USING TRANSGENIC MICE

To study the metabolism of chylomicron and VLDL remnants in greater detail, we introduced defective apoE variants into transgenic mice. This approach permitted us to study this aspect of lipoprotein metabolism under more standardized conditions, since 1) transgenic mice have a more homogeneous genetic and environmental background; 2) the number of animals per condition to be studied can be made as large as possible; and 3) by crossbreeding, all kinds of (rare) genetic combinations can be studied. We generated *apo*E*3-Leiden transgenic mice in order to study the dominant behavior of this variant in greater detail and to study the effect of subtle environmental factors such as different diets and the effect of age.

*Apo*E*3-Leiden transgenic mice express hyperlipoproteinemia even with a regular chow diet. This hyperlipidemia is confined to the VLDL/LDL-sized lipoprotein fractions and is dependent on the level of expression of the *apo*E*3-Leiden gene. The high-expressor mouse lines were more hyperlipidemic than a low-expressor line. This indicates that, in the mouse as well, the *apo*E*3-Leiden gene behaves in a dominant fashion in impairing chylomicron and VLDL remnant metabolism (Van den Maagdenberg *et al* 1993a).

When given high-cholesterol, high-fat diets, *apo*E*3-Leiden transgenic mice developed severe hypercholesterolemia. Again, this hyperlipidemia was confined to the VLDL fraction and was highly dependent on the level of expression of the transgene. We also found that the level of hypercholesterolemia could easily be modulated by varying the amounts of cholesterol and fat in the diet (Van Vlijmen *et al* 1994).

We also observed that, after receiving high-cholesterol, high-fat diets, the transgenic mice developed atherosclerotic lesions, particularly in the aortic arch. These atherosclerotic lesions ranged from mild fatty streaks containing some cholesterol-laden foam cells to severe atherosclerotic plaques containing cellular necrosis and typical cholesterol crystals. The development of atherosclerotic lesions also depends on the level of expression of the transgene and the amounts of cholesterol and fat administered in the diet (Van Vlijmen *et al* 1994).

SUMMARY

FD is a genetically heterogeneous disease. In cases with E2E2 homozygosity, FD is recessively inherited, whereas additional factors not related to the *apo*E gene are required for expression (i.e., expression shows low penetrance or is multifactorial). In cases of heterozygosity for rare apoE variants such as E2 (*lys*146 → *gln*) and E3-Leiden, the disease is dominantly inherited with high or almost complete penetrance. By using DGGE techniques, we found four new mutants in the *apo*E gene that were not clearly associated with the expression of any form of hyperlipoproteinemia.

In order to study the factors involved in remnant metabolism under more standardized conditions, we introduced a technique employing transgenic mice. Mice expressing the dominant apoE3-Leiden variant displayed hyperlipoproteinemia on a regular chow diet. Upon receiving a high-cholesterol, high-fat diet, these mice developed severe hypercholesterolemia dependent on the level of expression of the transgene. In parallel with the degree of hypercholesterolemia, these mice also developed atherosclerotic lesions. We conclude that the use of *apo*E*3-Leiden transgenic mice makes it possible for us to study subtle environmental factors influencing chylomicron and VLDL remnant metabolism.

REFERENCES

De Knijff P, Van den Maagdenberg AMJM, Stalenhoef AFH *et al* 1991 Familial dysbetalipoproteinemia associated with apolipoprotein E3-Leiden in an extended multigeneration pedigree. J Clin Invest 88: 643

Havekes LM, De Knijff P, Beisiegel U, Havinga J, Smit M, Klasen E 1987 A rapid micromethod for apolipoprotein E phenotyping directly in serum. J Lipid Rese 28: 445–463

Hixson SA, Vernier DT 1990 Restriction isotyping of human apolipoprotein E by gene amplification and cleavage with HhaI. J Lipid Res 31: 545–548

Mahley RW, Rall SC 1989 Type III hyperlipoproteinemia (dysbetalipoproteinemia): The role of the apolipoprotein E in normal and abnormal lipoprotein metabolism. *In*: Scriver CR, Beaudet AL Sly WE, Valle D (Eds) The Metabolic Basis of Inherited Disease, 6th Edition. McGraw-Hill, New York, pp 1195–1213

Rall SC, Weisgraber KH, Innerarity TL, Bersot TP, Mahley RW, Blum CB 1983 Identification of a new structural variant of human apolipoprotein E, E2 (Lys146 → Gln), in a type III hyperlipoproteinemic subject with the E3/2 phenotype. J Clin Invest 72: 1288–1297

Sheffield VC, Cox DR, Lerman LS, Myers RM 1989 Attachment of a 40-base-pair G+C-rich sequence (GC-clamp) to genomic DNA fragments by the polymerase chain reaction results in improved detection of single-base changes. Proc Natil Acad Sci USA 86: 232–236

Smit M, De Knijff P, Van der Kooij-Meijs E *et al* 1990 Genetic heterogeneity in familial dysbetalipoproteinemia: the E2 (lys146 Æ gln) variant results in a dominant mode of inheritance. J Lipid Res 31: 45–53

Van den Maagdenberg AMJM, De Knijff P, Stalenhoef AFH, Gevers Leuven JA, Havekes LM, Frants RR 1989 Apolipoprotein E*3-Leiden allele results from a partial gene duplication in exon 4. Biochem Biophys Res Commun 165: 851–857

Van den Maagdenberg AMJM, Hofker MH, Krimpenfort PJA *et al* 1993a Transgenic mice carrying the apolipoprotein E3-Leiden gene exhibit hyperlipoproteinemia. J Biol Chem 268: 10540–10545

Van den Maagdenberg AMJM, Weng W, de Bruijn IH *et al* 1993b Characterization of five new mutants in the carboxy-terminal domain of human apolipoprotein E: no cosegregation with severe hyperlipidemia. Am J Human Genet 52: 937–946

Van Vlijmen B, Van den Maagdenberg AMJM, Gijbels MJJ *et al* 1994 Diet-induced hyperlipoproteinemia and atherosclerosis in apolipoprotein E3-Leiden transgenic mice. J Clin Invest 4: (in press)

Wardell MR, Weisgraber KH, Havekes LM, Rall SC 1989 Apolipoprotein E3-Leiden contains a seven-amino acid insertion that is a tandem repeat of residues 121–127. J Biol Chem 264: 21205–21210

Multiple Risk Factors in Cardiovascular Disease, ed. by A. Yamamoto, Churchill Livingstone Japan, Tokyo, pp. 173–179 (1994)

MED PED: PREVENTIVE MEDICINE FOR HIGH RISK PEDIGREES[§]

Roger R. WILLIAMS,[*1] Steven C. HUNT,[*1] Gary K. BARLOW,[*1] Paul N. HOPKINS,[*1] Joan L. WARE,[*2] and Victor BOULYJENKOV[*3]

[*1] *Cardiovascular Genetics Research Clinic, Department of Internal Medicine, University of Utah Medical School,* [*2] *Bureau of Chronic Disease Control, Utah Department of Health, and* [*3] *Hereditary Diseases Program, World Health Organization*

Key words: prevention, genetics, atherosclerosis cholesterol, heart disease, family history

Practical Relevance for the Human Genome Project

An astounding explosion of new discoveries in genetics and molecular biology is rapidly capturing the attention of virtually every serious medical professional. An estimated 3 billion dollars are being spent world-wide to "map the human genome." What do we hope to gain from this massive investment in molecular genetics? Most of us hope it will lead to a better understanding of disease causation and set the stage for more effective detection and treatment of genetically promoted diseases and for the prevention of their serious consequences.

Chronic Diseases, the New Challenge for Genetics

Chronic diseases like early familial coronary heart disease and underlying genetic causes like *heterozygous familial hypercholesterolemia* (FH) present a new challenge for those interested in applying genetic principles to prevent disease consequences. For many years, genetic counselors have applied the principles of their discipline to help families with inborn errors of metabolism like phenylketonuria and hemophilia. These diseases have striking manifestations in young children and rarely (if ever) escape diagnosis in places like Utah with a well organized prenatal screening program and abundant supply of vigilant medical professionals. In contrast, the gene for FH acts like a time-bomb, often ticking too softly to be heard from birth until sudden death from myocardial infarction at age 45 in an asymptomatic male or 10–15 years later in an unsuspecting otherwise healthy female.

150 Mutations That Double Serum Cholesterol

Heterozygous FH is a dominantly inherited defect in low density lipoprotein (LDL) receptors carried on the short arm of chromosome 19. With one normal gene and one

[*1,2] Salt Lake City, UT, USA.
[*3] Geneva, Switzerland.
Address for reprints: MED PED FH Coordinating Center, Univ. of Utah CV Genetics, 410 Chipeta Way, Room 161, Salt Lake City, UT 84108, USA.
[§] MED PED FH is supported in part by a cooperative agreement (U58/CCU803454-05) with the U.S. Centers for Disease Control, Atlanta, Georgia; by the Utah Department of Health; by grants from Merck Human Health Inc. and international affiliates; by local affiliates of the American Heart Association; and by a grant from the World Health Organization, Geneva, Switzerland.

defective gene at the LDL receptor locus, single gene carriers have only half the normal number of receptors in the liver that recognize and remove circulating LDL-cholesterol from the blood stream. As a result, these heterozygotes typically have twice the normal LDL-cholesterol levels by age 2, and without treatment for the rest of their shortened lives (Yamamoto *et al* 1989).

FH is one of the most common single severe gene determinants of cardiovascular disease. In most countries it is estimated to occur once in every 500 persons (about 500,000 in the US, about 1.5 million in Europe, about 10.6 million in the world). Founder effects have led to much higher rates of FH in French Canadians, Afrikaners, Lebanese, and Finns. In 1985 Brown and Goldstein received the Nobel Prize for discovery of the LDL receptor defects that cause FH. To date 150 different causal mutations at the LDL receptor locus have been reported (Hobbs e*t al* 1992).

Now "genetic cousins" of FH are also emerging. *Familial defective apoprotein B 3500* (FDB) also appears to be a relatively common gene that can cause very high cholesterol and early death. If classic FH due to defective LDL receptors can be thought of as a deformed lock, then the gene for FDB can be thought of as a deformed key for this same lock. The net result is similar if defects are present in half of the keys (apoprotein B) or half of the locks (LDL receptors). Twice normal LDL-cholesterol level in blood results from half the normal rate of receptor-mediated removal of LDL-cholesterol by the liver.

Because FH is a dominant gene, 50% of first degree relatives will also be affected (parents, offspring, and siblings) and *on the affected side of the family*, 50% of second degree relatives on average will also have FH (aunts, uncles, nieces, nephews) as well as 25% of first cousins. It should be a high priority to screen all of these close relatives in a family with FH because they have such a high risk of a treatable fatal disease.

Early Deaths from FH — A Preventable Tragedy

Diffuse coronary atherosclerosis, often accelerated by other interacting factors like smoking, can lead to death from myocardial infarction in the 20's in some male and female FH heterozygotes, and typically in men aged 35–55 and women 10–15 years later. Until recent advances in cholesterol lowering medications, normal cholesterol levels could not be expected from even the most severe low fat diet, and the prognosis for FH heterozygotes was often reflected in the common advice given by physicians: "go write your will".

The Good News

The outlook has now changed! HMG Co-A Reductase inhibitors (nicknamed HMG's) were introduced a few years ago, and have proven to be true "miracle drugs" for FH. HMG's work by upregulating LDL-receptors, helping persons with FH to compensate for the half that are defective by getting better productivity out of the half that are normal. FH heterozygotes taking HMG's in combination with very strict diet and/or other agents such as resin binders and nicotinic acid can often achieve normal or near normal cholesterol-levels (Illingworth 1993) even though some of them started out with very high levels as illustrated in Fig. 1. In a study of such effective cholesterol-lowering therapy for 3 years, coronary angiograms before and after therapy showed significant delay or even regression of atherosclerotic lesions (Kane *et al* 1990). Moreover, primary prevention of coronary disease by treating cholesterol levels can save money as well as lives in contrast to the controversial expense versus benefit of primary prevention treatment of cholesterol in many other settings (Goldman *et al* 1993).

The Bad News

While performing genetic studies of coronary-prone pedigrees in Utah, we were surprised to see that many of the FH par-

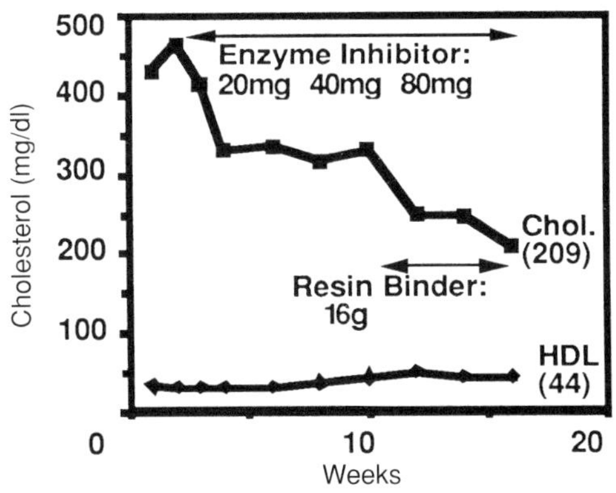

Fig. 1. Response to 2 medications in a male age 49.
One or more prescription medications can usually drop even extremely high cholesterol levels to normal as shown in this figure. Usually a low fat diet is helpful together with medications to achieve even lower cholesterol levels.

ticipants were still untreated and hypercholesterolemic, even though their physicians knew they had severely elevated cholesterol levels and a diagnosis of "FH." Furthermore, as we traced and tested their relatives as illustrated in Fig. 2, we found most of them had never been previously tested or diagnosed. Over the 17 years we have followed FH pedigrees we have often relived the tragedy of seeing the familiar faces of FH friends from our study pedigrees appearing in the obituary column of the local newspaper announcing another early coronary death and listing the names of the new widow and surviving children. Motivated by this human tragedy, and knowing that it could now be abated with proper treatment, we vowed to document the magnitude of the problem and to begin an effort to find and help FH heterozygotes avoid early deaths.

Under a cooperative agreement with the Centers for Disease Control and the Utah Department of Health we began a 5 year project to find and help as many FH cases in Utah as possible during the period 1989–1994. We decided to call the project "MED PED FH", standing for Make Early Diagnoses to Prevent Early Deaths

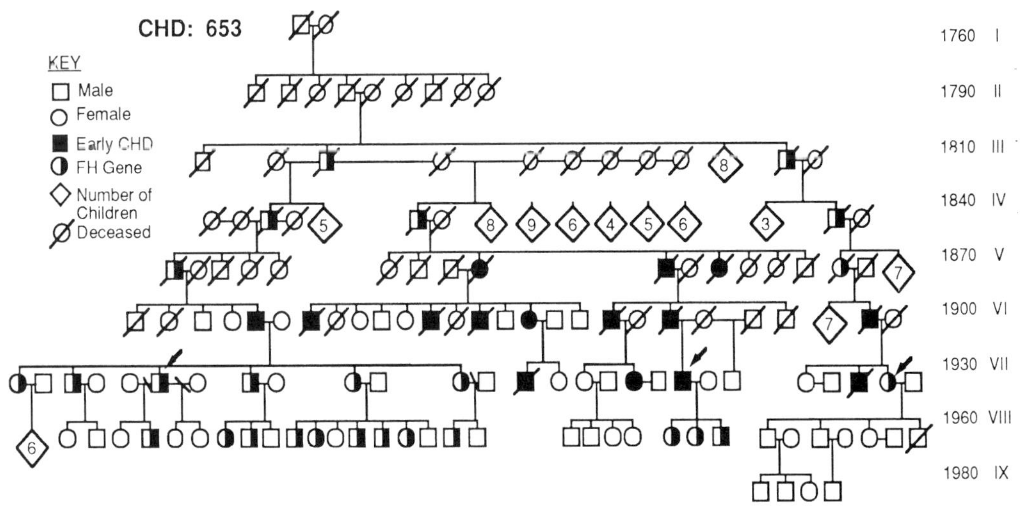

Fig. 2. CHD 653 is one of many large pedigrees being traced and followed by Utah Cardiovascular Genetics (CVG).
Among 9 generations of descendants from 1760 to the present, 43 persons have been found so far with familial hypercholesterolemia (FH) who have cholesterols of 350–450 and heart attacks (CHD = coronary heart disease) in their 30's to 50's. A DNA marker has already been found locating the gene on chromosome 19. As Utah CVG communicates with relatives in 10 states, hundreds more will be found and helped.

in MEDical PEDigrees with Familial Hypercholesterolemia.

METHODS DEVELOPED FOR MED PED FH IN UTAH

Finding Index Cases with FH

In the first year of our effort we tried several different methods for finding FH patients and identified a total of 101 different families. We already knew 12 different FH families from our past research studies and another 39 from our referral clinic for familial lipid disorders.

Two projects of the State Health Department yielded more cases. From a computerized file of 40,000 family questionnaires collected from parents of high school students, we evaluated about 200 families with a very strong family history of early heart attacks (2 + siblings with coronary events under age 55) and found another 20 FH cases. From a computer file of 75,000 persons tested for cholesterol by the Health Department, follow-up evaluation with those listed with cholesterol above 300 mg/dl yielded another 9 patients.

Three community-based efforts also contributed to this effort. A letter was sent to 720 primary care physicians in Utah yielding many referrals for possible FH of whom 14 were eventually confirmed to be FH heterozygotes. Local hospitals cooperated by sending a letter and questionnaire to patients discharged with early coronary events. Follow-up evaluation of these persons led to 5 more FH cases. The final contribution of 2 more cases came from follow-up of questionnaires filled out by 117 persons having a cholesterol result over 300 mg/dl when tested by a local pediatrician in several shopping malls.

Tracing FH Families to Find Many Other Relatives with FH

We applied methods from our pedigree research studies. Once we found a confirmed index case with FH, we identified more with FH by contacting *close relatives* as illustrated in Fig. 2 (offspring, parents, aunts, uncles, nieces, nephews, and first cousins). We also merged computerized data on known ancestors in 4–5 generations finding that some of the 101 independently ascertained families descended from about 50 unrelated 5 generation pedigrees. Contacting close relatives usually yielded about 5–10 new cases.

After two years of tracing FH families, the pool of *close relatives* began to run out and we found a much larger pool of *distant relatives* (2nd and 3rd cousins, etc.) from multigenerational pedigrees expanded with the help of local resources and expertise in genealogical record searches. This was done by sequential pedigree expansion and by finding common ancestors. For each generation back we could extend an FH pedigree the number of affected descendants is multiplied 3 or 4 times (the number of siblings in the FH grandparents family divided by 2). Thus, from 5–10 cases in a grandparent family (3 generations), extending up one generation to a great-grandparent carrier and back down to second cousins will find about 15–40 persons with FH. Going up one more generation and back down to 3rd cousins can lead to 45–160 new FH cases in a 5–6 generation pedigree. In Utah the work of 2 full-time staff members tracing about 30 large pedigrees seems to have no end in sight. The largest one goes back 7 generations and has led to over 100 FH heterozygotes so far (with an estimated 2,000 to 5,000 possible if we found all FH descendants). It should be no surprise that relatives in large pedigrees have led us to 35 states and several countries.

DNA-validated Clinical Criteria for Diagnosing FH

It may seem strange to develop diagnostic criteria in the middle of a screening program. But in our case "necessity was the mother of invention". We soon recognized that the same cholesterol cut-point should not be used to diagnose FH in general population screening and FH family screening. For example we found that 310 mg/dl was too low for diagnosing FH in the general population (only 5% above 310 had FH), but in first degree relatives of FH probands 95% of those above 310 had FH. We recognized that the probability of FH at a given cholesterol level depended highly on the probability of having FH before testing. We reasoned further that lower criteria should be developed for first degree relatives of a known FH proband, since they had a 50% chance of FH before testing, and that higher criteria should be used for general population testing when the initial probability before screening is only 1 in 500 for FH and even higher for familial combined or polygenic hypercholesterolemia.

We first used distributional mathematics to derive age-specific cholesterol screening criteria separately for population or family screening. Next we tested the accuracy of diagnosing FH from our new clinical screening criteria with the results of DNA testing for LDL receptor gene markers in 300 persons in FH families. Our clinical criteria showed 98% specificity and 87% sensitivity. They are presented in Table I (Williams *et al* 1993a).

RESULTS OF UTAH MED PED FH

Tracing Relatives, The Most Efficient Approach Using the relative tracing methods the total cost per new FH case found was about $400. This was about 5 times more efficient than any of the other methods tested for finding new cases (following-up on persons selected from existing computer files of cholesterol testing, family histories, hospital discharges, and referrals from primary care physicians) (Williams *et al* 1993b). The main reason seems to be "a priori probabilities". No matter how high the risk of FH seemed from these computer-assisted population screening methods, the majority of persons indexed did not have FH, and a lot of effort was expended evaluating a large number of non-FH persons using the population ascertainment criteria listed at the top of Table I. In the family tracing approach, most contacts are made with individuals whose chance of FH was either 50% or 25% and whose diagnosis requires only a simple cholesterol test (see the bottom of Table I).

TABLE I. Validated Criteria for the Diagnosis of Heterozygous Familial Hypercholesterolemia

1. DNA diagnosis of an accepted functional LDL-receptor defect.
2. Without a gene maker, use these clinical criteria for the index case.

(All 5 criteria must be met)	age 40	age 30	age 20	under 18
a. Very high total chol. (mg/dl)	> 360	> 340	> 290	> 270
b. Normal triglycerides (mg/dl)	< 200	< 180	< 150	< 100
or very high LDL chol. (mg/dl)	> 260	> 240	> 210	> 200

c. No secondary cause of high cholesterol (nephrotic syndrome, pregnancy, etc.)
d. At least one pediatric relative (child, grandchild, niece or nehew, etc. > 18 years of age with very high cholesterol (total cholesterol > 220) or at least one close relative with tendon xanthomas.
e. Dominant expression in the family:
   about half of siblings and offspring affected.
   bimodal (clear separation between normal and abnormal in relatives).

3. Among close relatives of confirmed FH index cases use these criteria:

(Both criteria must be met)	age 40	age 30	age 20	under 18
a. High total chol. (mg/dl)	> 300	> 280	> 240	> 220
or high LDL chol. (mg/dl)	> 215	> 195	> 175	> 165

b. No secondary cause of high cholesterol (nephrotic syndrome, pregnancy, etc.)

These clinical criteria were validated using DNA diagnoses and shown to have 98% specificity and 87% sensitivity in FH families. (From Am J Cardiol 72: 171–176, 1993.)

Most FH Heterozygotes Were NOT DIAGNOSED or NOT TREATED

Among 502 FH relatives found, only 31% reported being told by their physician that they had an inherited cholesterol problem, only 42% reported they were taking ANY prescription medication to lower cholesterol, and only 23% reported post-treatment cholesterol levels below the 90th percentile for their age (Williams *et al* 1993b).

Most FH Heterozygotes WANT HELP and CAN BE HELPED

Most FH patients have been eager to have us enter them and their physicians into the MED PED FH computer registry to facilitate the conduct and evaluation of a long-term educational intervention. We have developed educational materials that we mail to patients and their primary care physicians. We follow up with phone calls to encourage the patients to see their doctor regularly. A Pharm D and MED PED physicians provide telephone backup to primary care physicians who receive very practical and specific written guidelines from FH experts regarding the diagnosis, treatment, and laboratory follow-up of FH patients. Practical issues covered include side-effects of medications, factors improving compliance, cardiovascular testing, insurance matters, diet, special needs of women and children, etc.

In just the first follow-up questionnaire from 106 MED PED FH participants, 79% are now taking medication, 49% are below the 50th percentile, and 17% have cholesterol levels below the 50th percentile! We conclude that most patients with FH want help and can be helped.

EXPANSION OF MED PED FH TO OTHER STATES AND COUNTRIES

Initial encouragement and the first pilot support for international expansion of MED PED FH came from Victor Boulyjenkov, director of the Genetic Diseases Program of the World Health Organization (WHO) in Geneva. Physicians with special interest in FH began talking to each other about MED PED during coffee breaks at international meetings and followed with telefax letters to each other to share ideas. Several countries already had FH family tracing, patient registration, physician networking, and educational programs in place (Hayden & Josephson 1993). We met in Munich in February 1993 and in Israel in September 1993 to share ideas and to begin organizing an international MED PED FH network with start-up support of Merck Human Health. Collaborating countries include (in alphabetical order) Australia, Austria, Canada, Denmark, Germany, Hungary, Israel, Netherlands, Norway, South Africa, Sweden, Switzerland, United Kingdom, and the United States (California, Maryland, Massachusetts, Ohio, Oregon, Utah).

Our international MED PED FH goals include: 1) uniting our voices to demand that our societies stop neglecting FH and invest more to support FH diagnosis, treatment, and research; and 2) sharing our resources and expertise (PC programs for pedigree data, DNA testing, genealogical methodology and archives, lipid clinic management techniques); and 3) standardizing our approaches and data collection to facilitate future collaborative reporting of results. Many of the FH pedigrees lead from current members in one country to ancestors and distant cousins in other countries. We hope to facilitate the long-term success in case finding that merging such international pedigrees will foster.

MED PED FOR OTHER GENETIC DISEASES

Any dominantly inherited disease that a) can be found using a screening test (biochemical or genetic), and b) has treatable or preventable serious consequences is potentially a candidate for the MED PED approach. We are already talking about this approach for the "Long QT Syndrome," a dominant trait with DNA linkage established, and for which sudden death in youth can be prevented by diagnosis and treatment with beta-blocker medications. "Glucocorticoid Remediable Aldosteronism" (GRA) is a dominantly inherited disorder from well-defined causal mutations. It leads to severe hypertension and early stroke deaths but does not respond to the usual antihypertensive medications. When properly diagnosed, treatment with a glucocorticoid hormone can normalize blood pressures and likely prevent early stroke deaths. Pedigrees with Long QT sudden death or GRA hypertension with stroke are being extended to find persons who can benefit from preventive measures. Other diseases will be candidates for the MED PED approach as gene or biochemical markers are discovered for dominantly inherited breast cancer, colon cancer, and similar familial chronic diseases.

SUMMARY

MED PED stands for Make Early Diagnosis to Prevent Early Death in MEDical PEDigrees. It is a genetic approach to prevention for dominantly inherited disorders for which screening tests and methods for treatment or prevention have been developed. In its first application, persons with heterozygous FH have been traced in Utah from both close and distant relatives of a few known index cases. Compared with the most efficient alternative methods for finding new FH cases, tracing relatives in FH families was 5 times more cost efficient. Among 502 FH heterozygotes detected in 3 years of family tracing in Utah, only 31% had been diagnosed, only 42% were taking any medication to lower cholesterol, and only 23% had post-treatment cholesterol levels below the 90th percentile. Early follow-up of some registered FH patients and their primary care physicians are encouraging. Among 106 returning the first follow-up questionnaire, 79% are on medication and 49% are below the 90th percentile. A MED PED FH network is being formed by physicians with special interest in FH from 14 countries where this basic MED PED approach is already in use or beginning.

REFERENCES

Goldman L, Goldman PA, Williams LW *et al* 1993 Cost-effectiveness considerations in the treatment of heterozygous familial hypercholesterolemia with medications. Am J Cardiol 72: 75D–79D

Hayden MR, Josephson R 1993 Development of a program for identification of patients with familial hypercholesterolemia in British Columbia: A model for prevention of coronary disease. Am J Cardiol 72: 25D–29D

Hobbs HH, Brown MS, Goldstein JL 1992 Molecular genetics of the LDL receptor gene in familial hypercholesterolemia. Hum Mutat 1: 445–466

Illingworth RD 1993 How effective is drug therapy in heterozygous familial hypercholesterolemia? Am J Cardiol 72: 54D–58D

Kane JP, Malloy MJ, Ports TA *et al* 1990 Regression of coronary atherosclerosis during treatment of familial hypercholesterolemia with combined drug regimens. JAMA 264: 3007–3012

Williams RR, Hunt SC, Schumacher MC *et al* 1993a Diagnosing heterozygous familial hypercholesterolemia using new practical criteria validated by molecular genetics. Am J Cardiol 72: 171–176

Williams RR, Schumacher MC, Barlow GK, *et al* 1993b Documented need for more effective diagnosis and treatment of familial hypercholesterolemia according to data from 502 heterozygotes in Utah. Am J Cardiol 72: 18D–24D

Yamamoto A, Kamiya T, Yamamura T *et al* 1989 Clinical features of familial hypercholesterolemia. Arteriosclerosis 9 (suppl I): I-66–I-74

Multiple Risk Factors in Cardiovascular Disease, ed. by A. Yamamoto, Churchill Livingstone Japan, Tokyo, pp. 181–186 (1994)

PHYSIOLOGICAL ROLE OF HUMAN HEPATIC TRIGLYCERIDE LIPASE (HTGL): HTGL REGULATES THE MULTIPLE LIPOPROTEIN METABOLISM OF IDL, LDL, AND HDL_2

Yasuyuki IKEDA,[*1] Atsuko TAKAGI,[*1] Zenta TSUTSUMI,[*1] Akio TSURU,[*1] Atsuo MORI,[*1] Tomikazu FUKUOKA,[*1] Yasushi ASHIDA,[*1] Motoo TSUSHIMA,[*2] and Akira YAMAMOTO[*1]

[*1] *Department of Etiology and Pathophysiology, National Cardiovascular Center Research Institute, and* [*2] *Department of Medicine, National Cardiovascular Center Hospital*

Key words: hepatic triglyceride lipase, physiological role, deficiency, lipoprotein lipase, hypertriglyceridemia

Plasma lipoproteins are usually classified into five different fractions according to their density (Gotto 1987): chylomicrons and very-low-density lipoprotein (VLDL, $d < 1.006$), intermediate-density lipoprotein (IDL, $d = 1.006–1.019$), low-density lipoprotein (LDL, $d = 1.019–1.063$), high-density lipoprotein 2 (HDL_2, $d = 1.063–1.125$), and high-density lipoprotein 3 (HDL_3, $d = 1.125–1.21$). Lipoprotein metabolism is regulated by four enzymes and several receptors (Jackson 1983); these are lipoprotein lipase (LPL), hepatic triglyceride lipase (HTGL), lipid transfer protein (LTP), lecithin cholesterol acyltransferase (LCAT), remnant-receptor, LDL-receptor, and HDL-receptor.

HTGL is a lipolytic enzyme synthesized by hepatocytes and its gene is located on chromosome *15q21* with 9 exons that encode an mRNA of 1.6 kb (Cai *et al* 1989). HTGL is believed to be anchored to the surface of the liver endothelial cells and released into the circulation after intravenous injection of heparin (Jackson 1983). Human HTGL is catalytically active in monomeric form and its molecular weight is 65 kDa (Ikeda *et al* 1989). The physiological role of HTGL has been extensively studied by determining good substrates for HTGL using various lipoprotein fractions and investigating the nature of the physiological substrate for HTGL in patients with low HTGL activity or after inhibiting the HTGL activity *in situ* with anti-HTGL antibody (Kinnunen 1984). Although the results of these studies are not always entirely consistent, they suggest that HTGL may play a role in the catabolism of remnants of triglyceride-rich lipoproteins or in HDL metabolism. Patients with HTGL deficiency seem to be an important model for understanding the physiological role of HTGL. A few families with HTGL deficiency have been reported (Breckenridge *et al* 1982; Carlson *et al* 1986; Auwerx *et al* 1989; Hegele *et al* 1993), and they exhibit an accumulation of β-VLDL and the presence of triglyceride-rich LDL and HDL. However, the primary physiological function of human HTGL has not been clearly elucidated yet.

Recently, we developed a sandwich-enzyme immunoassay (EIA) to quantify the immunoreactive mass of HTGL (Ikeda *et al* 1990) and a selective immunoinactivation assay (SIIA) to measure the HTGL activity in human postheparin plasma (PHP) (Ikeda *et al* 1989, 1990). The EIA uses a combination of two distinct types of mouse anti-human

[*1,2] Fujishirodai, Suita 565, Japan.

HTGL monoclonal antibodies that recognize different epitopes on the HTGL molecule (Ikeda *et al* 1990). These assay systems enabled us to identify a patient with homozygous HTGL deficiency from a group of hypertriglyceridemic subjects.

In the present study, we have systematically investigated the physiological role of human HTGL by determining the immunochemical location of HTGL in human liver and by identifying the lipoproteins preferred by HTGL as physiological substrates *in vitro*. In addition, we also analyzed dyslipoproteins in the serum of a proband, MS, with homozygous HTGL deficiency. By this approach, we demonstrated that HTGL functions on the microvilli of hepatocytes and plays a role in the catabolism of multiple lipoproteins such as IDL, LDL, and HDL_2.

IMMUNOCHEMICAL LOCALIZATION OF HTGL IN HUMAN LIVER

The immunochemical localization of HTGL in human liver was examined by electron microscopy using mouse anti-human HTGL monoclonal antibody as the first antibody and goat anti-mouse IgG conjugated with 10-nm colloidal gold as the second antibody. A sample of human liver obtained by needle biopsy was fixed by immersion in 0.1 M sodium cacodylate buffer, pH 7.4, containing 0.5% glutaraldehyde, 2% formaldehyde, and 0.1% tannic acid. After rinsing with cacodylate buffer, the liver was dehydrated using a series of graded ethanol solutions, and embedded in Spurr. The Spurr-embedded liver was sectioned, and collected on nickel grids. The sections were incubated with mouse anti-human HTGL monoclonal antibody (2(4)F12C12) (200 µg IgG_1 in 1 ml of 10 mM glycine-phosphate buffer, pH 7.4), followed by goat anti-mouse IgG conjugated with 10 nm colloidal gold. The sections were stained with 1% OsO_4, 2% uranyl acetate and lead citrate, and examined under electron microscopy. The gold particles, representing HTGL, appeared on the microvilli of hepatocytes facing Disse's space, while only background levels of gold were detected on the surface of the sinusoidal endothelium, the same as those in a control experiment with nonimmune mouse IgG. These results indicate that human HTGL is initially synthesized in hepatocytes and translocated to the microvilli, while HTGL is neither secreted nor transferred to the surface of the sinusoidal endothelium. This is in sharp contrast to the observation that rat HTGL is located on the surface of the sinusoidal endothelium (Kuusi *et al* 1979). As liver sinusoidal endothelium has various sizes of fenestration, the appropriate size of lipoprotein could be utilized by HTGL located on the microvilli of hepatocytes, and then reaction products could be effectively incorporated into the hepatocytes.

DETERMINATION OF PREFERRED SUBSTRATES FOR HUMAN HTGL BY KINETIC ANALYSIS

Human lipoproteins (VLDL, IDL, LDL, HDL_2, and HDL_3) labeled with both [^{14}C] triolein and [^{14}C] phosphatidylcholine were used to determine the preferred substrates for HTGL purified from human PHP. The time course of degradation of both triolein and phosphatidylcholine in the above substrates was carried out in 0.3 ml of the reaction mixture containing 0.2 M Tris-HCl, 0.15 M NaCl, 5% bovine serum albumin, 390–600 ng pure human HTGL, and the radiolabeled lipoprotein. The mixture was incubated at 37°C for the indicated time (Fig. 1). The reaction was stopped by adding 2 ml of a 2 : 1 mixture of chloroform and methanol and lipids were extracted and analyzed by thin-layer chromatography (Merck, Kieselgel 60) as previously described (Ikeda *et al* 1989). As shown in Fig. 1, HTGL hydrolyzed about 60 % of triolein in IDL, LDL, and HDL_2 after 2 h incubation, whereas only 15% of the triolein in VLDL and a few percent of the triolein in HDL_3 were hydrolyzed by HTGL. In all lipoproteins, HTGL reaction produced free oleate as the main product, but mono-oleate

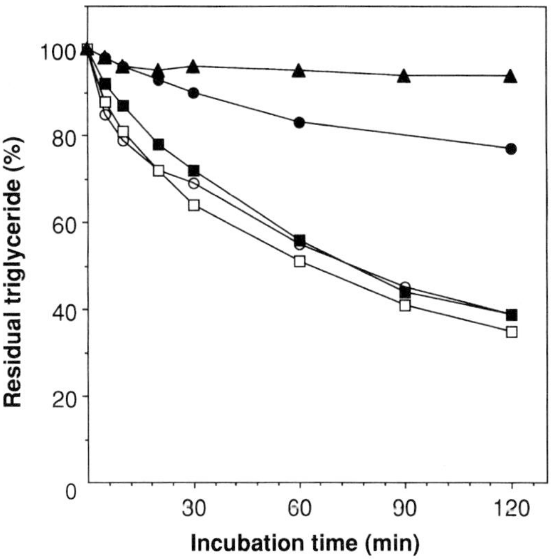

Fig. 1. Determination of lipoproteins preferred by human hepatic triglyceride lipase (HTGL). Individual lipoproteins labeled with [^{3}H] triolein were incubated for the indicated time at 37°C with HTGL. ●, VLDL; ○, IDL; ■, LDL; □, HDL_2; ▲, HDL_3.
HTGL, hepatic triglyceride lipase; VLDL, very-low-density lipoprotein; IDL, intermediate-density lipoprotein; LDL, low-density lipoprotein; HDL_2, high-density lipoprotein 2; HDL_3, high-density lipoprotein 3.

TABLE I. Determination of K_m, V_{max}, and V_{max}/K_m ratio of Human HTGL

Substrate		HTGL
VLDL	K_m (mM)	0.303
	V_{max} (mM/h/ml)	0.36
	V_{max}/K_m (h/ml)$^{-1}$	1.2
IDL	K_m	0.143
	V_{max}	0.09
	V_{max}/K_m	0.7
LDL	K_m	0.100
	V_{max}	0.18
	V_{max}/K_m	1.8
HDL_2	K_m	0.264
	V_{max}	0.27
	V_{max}/K_m	1.0
HDL_3	K_m	1.329
	V_{max}	0.14
	V_{max}/K_m	0.1

did not accumulate to such an extent in the LPL reaction, as previously reported by us (Ikeda *et al* 1989). The hydrolysis of phosphatidylcholine by HTGL was approximately ten times lower than that of triolein.

Kinetic parameters for the hydrolysis of triolein by purified human HTGL were determined using VLDL, IDL, LDL, HDL_2, and HDL_3 labeled with [^{3}H] triolein. The V_{max}/K_m ratio was used as an indicator to determine lipoproteins preferred by HTGL. As shown in Table I, the HTGL reaction exhibited a higher V_{max}/K_m ratio (1.8) for LDL, and its ratios were 1.2, 1.0, 0.7, and 0.1 for VLDL, HDL_2, IDL, and HDL_3, respectively. These biochemical studies suggest that human HTGL plays a role in the metabolism of multiple lipoproteins such as IDL, LDL, and HDL_2.

PHYSIOLOGICAL ROLE OF HTGL ILLUSTRATED BY ANALYSIS OF ABNORMAL LIPOPROTEINS IN A PATIENT WITH HOMOZYGOUS HTGL DEFICIENCY

We identified a proband-MS with homozygous HTGL deficiency from a group of unrelated hypertriglyceridemic patients (n = 500) by monitoring the HTGL immunoreactive mass in PHP using sandwich-EIA (Ikeda *et al* 1990), followed by an analysis of the HTGL gene aberrations using PCR-SSCP and direct sequencing methods. The proband, MS, had a missense mutation in exon 2 of the HTGL gene leading to no detectable HTGL in PHP. This was also confirmed by an experiment involving mutant HTGL expression in COS-1 cells. Laboratory analysis of the proband's serum showed that one of the most impressive findings was clear serum, even though the serum triglyceride concentration (320 mg/dl) of the proband was as high as that of type IV hyperlipoproteinemia, in which the serum is usually turbid. Analysis of the proband's fractionated lipoproteins (VLDL, IDL, LDL, HDL_2, and HDL_3) showed multiple dyslipoproteinemia: the accumulation of both

TABLE II. Multiple Dyslipoproteins of IDL, LDL, and HDL_2 in the Proband-MS, with Homozygous HTGL

Lipoproteins	Proband-MS	Control
IDL		
Size (mm)	24.88–27.05	25.44–27.05
Density (g/ml)	1.015	1.015 ± 0.01
LDL		
Size (nm)	24.08	24.06 ± 0.3
Density (g/ml)	1.032	1.059 ± 0.01
HDL_2		
Size (nm)	12.38	11.33 ± 0.2
Density (g/ml)	1.095	1.110 ± 0.01

small-sized IDL (IDL-remnant, 24.9–25.4 nm) and large-sized buoyant triglyceride-rich HDL_2, and normal-sized buoyant triglyceride-rich LDL (Table II), whereas VLDL triglyceride was within the normal range. Agarose-gel electrophoresis of VLDL from the proband did not show a broad β-band peculiar to type III hyperlipoproteinemia, and the ratio of VLDL-cholesterol to triglyceride (0.21) was within the normal range. This finding is in sharp contrast to the observation that the accumulation of ß-VLDL is one of the characteristics of compound heterozygous HTGL deficiency reported by a Canadian group (Hegele *et al* 1993). Demant *et al* (1988) reported that HTGL is involved in the formation of LDL from IDL based on their observation that accumulation of IDL and decreased LDL (only 10% of control) were found in patients with HTGL deficiency. However, this was not the case in the proband-MS, in whom the LDL concentration was normal or higher, suggesting that normal-sized buoyant triglyceride-rich LDL was produced by the actions of LPL and LTP. It should be noted that the particle size of buoyant (triglyceride-rich) LDL in the proband-MS, is not as large as that of a patient with HTGL deficiency reported by Auwerx *et al* (1989).

We further studied the correlation between the triglyceride concentration of LDL particles (LDL triglyceride/apoB ratio) and HTGL mass, and between HDL_2 triglyceride concentration and HTGL mass. As shown in Figs. 2A and 2B, HTGL mass concentration correlated inversely with either the LDL-triglyceride/apoB ratio ($r = 0.91$, $p = 0.0001$) or HDL_2 triglyceride concentration ($r = 0.96$, $p = 0.0001$). These results indicate that HTGL is primarily involved in the catabolism of triglyceride in multiple lipoproteins such as IDL, LDL, and HDL_2, as illustrated in Fig. 3.

SUMMARY

Human HTGL is synthesized by hepatocytes and is localized on the surface of the microvilli of hepatocytes, where it plays a variety of physiological roles. HTGL appears

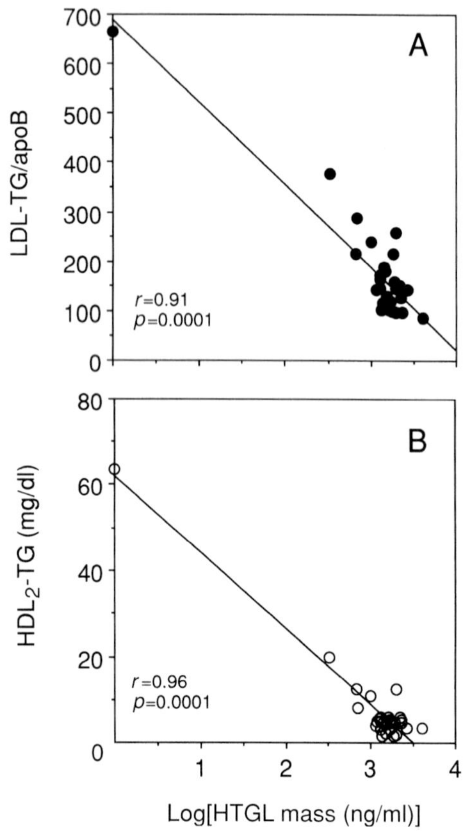

Fig. 2. Correlation between HTGL mass in PHP and LDL-triglyceride/apoB ratio (A), and HDL_2-triglyceride concentration (B). PHP, postheparin plasma.

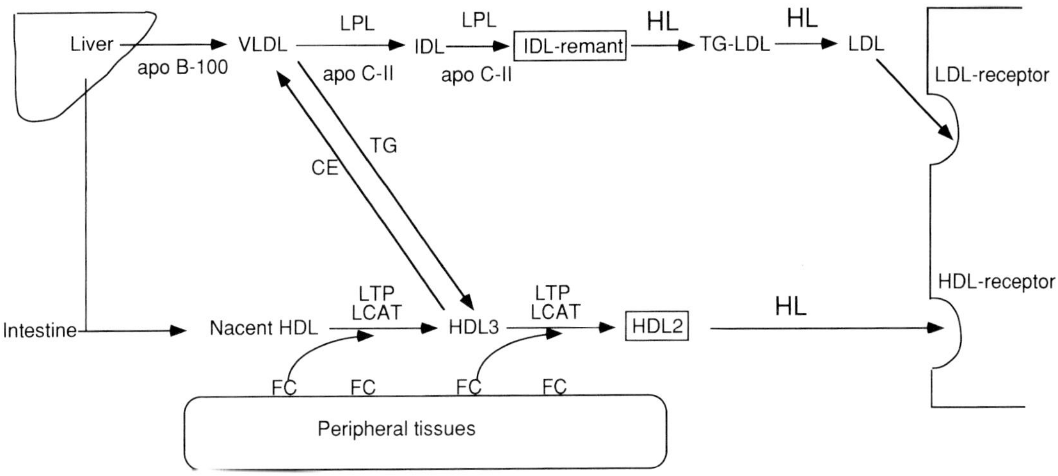

Fig. 3. Proposed physiological role of human HTGL.
LPL, lipoprotein lipase; LTP, lipid transfer protein; LCAT, lecithin cholesterol acyltransferase; FC, free cholesterol; CE, cholesterol ester; TG, triglyceride.

to be involved in multiple lipoprotein catabolism: 1) the conversion of remnant particles (IDL-remnant) initially formed by the action of LPL to triglyceride-rich LDL and then further to normal-density LDL by hydrolyzing the triglyceride of LDL; 2) the incorporation of HDL_2 into hepatocytes via the action of HTGL. We have demonstrated that HTGL plays roles in both reverse cholesterol transport via HDL_2 metabolism and effectively supplies cholesterol to peripheral tissues via the conversion of IDL to LDL.

REFERENCES

Auwerx JH, Marzetta CA, Hokanson JE, Brunzell JD 1989 Large buoyant LDL-like particles in hepatic lipase deficiency. Arteriosclerosis 9: 319–325

Breckenridge WC, Little JA, Alaupovic P *et al* 1982 Lipoprotein abnormalities associated with a familial deficiency of hepatic lipase. Atherosclerosis 45: 161–179

Cai SJ, Wong DM, Chen SH Chan L 1989 Structure of the human hepatic triglyceride lipase gene. Biochemistry 28: 8966–8971

Carlson LA, Holmquist L, Nilsson-Ehle P 1986 Deficiency of hepatic lipase activity in post-heparin plasma in familial hyper-a-triglyceridemia. Acta Med Scand 219: 435–447

Demant T, Carlson LA, Holmquist L *et al* 1988 Lipoprotein metabolism in hepatic lipase deficiency: studies on the turnover of apolipoprotein B and on the effect of hepatic lipase on high density lipoprotein. J Lipid Res 29: 1603–1611

Gotto AM Jr 1987 Plasma lipoproteins. New comprehensive biochemistry, vol. 14, Elsevier, Amsterdam

Hegele RA, Little JA, Vezina C *et al* 1993 Hepatic lipase deficiency. Clinical, biochemical. and molecular genetic characteristics. Arterioscler Thromb 13: 720–728

Ikeda Y, Takagi A, Yamamoto A 1989 Purification and characterization of lipoprotein lipase and hepatic triglyceride lipase from human postheparin plasma: production of monospecific antibody to the individual lipase. Biochim Biophys Acta 1003: 254–269

Ikeda Y, Takagi A, Ohkaru Y *et al* 1990 A sandwich-enzyme immunoassay for the quantification of lipoprotein lipase and hepatic triglyceride lipase in human postheparin plasma using monoclonal antibodies to the corresponding enzymes. J Lipid Res 31: 1911–1924

Jackson RL 1983 Lipoprotein lipase and hepatic

lipase. *In* Boyer PD (Ed) The Enzymes. Academic Press, New York, vol.16, pp 141–181

Kinnunen PKJ 1984 Hepatic endothelial lipase: Isolation, some characteristics, and physiological role. *In* Borgstrom B, Brockman HL (Eds) Lipase. Elsevier, Amsterdam, pp 307–328

Kuusi T, Nikkla EA, Virtanen I, Kinnunen PK 1979 Localization of the heparin-releasable lipase in situ in the rat liver. Biochem J 181: 245–246

SECTION 5.

OBESITY & HYPERINSULINEMIA

Multiple Risk Factors in Cardiovascular Disease, ed. by A. Yamamoto, Churchill Livingstone Japan, Tokyo, pp. 189–192 (1994)

METABOLIC BASIS FOR CORONARY HEART DISEASE RISK IN CENTRAL OBESITY AND GLUCOSE INTOLERANCE[§]

Wilfred Y. FUJIMOTO, Steven E. KAHN, and John D. BRUNZELL

*Division of Metabolism, Endocrinology, and Nutrition, University of Washington School of Medicine**

Key words: insulin resistance, visceral adiposity, lipoproteins

Japanese Americans have an increased prevalence of non-insulin-dependent diabetes mellitus (NIDDM) and coronary heart disease (CHD) compared with native Japanese (Fujimoto et *al* 1989). This has been associated with fasting hyperinsulinemia, hypertriglyceridemia, and low plasma levels of high density lipoprotein (HDL). Furthermore, all of these metabolic abnormalities are related to visceral adiposity assessed by computed tomography (CT) of the abdomen (Fujimoto *et al* 1989). Of interest is the metabolic basis for these associations which has been called the insulin resistance syndrome, the metabolic syndrome, or "Syndrome X" (Reaven 1988).

* Seattle, Washington 98195, USA.

§ This work was supported in part by grants from the National Institutes of Health (P01 DK-02456 and R22 DK-31170) and the Department of Veterans Affairs, and by services provided by the Diabetes Endocrinology Research Center (P30 DK-17047), the Clinical Nutrition Research Unit (P30 DK-35816), the Northwest Lipid Research Lipoprotein Laboratory, and the General Clinical Research Center (M01 RR-00037).

OBESITY AND INSULIN RESISTANCE

Obesity is an important risk factor for NIDDM and for CHD and is usually centripetal, shown by CT to be intra-abdominal (Fujimoto *et al* 1989). Although centripetal obesity is roughly correlated with overall obesity, it is an important risk factor independent of total body fat mass. Moreover, neither body mass index (BMI) nor waist-to-hip ratio (WHR) can be used to reliably predict the amount of intra-abdominal fat. Elevated fasting plasma levels of insulin occur with centripetal obesity (Fujimoto *et al* 1989) and such levels are a marker of insulin resistance and have been used as a proxy for insulin resistance.

Various techniques are available for quantitative assessment of *in vivo* insulin sensitivity (S_I). One method is the minimal model devised by Bergman *et al* (1979), used in the studies described here. By means of this method, S_I can be calculated.

Osei *et al* (1991) have reported that S_I was significantly lower in nondiabetic subjects with at least one parent who has NIDDM than in control subjects without any diabetic relatives. S_I exhibited a significant negative correlation with WHR in control subjects but not with body fat content. The correlation between S_I and WHR was not significant in offspring of NIDDM patients, although these offspring had significantly more body fat content than control subjects and a significant negative correlation between S_I and body fat content. It is possible that the increased body fat content in the offspring of NIDDM patients may have been mainly in a visceral location that could have been detected by CT.

LIPID ABNORMALITIES ASSOCIATED WITH OBESITY AND INSULIN RESISTANCE

Both hypertriglyceridemia and low HDL cholesterol are associated with obesity and insulin resistance. Hypertriglyceridemia has been atributed to both increased production and decreased clearance of very low density lipoprotein (VLDL). Hypertriglyceridemia is also often accompanied by low HDL levels, a well-recognized risk factor for atherosclerosis. In addition, high lipoprotein lipase (LPL) activity has been associated with high HDL levels while high hepatic lipase (HL) activity has been associated with low HDL levels.

Low density lipoprotein (LDL) cholesterol levels are not consistently abnormal in obesity or insulin resistance. LDL cholesterol levels, however, may not accurately reflect the number of LDL particles in the presence of hypertriglyceridemia. Moreover, centripetal obesity has been directly related to LDL particles that are small (assessed by nondenaturing polyacrylamide gradient gel electrophoresis) and dense (assessed by nonequilibrium density gradient ultracentrifugation using vertical rotor techniques). A pattern of smaller, denser LDL particles (pattern B) has been associated with a more atherogenic lipoprotein profile than a pattern of larger, more buoyant LDL (pattern A) (Austin *et al* 1988).

Barakat *et al* (1990) have reported that morbidly obese women with either impaired glucose tolerance or NIDDM had significantly smaller LDL peak density than either morbidly obese or lean nondiabetic women. Stewart *et al* (1993) have reported LDL particles to be smaller and denser in NIDDM patients when compared with control subjects matched for age, BMI, triglycerides, and HDL cholesterol. Reaven *et al* (1993) have reported that men and women with LDL subclass phenotype B were more glucose-intolerant and hyperinsulinemic and were more insulin-resistant than men and women with LDL subclass phenotype A matched by age, gender, and BMI. Body fat distribution was not assessed by these investigators.

Peeples *et al* (1989) have reported that 9 non-obese men with WHR > 1 (mean 1.05, range 1.01–1.07) matched by age and percentage body fat to 9 men with WHR < 1 (mean 0.94, range 0.88–0.96) had smaller and more dense LDL. Houmard *et al* (1991) have reported in 46 men that LDL size was negatively correlated with WHR, percentage body fat, and BMI. Furthermore, WHR was positively correlated with both percentage body fat and BMI.

RELATIONSHIP BETWEEN VISCERAL ADIPOSITY AND THE METABOLIC ABNORMALITIES OF THIS SYNDROME

The metabolic features of the insulin resistance syndrome are fasting hyperinsulinemia, hypertriglyceridemia, low HDL cholesterol, and small, dense LDL. Because Japanese Americans with NIDDM and CHD have many of the metabolic features of the insulin resistance syndrome, and because these seem to be strongly associated with visceral adiposity, we examined the relationship between visceral adiposity and S_I, plasma lipids and lipoproteins, LDL size and density, and post-heparin plasma HL and LPL activities in 6 second-generation (Nisei) Japanese-American men with NIDDM, each receiving an oral sulfonylurea. Each diabetic man was matched with 1 or 2 nondiabetic Nisei men, or a total of 9 nondiabetic men. Men were matched on the basis of age and

BMI. The amount of visceral adiposity was measured as intra-abdominal fat area by CT.

Diabetic subjects had significantly higher fasting plasma glucose ($p = 0.0007$) and lower SI ($p = 0.018$) than nondiabetic subjects. For all other characteristics, mean values between diabetic and nondiabetic subjects were not significantly different. Notably, mean BMI was 22.9 and 23.5 kg/m^2 ($p = 0.77$) and mean intra-abdominal fat area 121 and 78 cm^2 ($p = 0.11$) in NIDDM and nondiabetic men, respectively. Fasting plasma lipids and lipoproteins, LDL size and density, and post-heparin LPL and HL activities were likewise similar ($p = 0.11$ to 0.93).

Six men (2 with NIDDM) had LDL phenotype A and 8 (4 with NIDDM) had phenotype B. One nondiabetic man had an intermediate LDL pattern. Significantly greater amounts of intra-abdominal fat (121 vs 68 cm^2, $p = 0.045$) were found in men with phenotype B while fasting insulin (74 vs 46 pM, $p = 0.07$) and triglycerides (1.38 vs 0.91 mM, $p = 0.051$) tended to be higher. All other characteristics (BMI, fasting glucose, SI, lipids and lipoproteins, and post-heparin LPL and HL activities) were not significantly different ($p = 0.11$ to 0.95) between phenotypes A and B.

To examine more closely relationships between visceral adiposity and the metabolic variables, linear correlation analysis was performed for pairs of variables for all subjects combined. Intra-abdominal fat area was significantly correlated with SI ($r = -0.559$, $p = 0.030$), plasma triglycerides ($r = 0.541$, $p = 0.046$), LDL density measured as "relative flotation" ($r = -0.803$, $p = 0.001$), and plasma HDL cholesterol ($r = -0.717$, $p = 0.004$). Intra-abdominal fat was not significantly correlated with either HL or LPL, but SI tended to be correlated with HL ($r = -0.512$, $p = 0.061$). SI was not significantly correlated with any of the other variables.

SUMMARY

Japanese Americans have an increased prevalence of NIDDM and CHD when compared with native Japanese. This increase has been associated with fasting hyperinsulinemia, hypertriglyceridemia, and low plasma levels of HDL cholesterol.

Six Japanese-American men with NIDDM were matched for age and BMI with 9 nondiabetic Japanese-American men. Six men (2 with diabetes) had LDL phenotype A and 8 (4 with diabetes) had phenotype B. One nondiabetic subject had an intermediate LDL pattern. Significantly greater amounts of intra-abdominal fat ($p = 0.045$) measured by CT were found in the men with phenotype B while fasting insulin ($p = 0.070$) and triglycerides ($p = 0.051$) tended to be higher.

Linear correlation analysis was done for pairs of variables for all subjects combined. Intra-abdominal fat was significantly correlated with SI ($r = -0.559$), plasma triglycerides ($r = 0.541$), LDL density (relative flotation rate, $r = -0.803$), and plasma HDL cholesterol ($r = -0.717$). SI was not significantly correlated with any of the variables although it tended to be correlated with HL activity ($r = -0.512$, $p = 0.061$).

In conclusion, these observations indicate that in non-obese Japanese-American men, the metabolic features of the insulin resistance syndrome, including LDL phenotype B, are more strongly correlated with visceral adiposity than with insulin resistance. It may therefore be more appropriate to call this the visceral adiposity syndrome. Although questions concerning mechanisms still remain, we postulate that visceral adiposity plays a central role in the development of many of the metabolic abnormalities, including LDL subclass phenotype B, that occur in this metabolic syndrome (Fig. 1).

Acknowledgments

We are deeply indebted to the men who volunteered for this study. We thank Samuel Abbate, John Hokanson, Richard Chan, Ruth Hollingsworth, Carol Isaac, Alegria Aquino-Albers, Alem Nicodemis, Jennifer Cockburn, and the nursing staff of the General Clinical Research Center for their expert assistance. We also gratefully acknowledge the partici-

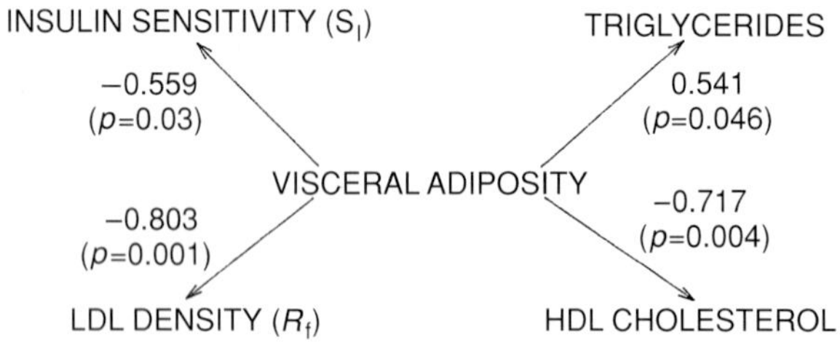

Fig. 1. Significant correlation of visceral adiposity with insulin sensitivity (S_I), fasting plasma levels of triglycerides and HDL cholesterol, and LDL density in Japanese-American men, suggesting a central role of visceral adiposity in the development of these metabolic abnormalities that are associated with coronary heart disease (CHD) and glucose intolerance.
Higher amounts of visceral fat are significantly related to lower S_I, higher triglycerides, lower HDL cholesterol, and higher LDL density (lower LDL relative flotation or R_f).

pation of Drs. Richard Bergstrom, Donna Leonetti, Laura Newell, and William Shuman in previous studies performed in these subjects from which the present study was developed.

REFERENCES

Austin MA, Breslow JL, Hennekens CH, Buring JE, Willett WC, Krauss RM 1988 Low-density lipoprotein subclass patterns and risk of myocardial infarction. JAMA 260: 1917–1921

Barakat HA, Carpenter JW, McLendon VD *et al* 1990 Influence of obesity, impaired glucose tolerance, and NIDDM on LDL structure and composition. Possible link between hyperinsulinemia and atherosclerosis. Diabetes 39: 1527–1533

Bergman RN, Ider YZ, Bowden CR, Cobelli C 1979 Quantitative estimation of insulin sensitivity. Am J Physiol 236: E667–677

Fujimoto WY, Bergstrom RW, Newell-Morris L, Leonetti DL 1989 Nature and nurture in the etiology of type 2 diabetes mellitus in Japanese Americans. Diabetes Metab Rev 5: 607–625

Houmard JA, Wheeler WS, McCammon MR *et al* 1991 An evaluation of waist to hip ratio measurement methods in reltion to lipid and carbohydrate metabolism in men. Int J Obesity 15: 181–188

Osei K, Cottrell DA, Orabella MM 1991 Insulin sensitivity, glucose effectiveness, and body fat distribution pattern in nondiabetic offspring of patients with NIDDM. Diabetes Care 14: 890–896

Peeples LH, Carpenter JW, Israel RG, Barakat HA 1989 Alterations in low-density lipoproteins in subjects with abdominal obesity. Metabolism 38: 1029–1036

Reaven GM 1988 Role of insulin resistance in human disease. Diabetes 37: 1595–1607

Stewart MW, Laker MF, Dyer RG *et al* 1993 Lipoprotein compositional abnormalities and insulin resistance in type II diabetic patients with mild hyperlipidemia. Arterioscler Thromb 13: 1046–1052

Multiple Risk Factors in Cardiovascular Disease, ed. by A. Yamamoto, Churchill Livingstone Japan, Tokyo, pp. 193–197 (1994)

CLUSTERS OF RISK FACTORS FOR CARDIOVASCULAR DISEASE IN ABDOMINAL OBESITY

Jean-Pierre Després

*Lipid Research Center, Laval University Medical Research Center**

Key words: visceral obesity, lipoproteins, insulin resistance, apolipoprotein B and E, genetic susceptibility

The concept of insulin resistance syndrome describing a cluster of metabolic disturbances which increases the risk of developing not only diabetes but also coronary heart disease (CHD) was first introduced by Reaven (1988) and has substantial public health implications. Indeed, Reaven (1988) has suggested that resistance to insulin-stimulated glucose uptake can be found in up to 25% of the non-diabetic population. This insulin resistance state which can be measured by the euglycemic hyperinsulinemic glucose clamp is associated with a dyslipidemic profile which includes not only elevated triglyceride and low high-density lipoprotein (HDL) cholesterol levels (Laakso *et al* 1990) but also an increased concentration of apolipoprotein B (apoB) as well as an elevated proportion of small dense low-density lipoprotein (LDL) particles (Després 1994). Epidemiological evidence indicates that the dyslipidemia associated with the insulin resistant-hyperinsulinemic state is associated with an increased CHD risk (Fontbonne *et al* 1989). Furthermore, the high prevalence of this condition has led to the suggestion that the insulin resistance syndrome may be the most frequent cause of CHD (Després 1993a, b). In this regard, we have been interested in studying the metabolic heterogeneity underlying fasting hypertriglyceridemia in the presence or absence of low HDL-cholesterol. In order to examine this issue, we have compared glucose tolerance and plasma insulin levels in individuals with elevated triglyceride concentrations but with either low or normal HDL-cholesterol (Lamarche *et al* 1993). We have reported that isolated hypertriglyceridemia was not associated with fasting hyperinsulinemia nor with any elevation in the insulin response to a standard 75 g oral glucose load. However, the dyslipidemic phenotype which includes fasting hypertriglyceridemia and low HDL-cholesterol, was associated with marked elevation in plasma insulin levels as well as with a greater insulin response to an oral glucose challenge, suggesting that this dyslipidemic profile is related to an impairment in insulin action. Thus, the high triglyceride low-HDL profile which has been reported to increase the risk of CHD (Assmann & Schulte 1992; Manninen *et al* 1992) is also associated with an insulin-resistant state (Laakso 1992).

* 2705 Laurier Blvd., S-102, Ste-Foy, Quebec, G1V 4G2 Canada

ABDOMINAL OBESITY: A COMPONENT OF THE INSULIN RESISTANT DYSLIPIDEMIC PHENOTYPE

It is now well accepted that a high proportion of abdominal fat is a risk factor for the development of Type II diabetes and that this association is independent of variations in the level of total body fat (Vague 1956; Björntorp 1988; Kissebah & Peiris 1989). Furthermore, prospective studies have shown that abdominal obesity is a major risk factor for cardiovascular disease and related mortality, this association also being independent of the level of obesity (Larsson *et al* 1984; Lapidus *et al* 1984; Stokes III *et al* 1985; Ducimetière *et al* 1986; Donahue *et al* 1987; Terry *et al* 1992). With the development of imaging techniques, it has been possible to more accurately measure the distribution of body fat. Computed tomography is a radiological technique that is able to assess not only the amount of subcutaneous fat but also the cross-sectional adipose tissue area located in the abdominal cavity, the so-called visceral adipose tissue, which includes omental, mesenteric, retroperitoneal, and perirenal adipose depots (Sjöström *et al* 1986). By measuring the amount of subcutaneous and visceral abdominal fat by computed tomography, we reported that the cross-sectional area of abdominal visceral adipose tissue was the best correlate of glucose tolerance as well as of the insulin response measured following a 75 g of glucose load in both men and women (Després *et al* 1989; Pouliot *et al* 1992). We have also compared two subgroups of obese subjects who were matched for their levels of total body fat but who had either low or high levels of visceral adipose tissue (Després *et al* 1990; Pouliot *et al* 1992). Obese men and women with low levels of visceral adipose tissue did not exhibit major alterations in their plasma lipoprotein lipid profiles in comparison with lean controls (Després *et al* 1990; Pouliot *et al* 1992). However, the subgroup of obese men and women with high levels of visceral fat exhibited alterations in glucose tolerance, hyperinsulinemia, and a marked dyslipidemic state which included hypertriglyceridemia, elevated plasma apoB, and marked reduction in HDL-cholesterol (Després *et al* 1990; Pouliot *et al* 1992). These results indicate that the visceral obese subjects represent a subgroup of obese patients clearly at greater risk of developing Type II diabetes and premature CHD (Després 1991).

ANTHROPOMETRIC ASSESSMENT OF ABDOMINAL VISCERAL OBESITY

As visceral obesity is clearly a component of the insulin-resistant dyslipidemic phenotype (Després 1993a), we were also interested in predicting visceral adipose tissue accumulation from simple anthropometric measurements. In this regard, we found that the waist circumference was a better correlate of the amount of cross-sectional visceral adipose tissue area measured by computed tomography than the commonly used ratio of waist-to-hip circumference (waist/hip ratio) (Pouliot *et al* 1994). Furthermore, we could explain up to 90% of the variance in the waist girth by using as independent variables the total adipose tissue mass and the cross-sectional visceral adipose tissue area (Pouliot *et al* 1994). Thus, it appears that the individual variation in waist circumference may depend upon variations in the level of total body fat as well as on the differences in the amount of visceral adipose tissue. We then became interested in finding out whether there would be a threshold of waist circumference above which we would observe a deterioration in the overall metabolic profile. It appears that a waist girth of approximately 1 m may delineate a gray zone above which metabolic disturbances associated with excess abdominal adipose tissue are more likely to be found. Therefore, measurement of a 1 m waist girth in an obese patient is a clear indication for undertaking further investigations of potential impairments in carbohydrate and lipid metabolism (Pouliot *et al* 1994b).

Furthermore, abdominal obesity combined with a high accumulation of visceral adipose tissue is frequently associated with cholesterol and LDL-cholesterol levels in the normal range. However, studies that have used additional techniques to assess potential changes in the composition and density of LDL have reported that abdominal obesity is associated with an elevated proportion of small dense LDL particles in the plasma (Harris Peeples *et al* 1989; Terry *et al* 1989). This greater proportion of dense LDL particles in the plasma may result from the hypertriglyceridemic state that is linked to abdominal visceral obesity (Després 1991). In addition, a reduced lipoprotein lipase is found in the heparinized plasma of abdominal obese patients (Després 1994). Therefore, from the insulin-resistant hyperinsulinemic state, an increased hepatic output of very-low density lipoprotein (VLDL) and apoB is observed which, when combined with the reduced clearance of triglyceride-rich lipoproteins (due to reduced lipoprotein lipase (LPL) activity), leads to a marked elevation in the concentration of triglyceride-rich lipoproteins. The resulting elevated concentrations of triglyceride-rich lipoproteins favor lipid exchange among lipoprotein fractions, resulting in a triglyceride enrichment of LDL and HDL particles. Furthermore, this triglyceride enrichment of LDL leads through the action of hepatic lipase to the formation of small dense-LDL particles (Després 1991). Therefore, the clinician will be misled by the measurement of plasma LDL-cholesterol concentrations in the insulin resistant visceral obese patient as these apparently normal levels are likely to mask marked alterations in LDL composition and a substantial increase in the proportion of atherogenic dense LDL particles.

THE INSULIN RESISTANCE DYSLIPIDEMIC SYNDROME: CONTRIBUTION OF GENETIC SUSCEPTIBILITY

Finally, although there are significant associations between visceral adipose tissue accumulation, impairment in insulin action, and a dyslipidemic profile predictive of an increased risk of CHD, not every visceral obese patient is at high risk of premature CHD. We have therefore postulated that some genes involved in lipoprotein metabolism may modulate the relationship between visceral obesity and dyslipidemias and ultimately determine susceptibility to premature CHD. For example, we have reported that apoE and apoB polymorphisms are important modulators of the relationship between visceral adipose tissue accumulation and plasma lipoprotein-lipid levels. Indeed, we have reported that visceral obese patients who were also carriers of the apoE $\in$ 2 allele were characterized by having significantly higher plasma triglyceride levels in comparison with apoE $\in$ 2 carriers with low levels of visceral fat, whereas we could not find any difference in plasma triglycerides between apoE $\in$ 4 carriers with either low or high levels of visceral fat (Pouliot *et al* 1990). We have also found an apoB polymorphism that can modulate the magnitude of the increase in plasma apoB levels in visceral obesity (Pouliot *et al* 1994a). Therefore, the polymorphism observed for some candidate genes relevant to lipoprotein-lipid metabolism may substantially affect the relationship between abdominal visceral fat accumulation and metabolic complications. It is therefore of paramount importance to identify those genetic markers of susceptibility to dyslipidemia and premature CHD in order to be able to tailor therapeutic approaches that are adapted to the genetic profile of each abdominally obese and insulin-resistant patient.

SUMMARY

It appears that visceral obesity and insulin resistance are two important features of a highly prevalent dyslipidemic profile which includes elevated plasma triglyceride and apoB levels and reduced HDL-cholesterol. Although the relationship between visceral obesity, insulin resistance and dyslipidemia is highly significant, there is still considerable metabolic heterogeneity among visceral obese patients. In this regard, the variation in the genes involved in lipoprotein metabolism is an important factor to take into account in the ultimate estimation of CHD risk in the visceral obese patient. Better knowledge of the interaction between genetic susceptibility to dyslipidemia and visceral adipose tissue accumulation will allow the development of individualized approaches for the prevention of CHD in the abdominal obese patient.

REFERENCES

Assmann G, Schulte H 1992 Relation of high-density lipoprotein cholesterol and triglycerides to incidence of atherosclerotic coronary heart disease (the PROCAM experience). Am J Cardiol 70: 733–737

Björntorp P 1988 Abdominal obesity and the development of non-insulin dependent diabetes mellitus. Diabetes Metab Rev 4: 615–622

Després JP 1991 Obesity and lipid metabolism: relevance of body fat distribution. Curr Opin in Lipidol 2: 5–15

Després JP 1993a Abdominal obesity as important component of insulin-resistance syndrome. Nutrition 9: 452–459

Després JP 1993b The insulin resistance-dyslipidemia syndrome: The most prevalent cause of coronary artery disease? Can Med Assoc J 148: 1339–1340

Després JP 1994 Dyslipidaemia and obesity. Baillières Clin Endocrinol Metab B:629–660

Després JP, Nadeau A, Tremblay A *et al* 1989 Role of deep abdominal fat in the association between regional adipose tissue distribution and glucose tolerance in obese women. Diabetes 38: 304–309

Després JP, Moorjani S, Lupien PJ e*t al* 1990 Regional distribution of body fat, plasma lipoproteins, and cardiovascular disease. Arteriosclerosis 10: 497–511

Donahue RP, Abbott RD, Bloom E *et al* 1987 Central obesity and coronary heart disease in men. Lancet April: 822–824

Ducimetière P, Richard J, Cambien F 1986 The pattern of subcutaneous fat distribution in middle-aged men and the risk of coronary heart disease: The Paris Prospective Study. Int J Obes 10: 229–240

Fontbonne A, Eschwège E, Cambien F *et al* 1989 Hypertriglyceridemia as a risk factor of coronary heart disease mortality in subjects with impaired glucose tolerance or diabetes. Results from the 11-year follow-up of the Paris Prospective Study. Diabetologia 32: 300–304

Harris Peeples L, Carpenter JW, Israel RG, Barakat HA 1989 Alterations in low-density lipoproteins in subjects with abdominal obesity. Metabolism 38: 1029–1036

Kissebah AH, Peiris AN 1989 Biology of regional body fat distribution: Relationship to non-insulin-dependent diabetes mellitus. Diabetes Metab Rev 5: 83–109

Laakso M 1992 Dyslipidaemias, insulin resistance and atherosclerosis. Ann Med 14: 505–509

Laakso M, Sarlund H, Mykkanen L 1990 Insulin resistance is associated with lipid and lipoprotein abnormalities in subjects with varying degrees of glucose tolerance. Arteriosclerosis 10: 223–231

Lamarche B, Després JP, Pouliot MC *et al* 1993 Metabolic heterogeneity associated with high plasma triglyceride or low HDL-cholesterol levels in men. Arterioscler Thromb 13: 33–40

Lapidus L, Bengtsson C, Larsson B *et al* 1984 Distribution of adipose tissue and risk of cardiovascular disease and death: a 12 year follow-up of participants in the population study of women in Gothenburg, Sweden. BMJ 289: 1261–1263

Larsson B, Svardsudd K, Welin L *et al* 1984 Abdominal adipose tissue distribution, obesity and risk of cardiovascular disease and death: 13 year follow-up of participants in the study of men born in 1913. BMJ 288: 1401–1404

Manninen V, Tenkanen L, Koskinen P *et al* 1992 Joint effects of serum triglyceride and LDL cholesterol and HDL cholesterol concentrations on coronary heart disease risk in the Helsinki Heart Study. Implications for treatment. Circulation 85: 37–45

Pouliot MC, Després JP, Moorjani S *et al* 1990 Apolipoprotein E polymorphism alters the association between body fatness and plasma lipoproteins in women. J Lipid Res 31: 1023–1029

Pouliot MC, Després JP, Nadeau A *et al* 1992 Visceral obesity in men. Associations with glucose tolerance, plasma insulin and lipoprotein levels. Diabetes 41: 826–834

Pouliot MC, Després JP, Dionne FT *et al* 1994a Apolipoprotein B-100 gene EcoRI polymorphism: Relations to the plasma liporptein changes associated with abdominal visceral obesity. Arterioscler Thromb 14:527–533

Pouliot MC, Després JP, Lemieux S *et al* 1994b Waist circumference and abdominal sagittal diameter: Best simple anthropometric indexes of abdominal visceral adipose tissue accumulation and related cardiovascular risk in men and women? Am J Cardiol 73:460–468

Reaven GM 1988 Role of insulin resistance in human disease. Diabetes 37: 1595–1607

Sjöström L, Kvist H, Cederblad A, Tylen U 1986 Determination of total adipose tissue and body fat in women by computed tomography, ^{40}K, and tritium. Am J Physiol (Endocrinol Metab) 250: E736–E745

Stokes J lll, Garrison RJ, Kannel WB 1985 The independent contributions of various indices of obesity to the 22-year incidence of coronary heart disease: The Framingham heart study. *In*: Vague J, Björntorp P, GuyGrand B *et al* (Eds) Metabolic complications of human obesities. Elsevier Science Publishers, Amsterdam, p 49–57

Terry RB, Wood PD, Haskell WL *et al* 1989 Regional adiposity pattern in relation to lipids, lipoprotein cholesterol, and lipoprotein subfraction mass in men. J Clin Endocrinol Metab 68: 191–199

Terry RB, Page WF, Haskell WL 1992 Waist/hip ratio, body mass index and premature cardiovascular disease mortality in US army veteran during a twenty-three year follow-up study. Int J Obesity 16: 417–423

Vague J 1956 The degree of masculine differentiation of obesities: a factor determining predisposition to diabetes, atherosclerosis, gout and uric-calculous disease. Am J Clin Nutr 4: 20–34

Multiple Risk Factors in Cardiovascular Disease, ed. by A. Yamamoto, Churchill Livingstone Japan, Tokyo, pp. 199–202 (1994)

THE ROLE OF HYPERINSULINEMIA IN THE DEVELOPMENT OF VISCERAL-TYPE OBESITY

Kohji SHIRAI,[*1] Hidekuni INADERA,[*2] Shunichi MURANO,[*2] Masaki SHINOMIYA,[*2] Sho YOSHIDA,[*2] and Yasushi SAITO[*3]

[*1] *Clinical Laboratory Medicine, Toho University, Sakura Hospital,* [*2] *The Second Department of Internal Medicine, Chiba University, and* [*3] *Clinical Laboratory Medicine, Yamagata University*

Key words: insulin, visceral fat, glucose uptake, triglyceride synthesis, insulinoma

Alteration in body fat distribution is one of the features of endocrine and metabolic disorders and is related to coronary heart disease (Nakajima *et al* 1989). In particular, visceral-type obesity is reported to accompany many coronary risk factors such as hypertension, glucose intolerance, and dyslipoproteinemia. However, the causes of visceral fat deposition are unknown.

Hormonal studies show that hyperinsulinemia is frequently observed in visceral-type obesity (Evans *et al* 1984). However, it is not known if the hyperinsulinemia directly causes the development of visceral adipose tissue, or is only an associated phenomenon.

In this report, to clarify the role of insulin in the development of visceral-type obesity, the body fat distribution of patients with insulinoma, where plasma insulin levels are primarily high, was studied. Furthermore, the effects of insulin on the proliferation of fibroblast-like cells, which originate in adipose tissues and are thought to be immature adipocytes, and on the triglyceride-synthesizing activities of the subcutaneous and visceral adipose tissues were studied.

BODY FAT DISTRIBUTION OF PATIENTS WITH INSULINOMA

The abdominal fat distribution in 7 patients with insulinoma was studied. The visceral fat (V) and subcutaneous fat (S) areas were measured by radiographic computed tomography (CT). The area with a CT value of –50

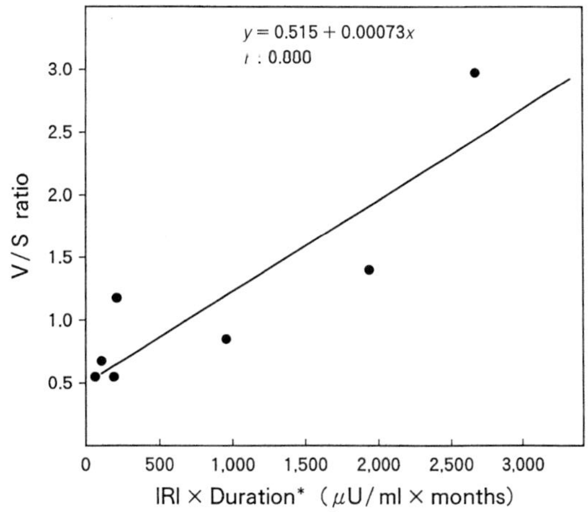

Fig. 1. The correlation between plasma insulin levels × disease duration (IRI × Duration) and the ratio of visceral and subcutaneous fat areas (V/S) in patients with insulinoma.
* Duration of insulinoma.

[*1] 564-1 Shimoshizu, Sakura 284, Japan.

to −100 was calculated as fatty tissue. The diagnosis of insulinoma was made from clinical signs such as a low blood glucose and a high insulin, and was confirmed by histological investigation of the tissue obtained during the operation.

The ratios of the area of visceral fat to subcutaneous fat (V/S) were all greater than the average value, 0.4 (Inadera et *al* 1993). Furthermore, as shown in Fig. 1, the plasma insulin level × disease duration (IRI × Duration) was significantly correlated with this V/S ratio. These results suggest that high levels of plasma insulin promote the development of visceral adipose tissue.

EFFECT OF INSULIN ON THE PROLIFERATION OF FIBROBLAST-LIKE CELLS FROM SUBCUTANEOUS ADIPOSE TISSUE AND EPIDIDYMAL ADIPOSE TISSUE IN RATS

Adipose tissue development is regulated by at least two factors: one is the proliferation of the adipocytes and the other is the accumulation of triglycerides in the cells. These properties and the effect of insulin were compared by studying subcutaneous adipose tissue and visceral adipose tissue in the rat.

In this study, we compared subcutaneous adipose tissue with epididymal adipose tissue as an example of one of the visceral adipose tissues.

At first, cell proliferation was compared. The fibroblast-like cells were obtained from both sites of adipose tissues by the ceiling culture method (Sugihara *et al* 1989). Fibroblast-like cells were cultured in DME medium containing 10% fetal calf serum in a CO_2 incubator. Cell proliferation was determined by counting the cell numbers using a Coulter counter (Counter Electronics, Luton, UK).

Proliferation of the fibroblast-like cells from subcutaneous adipose tissue was significantly faster than that from epididymal adipose tissue (data not shown). The population doubling times were 2.6 days and 4.1 days for subcutaneous and epididymal adipose tissues, respectively.

The addition of insulin (10 nM) enhanced the proliferation of subcutaneous fibroblast-like cells much more than that of epididymal fibroblast-like cells.

These results suggest that the proliferative abilities of adipocytes are different in the two types of adipose tissue, and the development of subcutaneous adipose tissue may be caused by cell proliferation due to insulin, while that of visceral adipose tissue is not.

EFFECT OF INSULIN ON [^{14}C] DEOXY-GLUCOSE UPTAKE AND TRIGLYCERIDE SYNTHESIS FROM [^{14}C] PALMITATE IN SUBCUTANEOUS AND EPIDIDYMAL ADIPOSE TISSUES

The effects of insulin on glucose uptake and triglyceride synthesis were compared between subcutaneous adipose tissue and visceral adipose tissue. Epididymal adipose tissue was used as one of the visceral adipose tissues in the Zucker-obese rat.

Glucose uptake was studied using [^{14}C] deoxy-glucose (Nishide *et al* 1987). After incubation, with or without insulin (10 nM) for 60 min, the tissues were washed and their radioactivity was counted.

Triglyceride synthesizing activity was evaluated using [^{14}C] palmitate (Matsuoka *et al* 1974). After incubation of the adipose tissues in the presence or absence of insulin (10 nM), the lipids were extracted. The radioactivity in the triglyceride fraction, separated by thin-layer chromatography, was counted.

As shown in Fig. 2, [^{14}C] deoxy-glucose uptake and triglyceride synthesizing activity from [^{14}C] palmitate were enhanced by the addition of insulin, much more in epididymal adipose tissue than in subcutaneous adipose tissue.

These results suggest that the development of epididymal adipose tissue may be induced by an increase in triglyceride synthesis by insulin.

DISCUSSION

Clinically, we investigated insulinoma patients, whose plasma insulin levels were primarily high. All patients exhibited visceral-type obesity and insulin level × duration correlated with V/S. These results indicate that high insulin levels may promote the development of a visceral-type obesity.

In a series of *in vitro* studies, we compared the properties of subcutaneous and epididymal adipose tissues in rats. The proliferation of fibroblast-like cells, which are thought to be immature adipocytes, was higher in subcutaneous adipose tissue than in epididymal adipose tissue, and their enhancement by insulin was also greater in subcutaneous adipose tissue. These results suggest that insulin is not involved in increasing epididymal adipose tissue by inducing cell proliferation.

Glucose uptake and triglyceride synthesis were enhanced by the addition of insulin, much more in epididymal adipose tissue than in subcutaneous adipose tissue.

It is controversial whether epididymal adipose tissue shares any common properties with typical visceral adipose tissue such as mesenteric adipose tissue. Considering that both types of adipose tissues exist in the peritoneal cavity and are commonly covered with peritoneum, the properties of these cells are generally supposed to be similar, although not identical. The above results are consistent with the idea that hyperinsulinemia can cause the development of visceral adipose tissue by enhancing triglyceride synthesis. Further studies on the properties of different parts of visceral adipose tissues are required.

Insulin insensitivity is supposed to underlie the visceral type of obesity (Fujioka *et al* 1987). If the adipose tissue is resistant to insulin, hyperinsulinemia would not affect triglyceride synthesis in adipose tissue. However, insulin resistance is mainly supposed to be due to muscle tissue and it is believed that adipose tissue retains insulin sensitivity (Cusin 1990). For this reason, we favor the hypothesis that hyperinsulinemia may cause the development of the visceral type of obesity.

More detailed studies of the insulin sensitivity of different parts of visceral adipose tissues are needed.

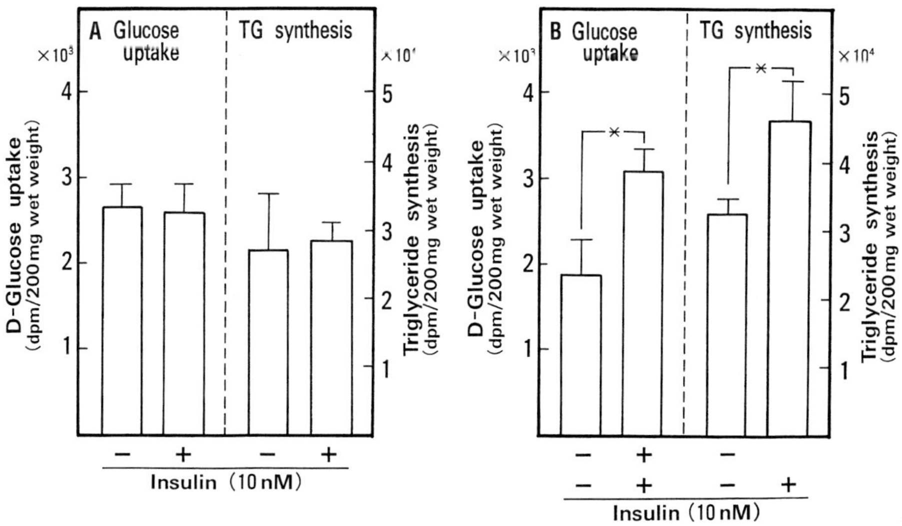

Fig 2. Effect of insulin on [14C] deoxy-glucose uptake and triglyceride (TG) synthesis from [14C] palmitate in subcutaneous and epididymal adipose tissues.
A, subcutaneous adipose tissues; B, visceral adipose tissues.

SUMMARY

The role of insulin on the formation of visceral-type obesity was investigated.

Patients with insulinoma exhibited a visceral type of obesity. The increase in glucose uptake and triglyceride synthesis from palmitate by the addition of insulin, were greater in epididymal adipose tissue than in subcutaneous adipose tissue.

These results suggest that hyperinsulinemia may be involved in the formation of the visceral type of obesity.

REFERENCES

Cusin I, Terrettaz J, Jeanrenaud RF, Jeanrenaud B 1990 Metabolic consequence of hyperinsulinemia imposed to normal rats on glucose handling by white adipose tissue, muscle and liver. Biochem J 267: 99–103

Evans DJ, Hoffman RG, Kalkhoff RK, Kissebah AH 1984 Relationship of body fat topography to insulin sensitivity and metabolic profiles in premenopausal women. Metabolism 33: 68–75

Fujioka S, Matsuzawa Y, Tokunaga K, Tarui S 1987 Contribution of intra-abdominal fat accumulation to the impairment of glucose and lipid metabolism in human obesity. Metabolism 36: 54–59

Inadera H, Ito S, Shinomiya M, Shirai K, Saito Y, Yoshida S 1993 Visceral fat deposition is seen patient with insulinoma. Diabetologia 36: 91–92

Matsuoka N, Saito Y, Okuda T, Fujii S 1974 Studies on triglyceride synthesis in lipid miscelles from adipose tissue. J Biochem 76: 359–364

Nakajima T, Fujioka Tokunaga K, Matsuzawa Y 1989 correlation of intraabdominal fat accumulation and left ventricular performance in obesity. Am J Cardiol 64: 369–373

Nishide T, Shirai K, Saito Y, Yoshida S 1987 Modification of intracellular glucose metabolism in human skin fibroblasts preincubated with *p*-chlorophenoxyisobutyrate. Br J Clin Pharmacol 24: 763–767

Sugihara H, Funatsumaru S, Yonemitu N, Miyabara S, Toda S, Hikichi Y 1989 A simple culture method of fat cells from mature fat tissue fragments. J Lipid Res 30: 1987–1986

Multiple Risk Factors in Cardiovascular Disease, ed. by A. Yamamoto, Churchill Livingstone Japan, Tokyo, pp. 203–207 (1994)

INSULIN RESISTANCE AND ATHEROSCLEROTIC VASCULAR DISEASE

Ryuichi FUJIWARA and Tsuguhiko NAKAI

*The Third Department of Internal Medicine, Fukui Medical School**

Key words: insulin resistance, coronary artery disease, apolipoprotein, vascular smooth muscle cells, Ca influx

In addition to the well-known association of obesity, diabetes mellitus (DM), and hypertension with coronary artery disease (CAD), recent prospective studies (Stout 1985) have shown that hyperinsulinemia is itself associated with an increased risk of CAD in non-diabetic subjects and this risk is independent of other CAD risk factors. Furthermore, it has been suggested that insulin resistance and hyperinsulinemia may be the common element accounting for the association of obesity, non-insulin-dependent diabetes mellitus (NIDDM), and hypertension play an important role in the pathogenesis and clinical course of CAD. There seems to be a substantial overlap of these conventional CAD risk factors in the general population. Our previous report (Fujiwara *et al* 1989a) demonstrated that endogenous hyperinsulinemia might be an important marker of an enhanced liability to develop CAD in normolipidemic borderline diabetic male patients.

This review will focus on the clinical and experimental aspects of the role of insulin in atherogenesis. The metabolic effect of hyperinsulinemia will be examined in normolipidemic male patients with varying degrees of glucose tolerance, particularly the relationship of angiographically-defined CAD to hyperinsulinemia, plasma lipids, or other CAD risk factors. We will also describe the effect of insulin on DNA synthesis (Fujiwara *et al* 1989b) and the activation of neutral cholesteryl ester hydrolase in cultured rat vascular smooth muscle cells (VSMC).

CLINICAL STUDY

Relationship of Endogenous Hyperinsulinemia to Angiographically-defined CAD in Normolipidemic Patients with Varying Degrees of Glucose Tolerance

The subjects were 127 normolipidemic (total cholesterol (T-Ch) < 230 mg/dl and triglycerides (TG) < 150 mg/dl) male patients aged 40 to 78 years who were referred to our clinic for coronary angiographic evaluations of chest pain suggestive of CAD. A stenosis of 75% or more of the cross-sectional area assessed by coronary cine angiography was considered indicative of significant CAD. The presence and severity of stenosis were determined by means of a separate classification system in 15 proximal coronary arterial segments which were defined according to the grading of the American Heart Associa-

* Matsuoka-cho, Fukui 910-11, Japan.

tion. The severity of atherosclerotic changes was also assessed by grading the stenotic lesions as follows: 0 = luminal reduction less than 25%; 1 = luminal reduction of 25–50%; 2 = luminal reduction of 50–75%; 3 = luminal reduction of 75–90%; 4 = luminal reduction of 90–95%; 5 = luminal reduction of 95–99%; 6 = total occlusion. The grading points for each branch of the coronary arteries were summed and a coronary score obtained. According to the results of coronary angiography, the patients were divided into two groups: those with normal coronary arteries (NCA) group ($n = 33$) and those with CAD group ($n = 94$). Plasma T-Ch and TG were measured by enzymatic methods. For high density lipoprotein (HDL)-Ch determination, very low density lipoprotein (VLDL) was first removed by ultracentrifugation at a density of 1.006 g/ml. Cholesterol was measured enzymatically in the supernatant after precipitation of low density lipoprotein (LDL) with sodium heparin and $MnCl_2$ using the VLDL free fraction. Plasma apolipoproteins (apo) A-I and B were determined by single radial immunodiffusion. Diagnosis of DM and impaired glucose tolerance (IGT) was based on a 75 g oral glucose tolerance test (OGTT). Venous blood samples were collected for determination of plasma glucose and insulin before, 30, 60, and 120 min after glucose ingestion. OGTT was assessed according to the criteria proposed by the WHO Expert Committee on Diabetes Mellitus. The glucose and insulin responses to the glucose load were calculated as the sum of the glucose values (ΣPG) and the sum of the plasma insulin levels (ΣIRI), respectively. The early glucose and insulin responses to glucose load were calculated as the differences between 0 and 30 min in the glucose (ΔPG) and insulin values (ΔIRI), respectively. The ratios of insulin over glucose concentration were also calculated (ΣIRI/ΣPG and ΔIRI/ΔPG). Hypertensive subjects were defined as those using antihypertensive medication, or whose systolic blood pressure was > 160 mmHg, or whose diastolic blood pressure was > 95 mmHg. All data were stored in a Statistical Analysis System (SAS) data base and were analyzed using the Mann-Whitney U test, chi-squared test with Yates' correction, Pearson's correlation coefficient, and stepwise multiple regression analysis. For statistical significance, a value of $p < 0.05$ was considered significant. All data were presented as means ± SEM.

Metabolic data of the study population are summarized in Table I. Of the 127 consecutive male patients undergoing coronary angiography, 94(74%) had significant CAD, and 33 patients(26%) were considered to be in the NCA group. Little differences in conventional risk factors for CAD were found between the NCA and CAD groups. The mean age, body mass index, and prevalence of hypertension were similar in the two groups. The prevalence of IGT and NIDDM was also similar in both groups. However, cumulative lifetime tobacco consumption

TABLE I. Concentrations of Plasma Lipids and Apolipoproteins and Insulin Response to the 75 g Oral Glucose Tolerance Test in NCA and CAD Groups

	Univariate comparison of plasma concentrations		
	NCA ($n = 33$)	CAD ($n = 94$)	p value
Total cholesterol	167 ± 5	186 ± 3	< 0.001
Triglyceride	100 ± 4	118 ± 3	< 0.001
HDL-cholesterol	47 ± 2	36 ± 1	< 0.001
Apolipoproteins			
A-1	114 ± 4	88 ± 2	< 0.001
B	89 ± 3	117 ± 2	< 0.001
Basal PG	96 ± 2	97 ± 1	NS
Basal IRI	9.4 ± 0.6	9.5 ± 0.4	NS
ΣPG	628 ± 17	632 ± 11	NS
ΣIRI	152 ± 13	229 ± 10	< 0.001
$\Sigma IRI/\Sigma PG \times 10^3$	249 ± 25	363 ± 15	< 0.001
ΔPG	81 ± 4	80 ± 3	NS
ΔIRI	24.4 ± 4.2	50.9 ± 3.6	< 0.001
$\Delta IRI/\Delta PG \times 10^2$	31.5 ± 5.5	67.6 ± 4.6	< 0.001

PG, plasma glucose; IRI, immunoreactive insulin; ΣPG, sum of glucose values; ΣIRI, sum of plasma insulin levels; ΔPG, differences between 0 and 30 min of glucose values; ΔIRI, differences between 0 and 30 min of plasma insulin values. Values are mean ± SEM.

was significantly higher in the CAD group ($p < 0.001$). T-Ch ($p < 0.001$) and TG ($p < 0.001$) levels were significantly higher in the subjects with CAD compared with those in the subjects without CAD. The HDL-Ch concentration in the CAD group was significantly lower than in the NCA group ($p < 0.001$). Plasma apoB levels were significantly higher in patients with CAD than in the patients without CAD ($p < 0.001$), whereas plasma apoA-I levels were significantly lower in the CAD group ($p < 0.001$). Of the 127 individuals, 41(32.3%) exhibited normal glucose tolerance (NGT), 41(32.3%) IGT, and 45(35.4%) were diabetic. A hyperinsulinemic response to the oral glucose load was observed in the subjects with CAD. The elevations of plasma insulin throughout the study and the early phase of OGTT were higher in the CAD group than in the NCA group. The ΣPG, basal glucose and insulin levels and the ΔPG were not significantly different between two groups. In the total patient group, graded reductions in HDL-Ch and apoA-I were observed with increasing tertiles of the sum of plasma insulin concentrations during the oral glucose challenge. Graded increases in T-Ch, TG, and apoB were also observed in the total patient group with increasing tertiles of the postglucose challenge and measures of insulinemia. These data indicate that endogenous hyperinsulinemia plays a crucial role in the pathogenesis of coronary atherosclerosis and is associated with adverse lipid, lipoprotein, and apolipoprotein changes favoring coronary atherosclerosis not only in nondiabetic patients but also in IGT and NIDDM.

EXPERIMENTAL STUDY

Effects of Insulin and Insulin-like Growth Factor-I on the DNA Synthesis of Cultured Rat VSMC

VSMC were isolated from rat aorta and cultured for several passages as described previously (Fujiwara *et al* 1993). The cells were subcultured in Dulbecco's modified Eagle's medium (DMEM) supplemented with 10% fetal calf serum (FCS). The cultured VSMC in confluent stages were dissociated by trypsinization and seeded into 35-mm plastic culture dishes in the same medium. For all experiments, VSMC in the synthetic phase were used between the fourth and eighth passages. VSMC in the logarithmic phase had their growth arrested by placing them in serum-free DMEM for 72 h. After VSMC had reached the G_0-arrested state, cells were exposed to insulin or insulin-like growth factor-I (IGF-I) for 48 h and incubated with [^{3}H]thymidine for the last 24 h. Cells were fixed with 10% trichloroacetic acid (TCA) and the TCA-insoluble counts were determined.

Both insulin and IGF-I stimulated [^{3}H]thymidine incorporation into the DNA of the cells in serum-free DMEM in a dose-dependent manner, especially in 0.5% FCS-containing medium. As shown in Fig. 1, VSMC in the logarithmic phase responded to insulin or IGF-I by exhibiting up to a 3-fold increase in the rate of DNA synthesis. The effect of IGF-I was approximately 10–100 times more potent in stimulating [^{3}H] thymidine incorporation than that of insulin. To investigate the role of intracellular Ca^{2+} in the mechanism of VSMC growth, VSMC were incubated with insulin or IGF-I with or without diltiazem, a Ca^{2+} channel blocker. At a concentration of 3×10^{-8} M diltiazem inhibited [^{3}H]thymidine incorporation stimulated by insulin and the average inhibitory effect at each concentration of insulin was approximately 17%.

Diltiazem inhibited DNA synthesis stimulated by insulin or IGF-I in a dose-dependent manner. Both insulin and IGF-I increased the unidirectional $^{45}Ca^{2+}$ uptake in a dose-dependent manner. These results suggest that the growth-promoting action of insulin and IGF-I on VSMC may be important for the development of atherosclerosis and that the effect of insulin and IGF-I on the growth of VSMC may be coupled to an increase in Ca^{2+} influx.

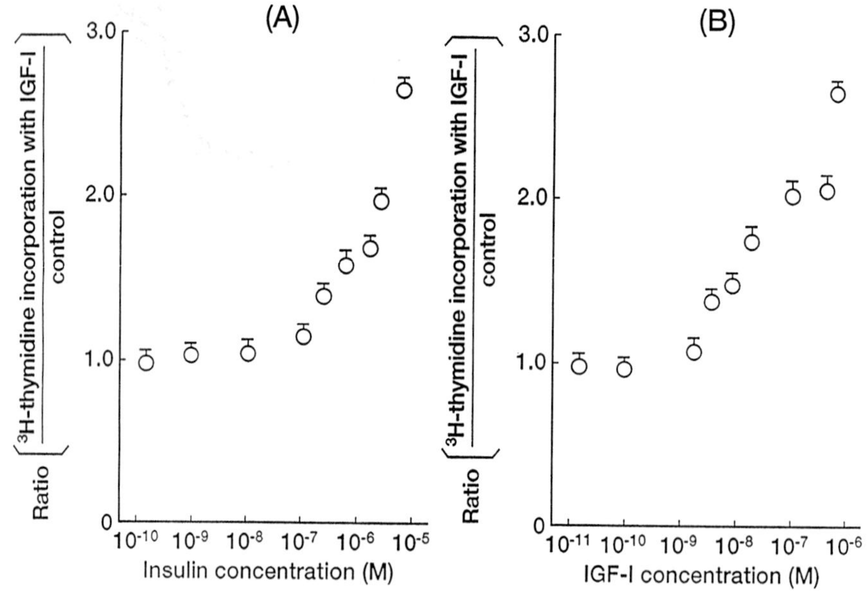

Fig. 1. Effects of insulin(A) and IGF-I(B) on [^{3}H]thymidine incorporation into DNA of VSMC.
Each point represents the means ± SEM of triplicate determinations. IGF-I, insulin-like growth factor-I; VSMC, vascular smooth muscle cells.

Effects of Insulin and IGF-I on the Activation of Neutral Cholesteryl Esterase in VSMC
When VSMC became confluent, they were washed in Hepes buffer and their growth arrested by placing them in serum-free DMEM for 48 h. Cells were exposed to insulin or IGF-I for 24 h and then cell homogenates were prepared. The neutral cholesteryl esterase (CEase) activity in VSMC was measured by the addition of cholesteryl-[1-^{14}C]oleate and the amount of liberated [1-^{14}C]oleate was counted.

Insulin over the range 10^{-8}–10^{-6} M significantly inhibited neutral CEase activity by 74% in VSMC in a dose-dependent manner. A similar selective inhibition of neutral CEase activity was exhibited by IGF-I. Incubation of cells with 10^{-8} M insulin for 24 h was found to reduce neutral CEase activity from 1,210 ± 30 to 920 ± 40 fmol/mg protein/min. These data suggest that both insulin and IGF-I participate in the regulation of processes leading to the accretion of cholesteryl ester in the arterial wall by modulating neutral CEase activity in VSMC.

SUMMARY

There are now various pieces of evidence to show that high insulin concentrations predispose patients to develop CAD (Fujiwara *et al* 1989a, 1990). The most plausible evidence comes from prospective epidemiological studies of CAD conducted in Helsinki, Paris, and Busselton, Western Australia (Stout 1985). In each study, there was a significant association between insulin concentration and the development of CAD and this was independent of other risk factors including plasma lipids, blood pressure and smoking. Recently, it has been suggested that insulin resistance, with its compensatory hyperinsulinemia unites with glucose intolerance, hypertension, dyslipidemia, and CAD to form a distinct syndrome (insulin resistance syndrome). Insulin resistance syndrome is a multifaceted syndrome that can express itself in many ways, depending on a particular individual's genetic background. Insulin resistance is a common disorder which occurs with high frequency in the general population. Within the normal healthy adult population there is a wide spectrum of insulin resistance. On the basis of our clinical data, we conclude that the basic defects in the subjects with CAD were insulin resistance and hyperinsulinemia, irrespective of the glucose tolerance status, with the changes observed in lipid metabolism and blood pressure resulting from abnormalities in insulin metabolism. Furthermore, our experimental evidence of the effects of insulin reported here can be used to form a concept linking hyperinsulinemia to the development of atherosclerosis. Studies in our laboratory have demonstrated that insulin appears to promote the development of atherosclerosis not only by stimulating the proliferation of VSMC but also by modulating lipid metabolism in VSMC. In addition, insulin could lead to increases in Ca^{2+} uptake which, in turn, would result in enhanced vascular responses to various agonists. This model provides a mechanism by which the hyperinsulinemia associated with clinical cardiovascular disease can promote the development of atherosclerosis.

REFERENCES

Fujiwara R, Kutsumi Y, Hayashi T *et al* 1989a Coronary risk factors in normolipidemic borderline diabetic patients with angiographically defined coronary artery disease. J Jpn Diabetes Soc 32: 853–857

Fujiwara R, Nakai T, Miyabo S 1989b Effect of calcium antagonist on DNA synthesis induced by insulin or IGF-I in cultured rat arterial smooth muscle cells. J Jpn Coll Angiol 29: 715–720

Fujiwara R, Kutsumi Y, Hayashi T *et al* 1990 Metabolic risk factors in the normolipidemic male patients with angiographically defined coronary artery disease. Jpn Circ J 54: 493–500

Fujiwara R, Hayashi T, Kutsumi Y *et al* 1993 Effects of nicorandil on cell proliferation and cholesteryl ester accumulation in arterial smooth muscle cells in culture. Cardiovasc Drugs Ther 7: 365–372

Stout RW 1985 Overview of the association between insulin and atherosclerosis. Metabolism 34 (suppl 1): 7–12

SECTION 6.

LIPOPROTEIN & THROMBOMODULATION SYSTEM

Multiple Risk Factors in Cardiovascular Disease, ed. by A. Yamamoto, Churchill Livingstone Japan, Tokyo, pp. 211–216 (1994)

RELATIONSHIP BETWEEN HYPERLIPIDEMIA AND TISSUE FACTOR-INDUCED BLOOD COAGULATION WITH EMPHASIS ON TISSUE FACTOR PATHWAY INHIBITOR

Per Morten SANDSET

*Haematological Research Laboratory, Medical Clinic, Ullevaal Hospital, University of Oslo**

Key words: tissue factor pathway inhibitor; tissue factor; factor VII, hyperlipidemia, atherosclerosis

Blood coagulation is triggered by the binding of circulating coagulation factor VII(a) to its membrane co-factor tissue factor (TF). The factor VIIa/TF complex formed then activates coagulation by proteolytic cleavage of zymogen factors X or IX, and is regulated by an important serine protease inhibitor called tissue factor pathway inhibitor (TFPI).[§] A schematic presentation of the TF-induced (or extrinsic) blood coagulation system is shown in Fig. 1. Recently, *in vivo* evidence was published showing that TFPI plays an important role in the regulation of TF-induced coagulation (Sandset *et al* 1991a). A pictorial description of the intravascular pools of TFPI and mode of action is shown in Fig. 2. There are several possible important links between TF-induced blood coagulation and hyperlipidemia: 1) TF is a membrane-anchored protein that requires the presence of particular phospholipids for its activity. Thus, variation in membrane lipid composition could play an important role in the regulation of TF activity. 2) The Northwick Park Heart Study (Meade *et al* 1986) identified factor VII as an important and independent risk factor for

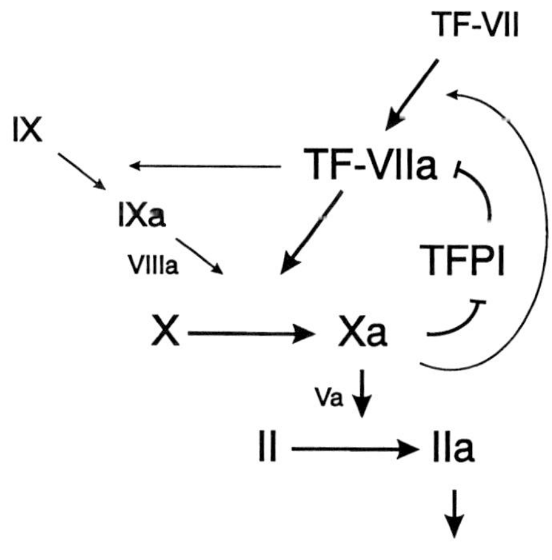

Fig. 1. A schematic presentation of tissue factor-induced blood coagulation with the generation of thrombin (IIa).
TF-tissue factor, TFPI-tissue factor pathway inhibitor. Zymogen forms of the clotting factors and their activated enzyme forms are denoted with Roman numerals, without or with the suffix *a* , respectively. →, activation pathway; ⊣, inactivation pathway.

* N-0407 Oslo, Norway.

§ A Scientific and Standardization Committee of the International Society of Thrombosis and Haemostasis (1991) recommended use of the name Tissue Factor Pathway Inhibitor. TFPI was earlier variously named anti-convertin, tissue factor inhibitor, extrinsic pathway inhibitor (EPI), or lipoprotein associated coagulation inhibitor (LACI).

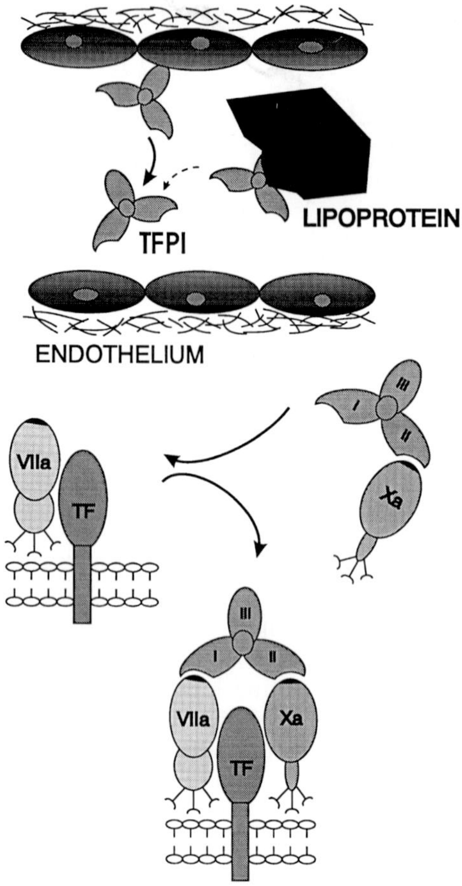

Fig. 2. The different intravascular pools and mode of action of TFPI.
TFPI is a Kunitz-type serine protease inhibitor with three inhibitory domains (denoted I, II, and III) and an estimated molecular weight of 32 kDa (based on the amino acid sequence). TFPI is found at least three intravascular pools (top part of the figure). A major pool (50–80%) is bound to the endothelial surface and may be released by the injection of heparin (Sandset *et al* 1988). The second pool is plasma TFPI. More than 90% of plasma TFPI is associated with lipoproteins (see text for details). A third pool of TFPI is located in platelets (not shown). The mode of action is a negative feedback loop (lower part of the figure). In the first step, TFPI binds to and inhibits factor Xa. In the second step, the TFPI-factor Xa complex binds to and neutralizes factor VIIa/TF activity by formation of a quaternary inhibitory complex. (For detailed reviews, see Rapaport 1989; Broze *et al* 1990; Sandset & Abildgaard 1991) Abbreviations, see Fig. 1. (Modified from Sandset & Abildgaard 1991, with permission)

cardiovascular disease. During the past decade, a number of studies have shown that factor VII activity is related to hypertriglyceridemia and to very low density lipoproteins (VLDLs) in plasma. 3) A major fraction of the circulating TFPI is associated with lipoproteins and TFPI activity is related to hypercholesterolemia. The present report will concentrate mainly on aspects related to TFPI.

TFPI IN PLASMA — THE ASSOCIATION WITH LIPOPROTEINS

Gel filtration of normal plasma allows the separation of TFPI activity into three different molecular weight forms. In our original report (Sandset *et al* 1987), more than 50% of the activity eluted in the void volume at a high molecular weight, about 40% at an intermediate molecular weight, and less than 10% at approximately 43 kDa (Fig. 3). These data were later confirmed using an antigen assay for the detection of TFPI (Novotny *et al* 1989). It was shown that the first high molecular weight fraction of TFPI coeluted with VLDLs and low density lipoproteins (LDLs), that the second intermediate molecular weight fraction coeluted with high density lipoproteins (HDLs) and that the third low molecular weight form was probably free TFPI. Thus, it appears that the major fraction of TFPI in plasma (>90%) is associated with lipoproteins and that combined VLDL/LDLs contain more than HDLs (50% vs 44%).

In another study of normolipemic subjects, precipitation of plasma VLDL and LDL by polyethylene glycol before gel filtration

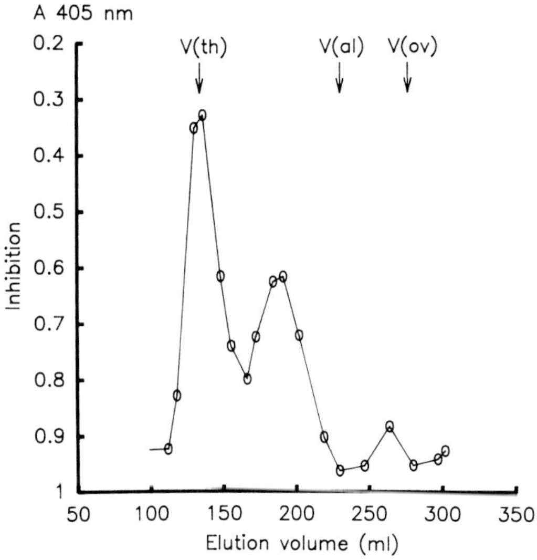

Fig. 3. Gel filtration of normal plasma separates TFPI activity in to three different molecular weight fractions.
It was later shown that the first high molecular weight fraction coelutes with VLDL/LDLs, the second fraction of intermediate molecular weight coelutes with HDLs, and the third low molecular weight fraction is carrier-free TFPI. (Reprinted from Sandset *et al* 1987, with permission)

almost completely removed the TFPI activity of the two high molecular weight fractions (Hansen *et al* 1994). Conversely, using the same column, gel filtration of isolated lipoprotein fractions prepared by ultracentrifugation showed that TFPI activity was recovered mainly from LDL and only minimally from VLDLs and HDLs. Immunoaffinity binding and precipitation of apolipoprotein-TFPI complexes in diluted plasma from normolipemic subjects showed a 76% reduction of TFPI activity after incubation with polyclonal immunoglobulin G against apolipoprotein B (anti-apoB), a non-significant 17% reduction after incubation with anti-apoA-I and no reduction after incubation with anti-apoA-II, suggesting again that TFPI is mainly associated with LDLs and only to a limited extent with HDLs.

In a recent report by Lesnik and colleagues (1993), the association of TFPI with lipoproteins was studied by ultracentrifugation of plasma from normolipemic subjects. These investigators found that LDL and HDL were the major lipoprotein carriers of TFPI activity (46% and 54% of the total lipoprotein-associated TFPI activity, respectively). Most of the activity was identified in small, dense subspecies of both LDL and HDL (34% and 36% respectively). Moreover, TFPI was also associated with lipoprotein (a) (Lp(a), a structural variant of LDL), but this association was related to Lp(a) particle size and phenotype.

Taken together, all the studies consistently identify LDLs as the major carriers of TFPI activity or antigen in plasma and very little activity is associated with VLDLs. Although the studies identify HDL as a carrier of TFPI activity or antigen, the fraction of TFPI associated with HDL varies.

NATURE OF THE TFPI-LIPOPROTEIN ASSOCIATION

TFPI purified from human plasma is heterogeneous when examined by sodium dodecyl sulfate-polyacrylamide gel electrophoresis (SDS-PAGE). Major bands of TFPI are detected at ~35 kDa and at ~41 kDa. In highly purified preparations of plasma TFPI at least 3–4 higher molecular weight bands can be isolated. These bands, as well as the 41 kDa form, probably contain TFPI associated with apoA-II through mixed disulfide linkages (Novotny *et al* 1989). By applying SDS-PAGE to isolated lipoproteins it appears that HDLs contain the 41 kDa form associated with apoA-II, which is thus covalently linked to HDLs, whereas LDLs contain the 35 kDa form (Novotny *et al* 1989; Lesnik *et al* 1993). The type of interaction involved in the interaction between TFPI and LDLs is currently unknown but is probably not due to ionic/polar interactions (Lesnik *et al* 1993).

TFPI IN HYPERCHOLESTEROLEMIA

Although gel filtration and ultracentrifugation identified lipoproteins as the major carriers of TFPI in plasma of normolipemic subjects, the regulation of TFPI levels in hyperlipidemia remained unknown. One possibility was that TFPI levels in plasma were maintained constant by other factors and independent of lipoprotein levels. Alternatively, TFPI levels could be dependent on lipoproteins and vary with changes in plasma lipoprotein composition. To test the latter hypothesis, a normal population and individuals with familiar hypercholesterolemia were studied. In a population of healthy blood donors TFPI activity gradually increased with age. Multiple regression analysis showed that the age-dependent increase in TFPI activity was to a large extent explained by an increase in total cholesterol (Sandset *et al* 1991b). Moreover, in 18 individuals with heterozygous hypercholesterolemia TFPI levels were elevated more than twice the standard deviation above the mean of the reference population in all the individuals. After dietary intervention and treatment with simvastatin, TFPI levels normalized and the relative change in TFPI activity was significantly correlated with the relative change in LDLs (Fig. 4). In a multiple regression analysis, LDL cholesterol and then HDL cholesterol were the major predictors of TFPI activity (Sandset *et al* 1991c). These data were confirmed in another study of patients with familial hypercholesterolemia (Hansen *et al* 1994) who were treated with lovastatin alone or in combination with fish oil concentrate. In this study, gel filtration of plasma demonstrated a specific drop in apoB-TFPI complexes, whereas TFPI not associated with lipoproteins remained unchanged. These data therefore suggest that plasma TFPI levels are to a great extent determined by lipoprotein levels.

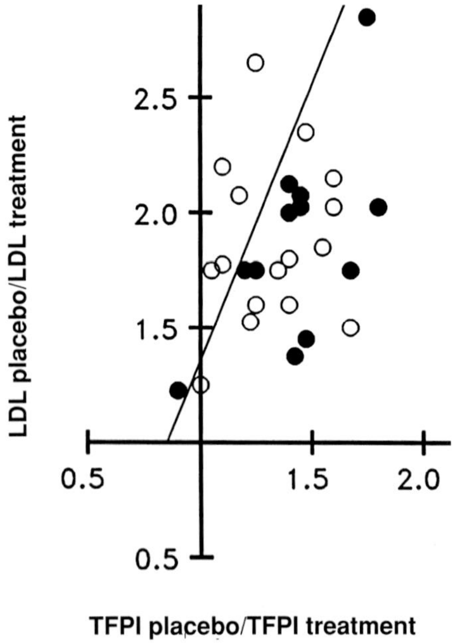

Fig. 4. Scatterplot showing the relative change in TFPI activity versus the relative change in LDL cholesterol in patients with familial hypercholesterolemia before and after treatment with simvastatin alone (○) or with simvastatin + n-3-fatty acids (●). $r = 0.55$, $p < 0.01$.
(Reprinted from Sandset *et al* 1991c, with permission)

THE ROLE OF THE TFPI-LIPOPROTEIN ASSOCIATION

The biological role of the TFPI-lipoprotein association is currently largely unknown. Lesnik and colleagues (1993) suggested that penetration of TFPI-bearing, dense LDLs into the subendothelial space might inhibit fibrin deposition in atherosclerotic plaques induced by TF expressed on the surface of lipid-laden macrophages. These investigators also suggested the interesting hypothesis that an elevated susceptibility of dense LDLs to oxidation coupled with subsequent inactivation of LDL-bound TFPI could result in neutralization of such an antiatherogenic and antithrombotic mechanism. The TFPI-lipoprotein association may therefore play an important role in atherogenesis.

Another possibility is that the TFPI-lipoprotein association merely serves as a reservoir for TFPI in plasma that would otherwise bind to the endothelium or rapidly leave the circulation. Recently, we provided evidence that TFPI associated with lipoproteins is functionally less efficient in a coagulant or kinetic assay of TFPI as compared with free or heparin-releasable TFPI

(Lindahl *et al* 1991). These results suggest that TFPI not complexed to lipoproteins, i.e. free TFPI in plasma or TFPI bound to endothelial cells, serves as the physiological anticoagulant of TF-induced coagulation, e.g. in disseminated intravascular coagulation. However, the data cannot rule out a specific antithrombotic and antiatherogenic role for TFPI-lipoprotein complexes in the development of atherosclerosis.

SUMMARY

TFPI is a potent and important physiological inhibitor of factor VIIa/TF as determined both *in vitro* and *in vivo*. TFPI is found in at least three intravascular pools. A major fraction (50–80%) consists of carrier-free TFPI molecules bound to the endothelium and releasable by heparin. The second blood plasma pool mainly contains TFPI associated with dense LDLs and HDLs with only minor amounts as carrier-free TFPI. The third pool (< 5%) consists of TFPI located in blood platelets. Apparently, TFPI is covalently linked to HDLs mediated by disulfide bridging to apoA-II. The nature of the TFPI-LDL association is currently unknown. Studies of normal individuals and individuals with familial hypercholesterolemia indicate that LDL is the major predictor of TFPI levels in plasma and that changes in LDL levels result in a similar change in TFPI activity. Although similar activity has been exhibited in capacity assays for TFPI, lipoprotein-associated TFPI preparations have considerably lower anticoagulant activity as determined in kinetic assays, compared with carrier-free and heparin-releasable TFPI. This suggests that only carrier-free and heparin-releasable TFPI are physiological anticoagulants *in vivo*. However, the TFPI-lipoprotein association may facilitate transportation of TFPI to the subendothelial space in atherosclerotic disease and may thus have a specific and important antithrombotic and antiatherogenic mechanism for neutralizing TF expressed on the surface of lipid-laden macrophages in atherosclerotic plaques.

REFERENCES

Broze GJ, Girard TJ, Novotny WG 1990 Regulation of blood coagulation by a multivalent Kunitz-type inhibitor. Biochemistry 29: 7539–7546

Hansen JB, Huseby NE, Sandset PM, Svensson B, Lyngmo V, Nordøy A 1994 Tissue-factor pathway inhibitor and lipoproteins. Arterioscler Thromb 14: 223–229

Lesnik P, Vonica A, Guerin M, Moreau M, Chapman MJ 1993 Anticoagulant activity of tissue factor pathway inhibitor in human plasma is preferentially associated with dense subspecies of LDL and HDL and with Lp(a). Arterioscler Thromb 13: 1066–1075

Lindahl AK, Jacobsen PB, Sandset PM, Abildgaard U 1991 Tissue factor pathway inhibitor with high anticoagulant activity is increased in post-heparin plasma and in plasma from cancer patients. Blood Coagul Fibrinolysis 2: 713–721

Meade TW, Brozovic M, Chakrabarti RR *et al* 1986 Haemostatic function and ischaemic heart disease: Principal results ofthe Northwick Park Heart Study. Lancet ii: 533–537

Novotny WF, Girard TJ, Miletich JP, Broze GJ 1989 Purification and characterization of the lipoprotein-associated coagulation inhibitor from human plasma. J Biol Chem 264: 18832–18837

Rapaport SI 1989 Inhibition of factor VIIa/tissue factor induced blood coagulation: With particular emphasis upon a factor Xa-dependent inhibitory mechanism. Blood 73: 359–365

Sandset PM, Abildgaard U 1991 Extrinsic pathway inhibitor: the key to feedback control of blood coagulation initiated by tissue thromboplastin. Haemostasis 21: 219–239

Sandset PM, Abildgaard U, Pettersen M 1987 A sensitive chromogenic substrate assay of extrinsic coagulation pathway inhibitor (EPI) in plasma and plasma fractions. Thromb Res 47: 389–400

Sandset PM, Abildgaard U, Larsen ML 1988 Heparin induces release of extrinsic coagulation pathway inhibitor (EPI). Thromb Resh 50: 803–813

Sandset PM, Warn-Cramer BJ, Rao LVM, Maki SL, Rapaport SI 1991a Depletion of extrinsic pathway inhibitor (EPI) sensitizes rabbits to disseminated intravascular coagulation induced with tissue factor: Evidence supporting a physiologic role of EPI as a natural anticoagulant. Proc Natl Acad Sci USA 88708–712

Sandset PM, Larsen ML, Abildgaard U, Lindahl AK, Odegaard OR 1991b Chromogenic substrate assay of extrinsic pathway inhibitor (EPI): levels in the normal population and relation to cholesterol. Blood Coagul Fibrinolysis 2: 425–433

Sandset PM, Lund H, Norseth J, Abildgaard U, Ose L 1991c Treatment with hydroxy-methyl-glutaryl-coenzyme A reductase inhibitors in hypercholesterolemia induces changes in the components of the extrinsic coagulation system. Arterioscler Thromb 11: 138–145

Multiple Risk Factors in Cardiovascular Disease, ed. by A. Yamamoto, Churchill Livingstone Japan, Tokyo, pp. 217–219 (1994)

MOLECULAR BASIS FOR THE PROTHROMBOTIC ACTION OF LP(a)[§]

Angelo M. SCANU

*Departments of Medicine, Biochemistry and Molecular Biology, and Committee on Genetics, University of Chicago**

Key words: Lp(a) polymorphism, apo(a) mutants, kringle 4-37, lysine binding pocket, apo(a) as risk factor

A functional property of human lipoprotein (a) (Lp(a)) is to bind to lysine/fibrin (Scanu 1993). It is known that this property resides in the kringle domain of apolipoprotein (a) (apo(a)), the specific glycoprotein of Lp(a), although the actual site for the interaction has not been established. We know, however, that kringle 4 class 2, whose number of repeats determines the apo(a) size, has no lysine binding function (Li *et al* 1992). Of the other classes of kringle 4s of apo(a), kringle 4-37 is the one predicted on structural considerations to have lysine binding properties (Guevara *et al* 1993). This prediction has been difficult to verify experimentally, although this information is critical for an understanding of the postulated prothrombotic function of Lp(a).

THE LYSINE BINDING POCKET

Structural studies on human plasminogen have shown that two of its five kringles, namely kringle 1 and 4, have the lysine binding pocket responsible for the lysine binding function of this zymogen. In this protein the lysine binding pocket consists of 7 amino acids, two anionic: asp55, asp57; two cationic: lys35, arg71 and three nonpolar: trp62, trp72, and phe64. In human apo(a) the lysine binding pocket, which is present in kringle 4-37, has arg instead of lys at position 35 (Scanu 1993). The conservative nature of this amino acid substitution is not expected to cause functional differences in lysine binding.

EVIDENCE THAT THE LYSINE BINDING POCKET IN APO(A) KRINGLE 4-37 IS INVOLVED IN THE BINDING OF APO(a) TO LYSINE

The rhesus monkey is one of the non-human primate species containing Lp(a) which is structurally similar to human Lp(a); however, in contrast, it exhibits defective lysine binding. An investigation of the mechanism of this functional defect has revealed that in rhesus apo(a) kringle 4-37, arginine 72 has replaced tryptophan, one of the key amino acids of the lysine binding pocket (Scanu *et al* 1993). This mutation has been found in all rhesus monkeys studied and, thus, it appears to be species-specific. These results

* 5841 South Maryland, MC 5041, Chicago, IL 60637, USA.

§ The work by the Author mentioned in this review was supported by NIH Program Project Grant HL18577.

support a dominant role for the lysine binding pocket of kringle 4-37 in the binding of apo(a) to lysine and also indicate that there is an important structural and functional difference between rhesus and human apo(a).

Further evidence for the role of kringle 4-37 in the lysine binding function of apo(a) has come from our recent studies (Scanu *et al* 1994) that have identified human subjects with a lysine binding-defective Lp(a). Interestingly, subjects who were 100% defective exhibited the trp72 → arg mutation as shown by sequence analysis of the amplified DNA segment coding for the lysine binding pocket of kringle 4-37. In the course of these studies we also observed that there are subjects who have a partial lysine binding defect without the trp72 → arg mutation, indicating a previously unsuspected important degree of functional polymorphism in lysine binding. Interestingly, the subjects in whom lysine binding was totally absent had neither personal nor family histories of atherosclerotic cardiovascular disease.

LYSINE BINDING POLYMORPHISM: RELEVANCE TO THE ATHEROTHROMBOGENIC POTENTIAL OF LP(a)

A number of studies have established that the apo(a) gene is highly polymorphic due to its several alleles that code for apo(a) isoforms varying between 300 and 800 kDa (Scanu 1993). A relationship between the size polymorphism of apo(a) and Lp(a) function has not been clearly established although apo(a) size has been shown to affect density heterogeneity and plasma concentrations of Lp(a).

Our results now show that there is a functional polymorphism of Lp(a) in terms of lysine binding function and that mutations at the level of the lysine binding pocket of apo(a) kringle 4-37 contribute to this polymorphism. This observation introduces the notion that apo(a) is mutable and leads to the prediction that other sequence changes, either functional or non functional, will be found in the future. Lysine binding can be equated with fibrin binding and may represent one of the mechanisms for the atherothrombotic action of Lp(a). Lysine binding-defective Lp(a) species may prove to be "benign" or "good" from the standpoint of cardiovascular pathogeneses. It follows that in assessing Lp(a) as a cardiovascular risk factor, it may be necessary to complement measurements of plasma concentrations of this lipoprotein with analyses of its lysine binding function. We may also speculate that the functional polymorphism of Lp(a) may account for the conflicting reports regarding the cardiovascular pathogenicity of this lipoprotein variant (Scanu 1993).

SUMMARY

The results of studies on rhesus monkey Lp(a) and a mutant form of human Lp(a) have shown that kringle 4-37 of apo(a) is involved in the lysine binding function via its lysine binding pocket. A mutation of one its amino acids, trp72 → arg, is associated with defective lysine binding of Lp(a). The functional polymorphism of apo(a) should be taken into account when assessing Lp(a) as a cardiovascular risk factor.

REFERENCES

Guevara JJ, Spurlino J, Jan AY *et al* 1993 Proposed mechanisms for binding of apo(a) kringle type 9 to apoB_{100} in human lipoprotein(a). J Biophys 64: 686–700

Li Z, Gambino R, Fless GM, Copeland, RA, Halfpenny AJ, Scanu AM 1992 Expression and purification of kringle 4-type 2 of human apolipoprotein(a) in *E. coli*. J Protein Expression 3: 212–222

Scanu AM 1993 Structural basis for the presumptive athero-thrombogenic action of Lp(a). Facts and speculations. Biochem Pharmacol 46: 1675–1680

Scanu AM, Miles LA, Fless GM *et al* 1993 Rhesus monkey Lp(a) binds to lysine Sepharose and U937 monocytoid cells less efficiently than human Lp(a). Evidence for the dominant role of Kringle 437. J Clin Invest 91: 283–291

Scanu AM, Pfaffinger D, Lee JC, Hinman J 1994 A single point mutation (Trp72Arg) in human apo(a) kringle 4-37 associated with a lysine binding defect in Lp(a). Biochim Biophys Acta (in press)

Multiple Risk Factors in Cardiovascular Disease, ed. by A. Yamamoto, Churchill Livingstone Japan, Tokyo, pp. 221–224 (1994)

HYPERLIPIDEMIA AND THE HEMOSTATIC SYSTEM

Eriko MORISHITA,*1 Hiroshi JOKAJI,*2 Tamotsu MATSUDA*1

*1 *Department of Internal Medicine (III), School of Medicine, Kanazawa University, and*
*2 *Department of Internal Medicine, Inami General Hospital*

Key words: factor VII, thrombin-antithrombin III complex, plasminogen activator inhibitor-1, hypercoagulable state, hypofibrinolytic state

The relationship between hyperlipidemia and atherosclerosis has been well established. The importance of thrombosis in the development of myocardial infarction is also well recognized. These observations suggest that prolonged hyperlipidemia may adversely affect the hemostatic system, leading to occlusive thrombosis. However, the precise relationship between blood lipids and thrombosis is not yet clear. For example, the effects of differing types or degrees of severity of hyperlipidemia on the expression of blood coagulation or fibrinolytic factors are not fully understood.

In this study, a statistical approach was employed to investigate the question of hemostatic system activation in patients with hyperlipidemia. The subjects (39 healthy controls and 75 patients with primary hyperlipidemia) were drawn from persons who were admitted for periodic health check-ups. Hyperlipidemic patients were classified as type IIa, IIb, or IV according to Fredrickson's classification for hyperlipidemia. The characteristics of the subjects are shown in Table I.

*1 13-1 Takara-machi, Kanazawa 920, Japan.
*2 Inami-machi, Toyama, 932-02 Japan.

COAGULATION SYSTEM

Evidence for the possible effects of hyperlipidemia on the coagulation system has been reported by a number of investigators (Bajaj *et al* 1976; Constantino *et al* 1977). We measured plasma levels of blood coagulation factors and observed that the mean activities of factors II, VII, and IX were elevated in subjects with all three types of hyperlipidemia, compared to normal controls (Table I). In particular, the levels of factor VII activity (FVIIc) in type IIb were markedly elevated. The concentrations of fibrinogen in hyperlipidemic patients were not significantly different from those in control subjects. Significant positive correlations were found between the levels of factor VII activity and serum triglyceride as well as serum cholesterol.

This increase in FVIIc in the hyperlipidemic subjects could be due either to an increase in the concentration of factor VII or to an increase in the reactivity of this protein. To clarify this matter, we assayed factor VII antigen (FVIIag), as measured by immunologic assay in the plasma. In the hyperlipidemic subjects, although levels of FVIIc were significantly increased compared to normal controls, the levels of FVIIag were

TABLE I. Characteristics and Blood Coagulation and Fibrinolytic Parameters of Normal Controls and Hyperlipidemic Patients

	Control	Type of hyperlipidemia		
		IIa	IIb	IV
	(n = 39)	(n = 31)	(n = 11)	(n = 33)
Age (years)	50 ± 11	51 ± 11	50 ± 12	48 ± 7
T-chol (mg/dl)	180 ± 22	249 ± 24**	289 ± 45**	195 ± 33*
TG (mg/dl)	95 ± 30	97 ± 25	246 ± 80**	245 ± 70**
Fibrinogen (mg/dl)	243 ± 50	277 ± 50	278 ± 51	239 ± 59
Factor II (%)	100 ± 16	121 ± 20*	107 ± 20	105 ± 15
VII (%)	100 ± 21	111 ± 24	137 ± 25**	119 ± 26**
IX (%)	100 ± 18	101 ± 26	124 ± 71	113 ± 16
X (%)	100 ± 18	100 ± 24	111 ± 11	110 ± 11
TAT (g/ml)	1.3 ± 0.6	1.9 ± 1.9	2.7 ± 2.2**	1.5 ± 1.2
F_{1+2} (nmol/l)	0.70 ± 0.42	0.97 ± 0.41*	1.05 ± 0.65*	0.89 ± 0.33
PAI-1 (ng/ml)	11.7 ± 9.5	14.8 ± 10.8	32.3 ± 23.8**	32.1 ± 21.1**
TM (ng/dl)	7.9 ± 2.8	11.0 ± 3.8*	12.8 ± 5.5*	12.8 ± 4.6**

Values are means ± SD. * $p < 0.05$; ** $p < 0.01$. T-chol, total cholesterol; TG, serum triglyceride; TAT, thrombin-antithrombin III complex; F_{1+2}, prothrombin fragment F_{1+2}; PAI-1, plasminogen activator inhibitor-1; TM, thrombomodulin.

almost the same as those of normal controls. These results suggest that the major part of the observed increase in FVIIc is due to increased reactivity of this protein. Negri *et al* (1993) showed that the increase in FVIIc is related to increases in both FVIIag and the activity of FVII, and that the increase in activity is dependent on an increase in FVII-phospholipid complex, which has a higher specific activity than normal zymogen factor VII, rather than activated FVII (FVIIa). The mechanism of the interaction between serum lipids and factor VII remains a subject of debate.

Recently, it has become possible to demonstrate the prethrombotic state by employing an assay for prothrombin fragment F_{1+2} (F_{1+2}). The plasma concentration of this fragment reflects the production of thrombin in the circulating blood. Another marker that has recently been introduced into clinical practice is thrombin-antithrombin III complex (TAT). TAT is a circulating complex of thrombin with its immediate inhibitor, antithrombin III. Therefore, TAT is also a specific marker of thrombin generation in the circulating blood.

We measured plasma concentrations of TAT and F_{1+2} in hyperlipidemic patients (Table I). The mean levels of F_{1+2} in the patients with type IIa or IIb hyperlipidemia were significantly increased, compared to normal controls. On the other hand, the mean level of TAT in the patients with type IIb was also significantly higher than that in normal controls. We found that 12% and 18% of 75 patients with hyperlipidemia had abnormally high levels of TAT and F_{1+2}, respectively, which suggests activation of the coagulation system in circulating blood.

FIBRINOLYTIC SYSTEM

One of the important defense mechanisms of the body against thrombosis is the fibrinolytic system. Endothelial cells synthesize and secrete tissue plasminogen activator (t-PA). Activation of endothelial cell surface-bound plasminogen by t-PA results in plasmin generation. Plasminogen activator inhibitor-1 (PAI-1) is the main inhibitor of t-PA. Recent findings have shown that deficient fibrinolysis is often due to either reduced t-PA activity or increased levels of PAI-1.

We showed that plasma levels of PAI-1 in patients with type IIb or IV were significantly higher than those in normal controls. There was a significant correlation between the levels of PAI-1 activity and triglyceride in hyperlipidemic patients (Fig. 1). However, there was no significant correlation between the levels of PAI-1 activity and total cholesterol. These findings suggest that fibrinolytic activity is impaired in patients with hypertriglyceridemia.

To clarify the relationship between PAI-1 activity and triglyceride, we investigated the response of this antifibrinolytic activity to changes in triglyceride levels after intravenous administration of fat emulsion. Administration of fat emulsion (10% intralipos) to 18 patients with various diseases resulted in the induction of artificial hypertriglyceridemia; the mean levels of plasma PAI-1 as well as triglyceride were significantly increased, while the mean level of TAT was unchanged. From these results, it is reasonable to speculate that serum triglyceride may regulate the plasma level of PAI-1, and that fibrinolytic capacity is reduced in patients with hypertriglyceridemia. Recently, an interesting study was reported by Stiko-Rahm *et al* (1990), who found that very low density lipoprotein (VLDL) stimulates the secretion of PAI-1 from human umbilical vein endothelial cells and that the VLDL-induced secretion of PAI-1 is dependent on the binding of VLDL particles to receptors on the cells. Their experiment may explain our clinical finding of a relationship between levels of triglyceride and PAI-1. On the other hand, Tremoli *et al* (1993) reported that cholesterol-rich lipoproteins such as low density lipoproteins (LDLs) affect PAI-1 release by endothelial cells *in vitro*, although our study showed no statistically significant correlations between levels of PAI-1 and serum cholesterol. At least, our clinical findings support the notion that hypertriglyceridemia may cause a tendency towards thrombosis due to impaired fibrinolysis.

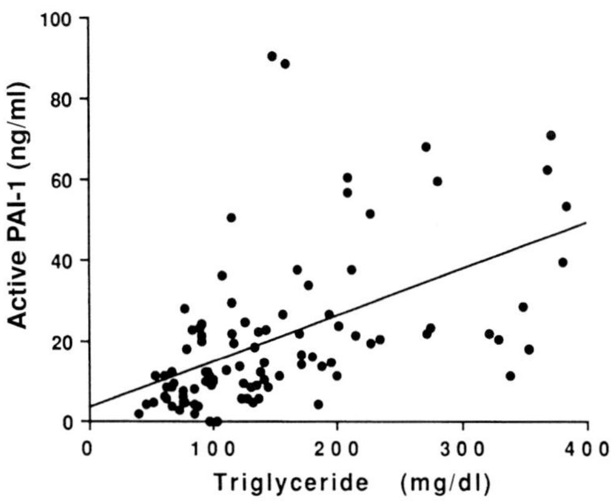

Fig. 1. Correlation between levels of active PAI-1 and triglyceride in normal and hyperlipidemic subjects.
PAI-1, plasminogen activator inhibitor-1. $n = 95$; $y = 0.11x + 3.34$; $r = 0.524$; $p < 0.0001$.

CONCLUSION

In conclusion, patients with hyperlipidemia are in a hypercoagulable and/or hypofibrinolytic state that could promote a tendency to thrombosis.

SUMMARY

Plasma levels of blood coagulation and fibrinolytic factors and serum levels of lipids were measured in 114 subjects (39 normal controls and 75 patients with primary hyperlipidemia) to investigate whether hyperlipidemia may affect the hemostatic system. Mean levels of prothrombin and the activities of factors VII and IX were elevated in subjects with all three types of hyperlipidemia, compared to normal controls. The levels of factor VII activity in patients with type IIb hyperlipidemia were particularly elevated. Significant correlations were observed between the levels of factor VII and serum triglyceride as well as serum cholesterol. Plasma levels of F_{1+2} and TAT were slightly but significantly higher in patients with type IIb hyperlipidemia than those in normal controls. These results suggest activation of the coagulation system in circulating blood in patients with hyperlipidemia.

Plasma levels of PAI-1 in patients with

type IIb and IV hyperlipidemia were significantly higher than those in normal controls. A significant correlation was found between triglyceride and PAI-1. After the administration of fat emulsion to 18 patients with various diseases, which induced artificial hypertriglyceridemia, levels of plasma PAI-1 as well as serum triglyceride were significantly increased. These results suggest that hypertriglyceridemia may increase the synthesis and/or release of PAI-1, inducing a hypofibrinolytic state. Since it leads to the decreased removal of fibrin deposits, hypofibrinolysis-induced hypertriglyceridemia would be a prime candidate for a role in the initiation and development of atherothrombosis.

REFERENCES

Bajaj SP, Harmony JAK, Martinez-Carrion M *et al* 1976 Human plasma lipoproteins as accelerators of prothrombin activation. J Biol Chem 25: 5233–5236

Constantino M, Merskey C, Kudzma DJ *et al* 1977 Increased activity of vitamin K-dependent clotting factors in human hyperlipoproteinemia — Association with cholesterol and triglyceride levels. Thromb Haemost 38: 465–474

Negri M, Arigliano PL, Talamini G *et al* 1993 Levels of plasma factor VII and factor VII activated forms as a function of plasma triglyceride levels. Atherosclerosis 99: 55–61

Stiko-Rahm A, Wiman B, Hamsten A *et al* 1990 Secretion of plasminogen activator inhibitor-1 from cultured human umbilical vein endothelial cells is induced by very low density lipoprotein. Arteriosclerosis 10: 1067–1073

Tremoli E, Camera M, Maderna P *et al* 1993 Increased synthesis of plasminogen activator inhibitor-1 by cultured human endothelial cells exposed to native and modified LDLs. Arterioscler Thromb 13: 338–346

Multiple Risk Factors in Cardiovascular Disease, ed. by A. Yamamoto, Churchill Livingstone Japan, Tokyo, pp. 225–229 (1994)

EFFECTS OF LIPOPROTEINS ON THE COAGULANT-FIBRINOLYTIC ACTIVITY OF HUMAN MONOCYTE-MACROPHAGES AND HUMAN UMBILICAL VENOUS ENDOTHELIAL CELLS

Hideo WADA, Toshihiro KANEKO, Yoshihiro WAKITA, Shyousaburou NAGAYA, Nobuyuki MINAMI, Katsumi DEGUCHI, and Shigeru SHIRAKAWA

*The Second Department of Internal Medicine, Mie University School of Medicine**

Key words: lipoprotein, monocyte-macrophages, human umbilical venous endothelial cells, tissue factor, plasminogen activator inhibitor

Ross (1986) has reported that monocyte-macrophages and endothelial cells play a very important role in forming atherosclerotic lesions; in particular, one of the key events in this process is the formation of the cholesterol-laden foam cells derived mainly from monocyte-macrophages. Under normal circumstances endothelial cells have anti-thrombogenic activity, however, in some abnormal states, such as sepsis and hypoxemia, the thrombogenic activity of endothelial cells exhibited via tissue factor (TF) (Colucci *et al* 1983) and plasminogen activator inhibitor (PAI)-I (Colucci *et al* 1985), for example, predominates over their anti-thrombogenic activity. In this study, we have investigated the effect of lipoproteins on monocyte-macrophages and human umbilical venous endothelial cells (HUVEC), with regard to their coagulant-fibrinolytic activity.

CULTURE OF MONOCYTE WITH LIPOPROTEINS

Mononuclear cells were obtained from the heparinized venous blood (100 ml) of healthy volunteers by means of Ficoll-Hypaque (Pharmacia Fine Chemicals) density separation. Purified monocyte monolayers were obtained by plating 10^5-mononuclear cells into the 6-mm collagen-coated wells of a 96-well plate (Corning). Monocytes were allowed to adhere for 120 min. HUVEC were obtained according to the method of Jaffe *et al* (1973), and all studies were performed on confluent HUVEC cultures at the third passage in 96-well plates. Each well contained $(2.47 \pm 0.34) \times 10^4$ cells. Low density lipoprotein (LDL), very low density lipoprotein (VLDL), and high density lipoprotein (HDL) were obtained from Sigma Chemical. Each lipoprotein sample contained 0.15 M NaCl and 0.01% EDTA, pH 7.4–7.5. Each of the materials contained less than 1×10^{-6} μg/μg of endotoxin. The content of these substances did not affect this experiment.

Monocytes (1×10^4/well) were incubated in 6-mm collagen-coated 96-well plates in RPMI-1640 (Gibco Laboratories)/10% fetal calf serum (FCS) with lipoprotein at 37°C in an atmosphere of 5% CO_2 in air. After incubation for the indicated times, culture medium was collected, clarified centrifuging for 8 min in a plastic tube and frozen at −80°C until use. After collection of the cul-

* 2-174 Edobashi, Tsu 514, Japan.

ture medium, the cells were also frozen at −80°C and, just before use, thawed, resuspended in 100 μl RPMI-1640 and sonicated (cell-lysate). HUVEC which reached confluence at 2.5×10^4/well in 6-mm collagen-coated 96-well plates were washed with serum-free RPMI-1640 three times; lipoproteins or the filtered culture medium of monocytes incubated with lipoproteins were then added, and the cells were incubated at 37°C in an atmosphere of 5% CO_2 in air. After incubation for the times indicated, the culture medium was collected, clarified by centrifuging for 8 min in a plastic tube, and frozen at −80°C until use. Following collection of the culture medium, the cells were also frozen at −80°C and just before use, thawed, resuspended in 100 μl RPMI-1640 and sonicated (cell-lysate).

The TF activity of the culture medium and lysate was determined using a modification of the method of Yvonne *et al* (1989). The 50 μl test samples were incubated for 120 min in 96-well plates with 25 μl 0.025 M $CaCl_2$ and 25 μl human coagulation factor IX complex 20 units/ml (Christmassin-HT; Midori-Juji) and 25 μl chromogenic substance S-2222 (Chromogenix AB). The change in optical density at 405 nm was quantitated using a microplate reader. Tissue-type plasminogen activator (t-PA), urokinase-type PA (u-PA), PAI-I, and PAI-II antigen levels in the samples were determined by enzyme immunoassays. The t-PA level was determined with Imuzain t-PA (Fuji-Rebio), u-PA with TintElize u-PA (Biopool), PAI-I with IMULYSE™ PAI-I (Biopool), and PAI-II with TintElize PAI-II (Biopool).

Results are expressed as means ± standard deviation. Statistical analysis was performed using Student's *t* test.

INCREASED TF ACTIVITY AND PAI ANTIGENS IN MONOCYTES AND HUVEC CULTURED WITH LIPOPROTEINS

Monocytes or HUVEC were incubated with 50 μg/ml VLDL, LDL, HDL and without lipoproteins. Figure 1A shows that within 6 h of stimulation, the lysate of monocytes incubated with VLDL increased more than 10-fold in terms of TF activity compared with that incubated with HDL or medium alone, and more than 2-fold compared with that incubated with LDL. There was no significant difference between t-PA antigen in the lysate of monocytes incubated with and without lipoproteins, and u-PA and PAI-I antigens were not detected in the monocyte lysate. PAI-II antigen in the monocyte lysate in the same experiment varied almost in parallel with the TF activity.

Figure 1B shows that within 12 h of stimulation, the lysate of HUVEC incubated with VLDL exhibited about a 4-fold increase in TF activity compared with that of control cells. The lysate of HUVEC incubated with LDL exhibited a small increase in TF activity, and there was no significant difference between the TF activity in HUVEC incubated with HDL and without lipoproteins. The t-PA and PAI-I antigens in the culture medium of HUVEC increased as the incubation times were prolonged, even without lipoproteins. The difference between t-PA antigen in the medium of HUVEC incubated with and without lipoproteins was not significant, but PAI-I antigen in the medium incubated with VLDL increased more than 3-fold compared with that incubated with HDL or LDL, and without lipoproteins within 30 h of incubation. u-PA and PAI-II antigens were not detected in the culture medium of HUVEC incubated with lipoproteins.

Table I shows that the concentrations of lipoprotein which induced maximum TF activity in monocytes were 1 μg/ml for VLDL, 100 μg/ml for LDL, and 500 μg/ml for HDL. TF activity increased in a dose-dependent manner with regard to lipoprotein concentration until it reached a peak. PAI-II antigen in monocyte lysate varied almost in parallel with TF activity. t-PA, u-PA, PAI-I, and PAI-II antigens were not detected in the medium of monocytes incubated with or without

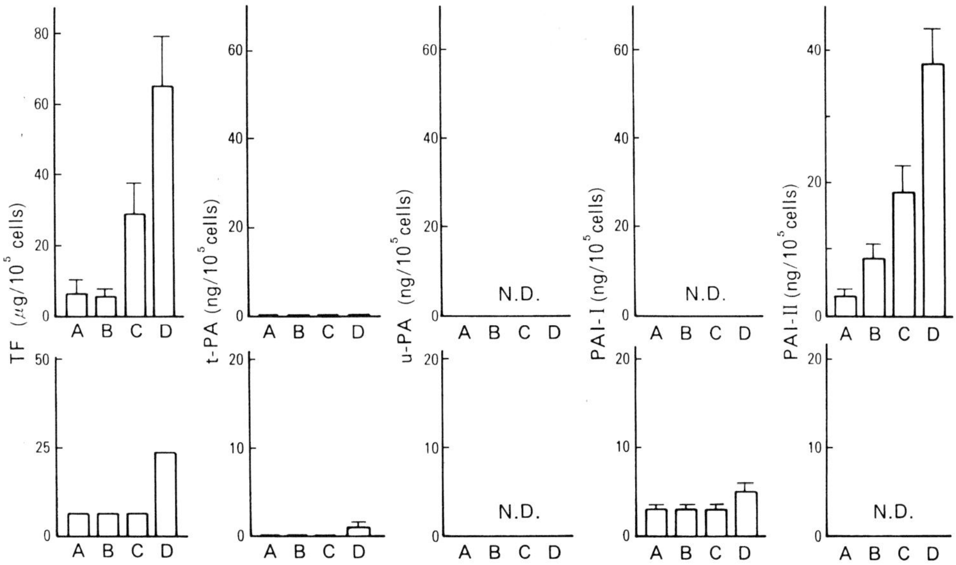

Fig. 1. Effects of lipoproteins on coagulant-fibrinolytic system in monocyte-macrophages and HUVEC.
HUVEC, Human Umbilical venous endothelial cells.
Upper column: monocyte-macrophages (6 h incubation with lipoprotein).
Lower column: HUVEC (12 h incubation with lipoprotein).
A, control; B, HDL (50 g/ml); C, LDL(50 g/ml); D, VLDL(50 μg/ml).

TABLE I. Maximum TF Activity and PAI Antigen in Monocytes and HUVEC Incubated with Lipoproteins

Monocytes	Concentration (g/ml)	TF activity (g/10^5 cells)	PAI-II antigens (ng/10^5 cells)
HDL	500	106.1 ± 2.7**	47.3 ± 1.1**
LDL	100	105.4 ± 3.7**	47.9 ± 1.9**
VLDL	1	100.0 ± 1.4**	53.0 ± 1.7**
Control	–	2.2 ± 0.3	6.7 ± 0.3
HUVEC	**Concentration (g/ml)**	**TF activity (g/2.5 × 10^5 cells)**	**PAI-I antigens (ng/2.5 × 10^5 cells)**
HDL	1000	20.5 ± 0.1	10.1 ± 0.3
LDL	1000	20.8 ± 0.4	14.8 ± 0.6
VLDL	50	68.5 ± 1.2**	28.1 ± 2.3**
Control	–	18.9 ± 1.1	9.8 ± 0.1

Data are means ± SD, ** $p < 0.01$.
TF activity and PAI-II antigen were measured in the lysate of monocytes incubated with lipoproteins for 18 h. TF activity in the lysates, and PAI-I antigen in the culture medium of HUVEC incubated with lipoproteins for 6 h, were measured. TF, tissue factor; PAI, plasminogen activator inhibitor; HUVEC, human umbilical venous endothelial cells.

lipoproteins. VLDL, at a concentration of 50 μg/ml, produced a more than 3-fold increase in the TF activity of HUVEC lysate compared with control cells. TF activity increased in a dose-dependent manner with regard to VLDL concentration until it reached its peak. However, LDL and HDL produced a little increase in TF activity at a concentration of even 1,000 μg/ml compared with the control. The addition of lipoproteins raised the level of PAI-I antigen in the culture medium of HUVEC almost in parallel with an elevation of TF. In particular, VLDL expressed maximum PAI-I antigen activity while the capacities of LDL and HDL to augment PAI-I antigen were negligible. t-PA antigen in the culture medium of HUVEC incubated with VLDL increased slightly in a dose-dependent manner; however, LDL and HDL did not have the capacity to augment t-PA antigen in HUVEC. u-PA and PAI-II antigens were not detected in the culture medium of HUVEC incubated with various lipoproteins (data not shown).

INCREASED LIPID LEVEL INDUCED A HYPERCOAGULANT-HYPOFIBRINOLYTIC STATE

Lipoproteins affected monocytes and HUVEC, and augmented TF activity in these cells. De Sousa *et al* (1988) have reported that coagulation factor VII and X are related to the concentration of plasma triglycerides, and Wada *et al* (1991) have reported that thrombin-antithrombin III complex was increased in patients with hyperlipidemia, suggesting that a hypercoagulable state exists in patients with this disease. Since TF is a lipoprotein cofactor that triggers blood coagulation, these findings suggest that TF may be related to plasma lipid levels and may produce a hypercoagulable state. Although TF is necessarily absent from the surfaces of cells in contact with plasma under normal circumstances, agents such as endotoxin (Niemetz *et al* 1977), immune complexes (Schwartz *et al* 1981) and lymphokines (Gregory *et al* 1986), can induce expression of TF in monocyte-macrophages and/or endothelial cells.

Lipoproteins also had the capacity to augment PAI-I (in HUVEC) and PAI-II (in monocyte-macrophages) production, but did not affect t-PA and u-PA. PAI-I is the major form of PAI found in plasma (Sprengers *et al* 1987) and is mainly released from vascular endothelial cells (Sakata *et al* 1988). In clinical studies, elevated PAI-I levels have been observed in patients with hypertriglyceridemia (Vague *et al* 1986) and in a variety of pathologic conditions associated with thrombosis (Juhan-Vague *et al* 1987; Emeis & Kooista 1986). PAI-II was first found in human placenta (Astedt *et al* 1985) and has since also been found in monocyte-macrophages (Stephens et *al* 1985). In monocytes, lipoproteins raised PAI-II antigen but did not affect PAI-I antigen; conversely, in HUVEC, they elevated PAI-I antigen and did not affect PAI-II antigen. These findings may be due to the organ-specificity of PAI. For example, PAI-I may exist in endothelial cells and function as an inhibitor of t-PA in the intravascular space, PAI-II may exist in monocyte-macrophages and function as an inhibitor of u-PA in the subendothelial space. Lipoproteins elevated PAI-I and PAI-II antigens, but did not affect t-PA and u-PA antigens; these findings show that lipoproteins may possibly induce a hypofibrinolytic state *in vivo*.

Our findings suggest that increased lipid levels effect both monocyte-macrophages and endothelial cells and directly induce a hypercoagulant-hypofibrinolytic state by augmenting the production of TF and PAI.

SUMMARY

The expression of TF and PAI was induced in cultured human monocyte-macrophages and HUVEC by incubation with lipoproteins. Although PAI-I was induced in HUVEC and PAI-II was induced in monocyte-macrophages, PA was induced in neither of these types of cell incubated with lipoproteins. VLDL had the strongest capacity to increase the expression of TF and PAI, followed by LDL, while the capacity of HDL in this regard was very weak. These findings indicate that lipoproteins affect both monocyte-macrophages and endothelial cells and cause a hypercoagulant-hypofibrinolytic state. It is thus possible that hyperlipidemia could be a direct risk factor for thrombotic disease.

Acknowledgment
We thank Dr. Yukio Nishiyama who kindly provided the umbilical cords for this study.

REFERENCES

Astedt B, Lecander I, Brodin T *et al* 1985 Purification of a specific placental plasminogen activator inhibitor by monoclonal antibody and its complex formation with plasminogen activator. Thromb Haemost 53: 122–125

Colucci M, Balconi G, Lorenzet R *et al* 1983 Cultured human endothelial cells generate tissue factor in response to endotoxin. J Clin Invest 71: 1893–1896

Colucci M, Paramo JA, Collen D 1985 Generation in plasma of a fast-acting inhibitor of plasminogen activator in response to endotoxin stimulation. J Clin Invest 75: 818–824

De Sousa J, Soria C, Ayrault-J M *et al* 1988 Association between coagulation factors VII and X with triglyceride rich lipoproteins. J Clin Pathol 41: 940 944

Emeis J J, Kooista T 1986 Interleukin 1 and lipopolysaccharide induce an inhibitor of tissue-type plasminogen activator in vivo and in cultured endothelial cells. J Exp Med 163: 1260–1266

Gregory SA, Kornbluth RS, Helin H *et al* 1986 Monocyte procoagulant inducing factor: a lymphokine involved in the T cell instructed monocyte procoagulant response to antigen. J Immunol 137: 3231–3239

Jaffe EA, Nachman RL, Becher CG, Minick CR 1973 Culture of human endothelial cells derived from umbilical veins. J Clin Invest 52: 2745–2756

Juhan-Vague I, Valadier J, Alessi MC *et al* 1987 Deficient tPA release and elevated PA inhibitor levels in patients with spontaneous or recurrent deep venous thrombosis. Thromb Haemost 57: 67–72

Niemetz J, Morrison C 1977 Lipid A as the biologically active moiety in bacterial endotoxin (LPS)-initiated generation of procoagulant activity by peripheral blood leukocytes. Blood 49: 947–956

Ross R 1986 The pathogenesis of atherosclerosis — An update. N Engl J Med 314: 488–500

Sakata Y, Okada M, Noro A *et al* 1988 Interaction of tissue-type plasminogen activator and plasminogen activator inhibitor 1 on the surface of endothelial cells. J Biol Chem 263: 1960–1969

Schwartz BS, Edgington TS 1981 Lymphocyte collaboration is required for induction of murine monocyte procoagulant activity by immune complexes. J Immunol 127: 438–443

Sprengers ED, Kluft C 1987 Plasminogen activator inhibitors. Blood 69: 381–387

Stephens RW, Golder JP, Fayle DRH *et al* 1985 Minactivin expression in human monocyte and macrophage populations. Blood 66: 333–337

Vague P, Juhan-Vaque I, Aillaud MF *et al* 1986 Correlation between blood fibrinolytic activity, plasminogen activator inhibitor level, plasma insulin level, and relative body weight in normal and obese subjects. Metabolism 35: 250–253

Wada H, Mori Y, Kita T *et al* 1991 Hypercoagulable state in Watanabe heritable hyperlipidemic rabbits and in patients with familial hypercholesterolemia. Atherosclerosis IX, Proceedings of the ninth International Symposium on Atherosclerosis. R&L Creative Communication, Tel Aviv, p 565–569

Yvonne MS, Zuckerman SH 1989 A novel microtiter plate assay for the quantitation of procoagulant activity on adherent monocytes, macrophage and endothelial cells. Thromb Res 53: 339–346

Multiple Risk Factors in Cardiovascular Disease, ed. by A. Yamamoto, Churchill Livingstone Japan, Tokyo, pp. 231–234 (1994)

PROSTAGLANDIN I_2 STABILIZING ACTIVITY REGULATED BY HIGH-DENSITY LIPOPROTEIN DECREASES IN ACUTE CORONARY EVENTS

Takeshi AOYAMA, Yoshiki YUI, Hiroshi MORISHITA, Chuichi KAWAI, and Shigetake SASAYAMA

*The Third Division, Department of Internal Medicine, Faculty of Medicine, Kyoto University**

Key words: prostaglandin I_2, high-density lipoprotein, apolipoprotein A-I, acute myocardial infarction, unstable angina pectoris

---

Prostaglandin I_2 (PGI_2) is a powerful vasodilator and inhibitor of platelet aggregation and has been thought to play an important role in the prevention of coronary thrombosis and atherosclerosis. PGI_2 is unstable in aqueous solution at physiological pH and is stabilized by binding to a serum factor. Reduced stability of PGI_2 has been observed in thrombotic disorders such as thrombotic thrombocytopenic purpura (Wu *et al* 1985) and ischemic stroke. We identified apolipoprotein (apo) A-I, a major apolipoprotein of high-density lipoprotein (HDL), as a serum PGI_2 stabilizing factor, which suggests that HDL or apoA-I may exert its antiatherogenic and antithrombogenic effects partly through stabilization of PGI_2.

EFFECT OF HDL ON STABILIZATION OF PGI_2

Serum PGI_2 stabilizing factor was purified from human serum to a single band with a molecular weight of 28 kDa by SDS-PAGE. Analysis of amino and carboxy terminal sequences and amino acid composition has disclosed its homology with human apoA-I (Yui *et al* 1988). When PGI_2 was incubated in lipoprotein-deficient serum (LPDS) or in LPDS with HDL (final apoA-I concentration: 140 mg/dl), the chemical half-life of PGI_2 was prolonged in HDL-supplemented serum. PGI_2 has several biological activities, such as inhibition of platelet aggregation, vasodilation, and stimulation of acid cholesterol ester hydrolase, which reduces cellular cholesterol content. These effects of PGI_2 were enhanced in HDL-supplemented serum (Aoyama *et al* 1990; Morishita *et al* 1990).

SERUM PGI_2 BINDING ACTIVITY IN PATIENTS WITH CORONARY ARTERY DISEASE

Serum PGI_2 binding activities in patients with angina pectoris, unstable angina pectoris, acute-phase myocardial infarction, and subacute-phase myocardial infarction were significantly lower than in control patients. PGI_2 binding activity in patients with unstable angina pectoris or acute-phase myocardial infarction was significantly lower than that in patients with angina pectoris or subacute-phase myocardial infarction (Table I) (Aoyama *et al* 1990). The reduced stability of PGI_2 in acute-phase myocardial infarction was not a secondary effect of myocardial

* 54 Kawara-machi, Shogoin, Sakyo-ku, Kyoto 606-01, Japan.

TABLE I. Prostaglandin I2 Binding Activities and Apolipoprotein A-I and A-II Levels

Group	PGI2 binding activities (%)	Total serum apoA-I (mg/dl)	Free apoA-I/ total apoA-I (%)	HDL-associated apoA-I (mg/dl)	Total serum apoA-II (mg/dl)	Total apo A-I/apoA-II (mol/mol)
Control	38.5 ± 3.5	137.3 ± 18.6	10.3 ± 1.7	124.4 ± 8.1	38.0 ± 5.1	2.25 ± 0.31
AP	31.8 ± 5.6#	105.7 ± 13.0#	8.3 ± 3.3	98.9 ± 13.9#	30.2 ± 4.4#	2.10 ± 0.29
UAP	26.2 ± 4.7#	101.4 ± 11.9#	22.1 ± 3.7#	76.9 ± 8.7#	33.0 ± 5.3*	1.96 ± 0.27*
MI-a	24.8 ± 3.2#	102.2 ± 11.5#	20.8 ± 3.2#	77.8 ± 8.8#	34.5 ± 5.0*	1.87 ± 0.28*
MI-s	33.3 ± 3.5#	103.9 ± 10.8#	11.5 ± 2.5	95.2 ± 8.3#	26.0 ± 3.5#	2.49 ± 0.45

Values are mean ± SD. PGI2, prostaglandin I2; apo, apolipoprotein; free apoA-I/total apoA-I, ratio of free apoA-I to total serum apoA-I; HDL, high-density lipoprotein; total apoA-I/total apoA-II, molar ratio of total serum apoA-I to total serum apoA-II; AP, angina pectoris; UAP, unstable angina pectoris; MI-a, acute-phase myocardial infarction (36 ± 1.7 h from onset); MI-s, subacute-phase myocardial infarction (75 ± 15 h from onset). * $p < 0.05$; # $p < 0.01$ vs control group. (Reprinted from Aoyama *et al* 1990, Circulation 81: 1787, with permission).

infarction because it was also decreased in unstable angina pectoris, which is considered to be a preinfarction state. In subacute-phase myocardial infarction, the stability of PGI2 was similar to that in angina pectoris. Decreased stability of PGI2 may lead to insufficient PGI2 activity at sites of vascular damage, resulting in excessive accumulation of platelet thrombi. The accumulation of microthrombi and the release of biological substances from platelets may lead to vasoconstriction and atherosclerosis in the coronary artery, and the accumulation of massive thrombi may lead to severe narrowing or obstruction of the coronary artery. This could result in unstable angina pectoris or acute myocardial infarction.

SERUM HDL-CHOLESTEROL, APO A-I, AND APO A-II LEVELS

The four age-matched groups with coronary artery disease (CAD) described above had significantly lower serum HDL-cholesterol and apoA-I levels, compared to the control group. However, there were no differences in the amount of HDL-cholesterol or apoA-I between groups. Epidemiological and clinical studies carried out in several countries have demonstrated an inverse association between the incidence of CAD and HDL-cholesterol and apoA-I concentrations. Several reports have revealed that apoA-I deficiency is closely related to premature CAD and severe coronary atherosclerosis. The decreased PGI2 binding activity in patients with acute-phase myocardial infarction or unstable angina pectoris could not be fully explained by the total serum apoA-I levels.

To examine the mechanism of this reduction in PGI2 binding activity in patients with acute coronary events, we investigated the serum apoA-II and HDL-associated apoA-I levels. The ratio of free apoA-I to total serum apoA-I was increased in patients with acute-phase myocardial infarction or unstable angina pectoris, compared with those in control patients, patients with angina pectoris, and patients with subacute-phase myocardial infarction. Specifically, HDL-associated apoA-I levels in groups with acute coronary events were lower than those in groups with angina pectoris or subacute-phase myocardial infarction. apoA-II levels in patients with CAD were lower than those in control patients. However, the level of apoA-II in patients with unstable angina pectoris or acute-phase myocardial infarction was higher than that in patients with angina pectoris or subacute-phase myocardial infarction. The molar ratio of total serum apoA-I to apoA-II was the lowest in patients with unstable angina pectoris or acute-phase myocardial infarction (Table I).

REDUCTION IN PGI2 BINDING ACTIVITY BY DISPLACEMENT OF APO A-I IN HDL BY APO A-II

The distribution of particles within HDL is heterogeneous not only with respect to hydrated density, but also in relation to apolipoprotein composition. It is recognized that HDL contains at least two types of apoA-I-containing lipoprotein particles that may have different metabolic functions and clinical significance. One species contains, as the major protein components, both apoA-I and apoA-II, whereas in the other species, apoA-II is absent. The amount of HDL-associated apoA-I is affected by the amount of apoA-II, which has a greater affinity than apoA-I for the HDL particle, and 2 mol of apoA-II is able to displace 1 mol of apoA-I from the HDL particle quantitatively. After incubation of HDL with increasing amounts of apoA-II, apoA-I in HDL was displaced by apoA-II, and free apoA-I was increased in parallel. PGI2 binding activity decreased with increasing concentrations of apoA-II. In this system, apoA-I was progressively displaced by apoA-II (Fig. 1). LPDS, which contains free apoA-I, did not stabilize PGI2. Thus, HDL-associated apoA-I, not free apoA-I, stabilizes PGI2. The HDL particles with apoA-I only appear to have a significant ability to stabilize PGI2.

CORRELATION BETWEEN PGI2 BINDING ACTIVITY AND HDL-ASSOCIATED APO A-I LEVELS

There was a positive correlation between PGI2 binding activity and HDL-associated

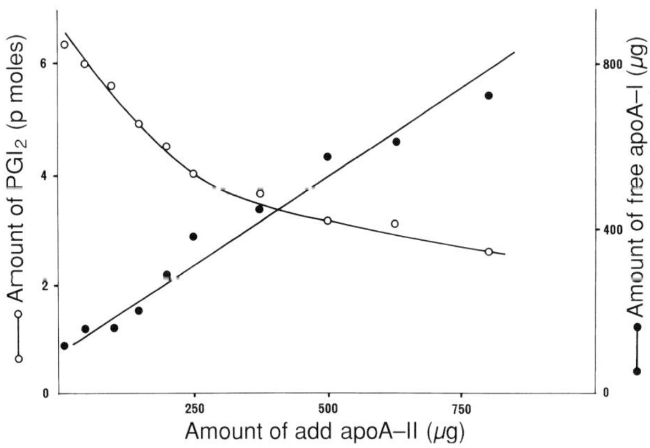

Fig. 1. Reduction in prostaglandin I2 (PGI2) binding activity as a result of displacement of apolipoprotein (apo) A-I in high-density lipoprotein (HDL) by apoA-II. Human serum HDL with an apoA-I concentration of 140 mg/dl and an apoA-II concentration of 40 mg/dl was prepared from normal fasting male donors. After incubation of 0.8 ml of an HDL sample with 0.2 ml of apoA-II solution at concentrations of 0–400 mg/dl, apoA-I in HDL was displaced by apoA-II. The amount of free apoA-I (closed circles) increased and the PGI2 binding activity (open circles) of the mixture decreased as the concentration of apoA-II was increased. (Reprinted from Aoyama *et al* 1990, Circulation 81: 1787, with permission)

apoA-I levels ($n = 35$, $r = 0.83$, $p < 0.01$). However, PGI_2 binding activities in patients with acute-phase myocardial infarction were lower than the values estimated from the regression curve, and activities in subacute-phase myocardial infarction were higher than the estimated values. This phenomenon may be due to the difference in the topographic change of apoA-I-phospholipid cholesterol.

The control patients had the highest levels of apoA-II and also total serum apoA-I, resulting in the highest levels of HDL-associated apoA-I and hence the highest PGI_2 binding affinities. In patients with angina pectoris, total serum apoA-I levels were decreased, compared with those in control patients. However, the molar ratio of apoA-I to apoA-II and the ratio of free apoA-I to total apoA-I did not change, compared with those in control patients. Decreased HDL-associated apoA-I levels were due to the reduction in total serum apoA-I levels. In patients with unstable angina pectoris or acute-phase myocardial infarction, the molar ratio of apoA-I to apoA-II, as well as total serum apoA-I levels, were decreased. The ratio of free apoA-I to total apoA-I was increased. Decreased HDL-associated apoA-I levels were due to the decreased total serum apoA-I levels and the increased free apoA-I levels.

SUMMARY

The serum PGI_2 half-life and total serum apoA-I levels were lower in the CAD group than in the control group. PGI_2 was least stable in patients with unstable angina pectoris or acute-phase myocardial infarction. In these patients, the molar ratio of apoA-I to apoA-II and HDL-associated apoA-I levels were decreased, and free apoA-I levels were increased. After *in vitro* incubation of HDL with increasing amounts of apoA-II, apoA-I in HDL was displaced by apoA-II, with a parallel decrease in the stability of PGI_2. Free apoA-I cannot stabilize PGI_2. HDL-associated apoA-I, the amount of which is affected by apoA-II, stabilized PGI_2 and correlated well with the stability of PGI_2 in patients with CAD and control patients. A decreased PGI_2 half-life may play an important role in the pathogenesis of atherosclerosis and thrombus formation in the coronary arteries, especially thrombus formation during an acute coronary event.

REFERENCES

Aoyama T, Yui Y, Morishita H, Kawai C 1990 Prostaglandin I_2 half-life regulated by high density lipoprotein is decreased in acute myocardial infarction and unstable angina pectoris. Circulation 81: 1784–1791

Morishita H, Yui Y, Hattori R, Aoyama T, Kawai C 1990 Increased hydrolysis of cholesterol ester with prostacyclin is potentiated by high density lipoprotein through prostacyclin stabilization. J Clin Invest 86: 1885–1891

Wu KK, Hall ER, Rossi EC, Papp AC 1985 Serum prostacyclin binding defects in thrombotic thrombocytopenic purpura. J Clin Invest 75: 168–174

Yui Y, Aoyama T, Morishita H, Takahashi M, Takatsu Y, Kawai C 1988 Serum prostacyclin stabilizing factor is identical to Apolipoprotein A-I (Apo A-I) a novel function of Apo A-I. J Clin Invest 82: 803–807

SECTION 7.
SMOKING CONTROL

Multiple Risk Factors in Cardiovascular Disease, ed. by A. Yamamoto, Churchill Livingstone Japan, Tokyo, pp. 237–241 (1994)

CIGARETTE SMOKING AND CORONARY HEART DISEASE: AN UPDATE

Lewis H. Kuller

*University of Pittsburgh, Graduate School of Public Health**

Key words: smoking, coronary heart disease, thrombosis, women, trends

Cigarette smoking is a major risk factor for coronary heart and other vascular diseases. Cigarette smoking probably increases the risk of vascular disease by several mechanisms. First, injury to the endothelium of blood vessels by cigarette smoke enhances the initial development and progression of atherosclerosis (U.S. Department of Health and Human Services 1989). Second, smoking increases the risk of thrombosis and platelet aggregation (Krobot et *al* 1992). Third, smoking probably increases the likelihood of oxidation of lipoprotein fatty acids that may be particularly important in the early development of the atherosclerotic lesions (Ames *et al* 1993). Fourth, smoking may have a direct effect on endothelial function, independent of the development of atherosclerosis (Celermajer *et al* 1993).

The effects of cigarette smoking on the coronary arteries may differ from those on peripheral blood vessels (Tell 1991; Bulpitt *et al* 1993). A critical level of saturated fat and cholesterol in the diet and a blood total cholesterol or low-density lipoprotein cholesterol (LDLc) level is probably necessary in order for cigarette smoking to have an important effect on coronary atherosclerosis and coronary heart disease (CHD). Peripheral blood vessels, especially in the lower extremities, may be directly injured by cigarette smoke. The lower blood cholesterol levels among populations in China and Japan, for example, is the most likely explanation of the paradox that there is a very high prevalence of cigarette smoking (especially among men) in these countries and consistently low rates of CHD; there is, however, increasing rates of lung cancer and other smoking related cancers.

In the United States, on the other hand, most of the population consumes a high saturated fat and cholesterol diet, especially compared with countries having lower rates of heart disease. The prevalence of atherosclerosis of the coronary arteries is high even in the relatively young. Smoking is a major risk factor for CHD, even among those with relatively low blood cholesterol by U.S. population criteria. For example, among those screened in the Multiple Risk Factor Intervention Trial (MRFIT), with blood cholesterol levels lower than 182 mg% (≤4.7 mmol%) and a diastolic blood pressure of <76 mmHg, the age-adjusted CHD death rate in those white men aged 35–57 years at entry was 3.6/10,000 per year for nonsmok-

* 130 DeSoto Street, Pittsburgh, PA 15261, USA.

ers, and 11.0/10,000 for smokers, almost a threefold difference. At the other extreme, a smoker with a cholesterol level ≥ 245 mg% (6.3 mmol%) and a diastolic blood pressure ≥ 92 mmHg, had a CHD death rate of approximately 60/10,000, about 20 times that for low risk nonsmokers (Neaton *et al* 1992).

The risk of CHD deaths among cigarette smokers is similar among ethnic groups in the United States (Table I). In the follow-up period of approximately 15 years in the MRFIT screened subjects, we were able to compare the CHD death rates among blacks, Hispanics, Orientals, and whites. The age-adjusted CHD mortality rates were higher among smokers than nonsmokers with relative risks varying from 2.34 ($p < 0.001$) for whites to 1.65 ($p < 0.05$) for Orientals.

Cigarette smoking was a risk factor for coronary artery disease deaths for both men in Japan and in Hawaii (Yano *et al* 1988) and the interquartile relative risk was approximately the same, 2.20 and 2.26. A study of Japanese physicians also noted a consistent and strong relationship between cigarette smoking and risk of CHD deaths (Kono *et al* 1985).

The continued low rates of CHD among Japanese men, even at relatively young ages, i.e. 35–44, is most likely due to the low saturated fat and cholesterol consumption and relatively low blood cholesterol levels. The cohort of Japanese men born after 1960 will probably be the first group to experience a post-World War II change in diet and high prevalence of cigarette smoking. At least some subgroups of men (in the 35–44 year age group) in Japan should have a substantial increase in CHD mortality, especially sudden deaths over the next 5–10 years. The consumption of both total fat and saturated fat, however, remains relatively low in Japan compared with that in the United States.

Cigarette smoking is also an important risk factor for CHD in women. A study by the American Cancer Society of approximately one million individuals noted a strong relationship between cigarette smoking and coronary artery disease mortality in both black and white women (Garfinkel

TABLE I. Age-Adjusted Rates per 10,000 Person-Years Excludes Other Races and Men Reporting Previous MI Screened MRFIT Participants Aged 35–57 (15 Year Follow-up)

Race	Cigs/day	CHD deaths	Adj. rate/ 10,000	Lung cancer deaths	Adj. rate 10,000
Black	0	289	17.1	64	3.8
	1–19	178	26.4	94	14.2
	20–39	280	36.5	208	27.2
	40+	36	27.3	71	61.8
Hispanic	0	68	13.0	6	1.1
	1–19	22	14.7	4	2.5
	20–39	44	30.9	17	12.9
	40+	12	27.2	7	15.1
Oriental	0	52	12.5	10	2.1
	1–19	9	14.5	3	5.7
	20–39	17	24.2	11	14.7
	40+	2	14.3	0	0.0
White	0	4973	15.2	946	2.9
	1–19	739	23.2	233	7.4
	20–39	3056	34.3	1641	18.7
	40+	1623	39.4	1136	28.3

MRFIT, the Multiple Risk Factor Intervention Trial; CHD, coronary heart disease.

1984). A recent report from the Framingham Study evaluated the health risks of smoking during the 34 years of follow-up. A strong relationship between CHD and smoking was reported only for men less than 65 years of age and a slight increase for women less than 65, and no relationship for men or women greater than 65. There was no consistent relationship between angina pectoris and cigarette smoking. When incident angina pectoris was excluded from the analysis, the relationship between cigarette smoking and CHD was consistent and strong for both men and women less than 65 years of age and also for women over the age of 65 years (Freund *et al* 1993).

The lack of an association between cigarette smoking and angina pectoris may be due to the specific effect of smoking on thrombosis, myocardial infarction, and sudden CHD deaths. The higher percentage of clinical coronary artery disease attributed to angina pectoris in women, as compared with men, may account for the lack of association between smoking and CHD among women sometimes reported.

Studies in Baltimore in the 1960's and early 1970's documented that practically all sudden CHD deaths under the age of 65 occurred among cigarette smokers. Similar studies of sudden death in the 1970's in Allegheny County, Pennsylvania, documented the strong association between cigarette smoking and sudden CHD death in women (Talbott *et al* 1983; Kuller *et al* 1986).

The sex differences in the characteristics of the epidemic of coronary artery disease deaths over time in the United States can be explained, in part, by the changing patterns of cigarette smoking.

Cardiovascular disease mortality began to increase among men but not women in the United States after World War I (Kuller *et al* 1986). The intake of total fat, saturated fat, and cholesterol was high, even in the early 1900's in the United States. Postmortem studies documented the prevalence of coronary atherosclerosis. The rise in the prevalence of cigarette smoking among men after World War I probably resulted in the substantial increase in CHD deaths in men and a rise in total cardiovascular mortality. During the same period many deaths due to other cardiovascular diseases such as renal disease, stroke, hypertension, and rheumatic heart disease declined. This resulted in an apparent decrease in cardiovascular disease among women, at the same time that there appeared to be an increase among men primarily related to CHD.

The epidemic of CHD deaths in the United States persisted until there was a decline in cigarette smoking in the late 1950's and 1960's. The decline was greater in the upper social class because of the earlier and greater reduction in risk factors, especially cigarette smoking (U.S. Department of Health and Human Services 1989).

The prevalence of smoking began to increase among women during and after World War II (U.S. Department of Health and Human Services 1989). The increase in CHD mortality, however, was modest and certainly not in proportion to the epidemic of smoking-related lung cancer among women. The reasons for this interesting phenomenon are two-fold. First, women develop atherosclerotic disease and clinical coronary artery disease at a much older age than men. At least part of this age difference between men and women is probably due to the effects of estrogens on atherosclerosis and arterial wall metabolism. The decrease in blood estrogens, peri- to postmenopause, is associated with an increase in LDLc among women and an increase in the prevalence of atherosclerosis, and later to the development of clinical CHD. Witteman documented the increased prevalence of abdominal atherosclerosis among postmenopausal women (Witteman *et al* 1993). She then followed 758 women, initially aged 45–64, for nine years. The development of new atherosclerotic plaques in the abdominal aorta was directly related to cigarette smoking while the rate of increase in atherosclerosis was reduced among the women who had stopped smoking.

The cohort of women who were in their early 20's in the 1940's would now be at a somewhat increased risk of CHD (i.e. at age 60–65+), i.e. those born after 1930. A large cohort of women should now be at risk. However, there is no evidence of a major increase in CHD among women in the United States.

The second key factor that precludes this epidemic of CHD is probably the effects of smoking cessation. By the age women are destined to develop atherosclerosis and a risk of CHD, many of them have already stopped smoking. The prevalence of smoking is high among young women, but only around 10–15% among older women in the United States (U.S. Department of Health and Human Services 1989).

Men are not as fortunate as women. The prevalence of atherosclerosis is higher among younger men at the same time as the percentage of cigarette smoking is still relatively high.

Smoking cessation has a substantial and fairly rapid effect on reducing the risk of heart attack and CHD deaths (Ockene *et al* 1990; Kawakchi *et al* 1994). The effect of smoking cessation may be present within months or, certainly, within a year or two. Differences in age at the development of substantial coronary atherosclerosis and smoking cessation probably count, in part, for the differences in the epidemic characteristics of CHD deaths between men and women.

Smoking cessation after a heart attack also significantly improves both short- and long-term prognosis (U.S. Department of Health and Human Services 1989). The continued decline in the prevalence of cigarette smoking, especially after a heart attack, probably accounts for part of the apparent improved short- and long-term prognosis after a heart attack. The improved treatment of hypertension, as well as a substantial decrease in blood total cholesterol level, especially among older women, also contributes to the decline in CHD.

The increase in lung cancer death rates, both among men and women in the United States as well in other countries including Japan and China, in spite of the lack of increase in CHD, is also related to the characteristics of the cigarette smoking epidemic.

The risk of lung cancer increases more sharply in relation to the degree of cigarette smoking than for CHD, especially among those who smoke 20 or more cigarettes per day (Table I). The percentages of those smoking cessation are inversely related to the degree of smoking. The percentage of heavy smokers who have stopped smoking will, therefore, be less than among lighter smokers. This difference in the percentage of smoking cessation has a much greater effect on lung cancer than CHD mortality rates. The reduction in the risk of heart attack is much more rapid on smoking cessation. The risk of lung cancer among ex-smokers probably never returns to the level of never smokers and even after six years of follow-up in the MRFIT, the risk of lung cancer was still substantial among former smokers compared with never smokers (Ockene *et al* 1990).

Smoking is probably an independent risk factor for lung cancer. The growing pool of older ex-cigarette smokers now at substantially reduced risk of dying from coronary artery disease swells the susceptible pool for lung cancer deaths. The change in tar content of cigarettes may have had a bigger effect on lung cancer than CHD.

SUMMARY

The continued decline in the prevalence of cigarette smoking, especially in the middle aged and elderly, in the United States and in some other countries is consistent with the continued decline in CHD and other vascular disease mortality. The prevalence of coronary atherosclerosis and non-fatal heart attacks may not be decreasing as rapidly as are deaths. The epidemic of sudden CHD deaths and the high rate of fatality after myocardial infarction may be replaced in the future by a more indolent chronic CHD, primarily among older men and women in the

United States. On the other hand, in several other countries such as China, Japan, and Southern Europe, the rising blood cholesterol levels and changes in diet should lead to an increase in the prevalence of atherosclerosis and the high prevalence of cigarette smoking could lead to a major epidemic of coronary artery disease similar to that seen in the United States after World War I.

REFERENCES

Ames BN, Shigenaga MK, Hagen TM 1993 Oxidants, antioxidants, and the degenerative diseases of aging. Proc Natl Acad Sci USA 90: 7915–7922

Bulpitt CJ, Shipley M, Fletcher AE *et al* 1993 Smoking and blood pressure in the leg. J Hypertens 11: 211–215

Celermajer DS, Sorensen KE, Georgakopoulos D *et al* 1993 Cigarette smoking is associated with dose-related and potentially reversible impairment of endothelium-dependent dilation in healthy young adults. Circulation 88: 2149–2155

Freund KM, Belanger AJ, D'Agostino RB, Kannel WB 1993 The health risks of smoking. The Framingham Study: 34 years of follow-up. Ann Epidemiol 3: 417–424

Garfinkel L 1984 Cigarette smoking and coronary heart disease in blacks: comparison to whites in a prospective study. Am Heart J 108: 802–807

Kawakchi I, Colditz GA, Stampfer MJ *et al* 1994 Smoking cessation and time course of decreased risks of coronary heart disease in middle-aged women. Arch Intern Med 154: 169–175

Kono S, Ikeda M, Tokudome S, Nishizumi M, Kuratsune M 1985 Smoking and mortalities from cancer, coronary heart disease and stroke in male Japanese physicians. J Cancer Res Clin Oncol 110: 161–164

Krobot K, Hense HW, Cremer P, Eberle E, Keil U 1992 Determinants of plasma fibrinogen: relation to body weight, waist-to-hip ratio, smoking, alcohol, age, and sex. Results from the second MONICA Augsburg survey, 1989–1990. Arterioscler Thromb 12: 780–788

Kuller LH, Perper JA, Dai WS, Rutan G, Traven N 1986 Sudden death and the decline in coronary heart disease mortality. J Chron Dis 39: 1001–1019

Neaton JD, Wentworth D, for the MRFIT Research Group 1992 Serum cholesterol, blood pressure, cigarette smoking, and death from coronary heart disease. Overall findings and differences by age for 316,099 white men. Arch Intern Med 152: 56–64

Ockene JD, Kuller LH, Svendsen KH, Meilahn E 1990 The relationship of smoking cessation to coronary heart disease and lung cancer in the Multiple Risk Factor Intervention Trial (MRFIT). Am J Public Health 80: 954–958

Talbott E, Kuller LH, Murphy PA 1983 The epidemiology of sudden coronary death. Journal — South Carolina Med Assoc Oct: 574–586

Tell GS 1991 Cigarette smoking, lipids, lipoproteins, and extracranial carotid artery atherosclerosis. Mayo Clinic Proc 66: Editorial 327–331

U.S. Department of Health and Human Services 1989 Reducing the health consequences of smoking: 25 years of progress. A report of the Surgeon General. U.S. Department of Health and Human Services, Public Health Service, Centers for Disease Control, Center for Chronic Disease Prevention and Health Promotion, Office on Smoking and Health. DHHS Publ No. (CDC) 89-8411, Prepublication version, January 11

Witteman JCM, Grobbee DE, Valkenburg HA, VanHemert AM, Stignen T, Hofman A 1993 Cigarette smoking and the development and progression of aortic atherosclerosis. A 9-year population-based follow-up study in women. Circulation 88: 2156–2162

Yano K, MacLean CJ, Reed DM *et al* 1988 A comparison of the 12-year mortality and predictive factors of coronary heart disease among Japanese men in Japan and Hawaii. Am J Epidemiol 127: 476–487

Multiple Risk Factors in Cardiovascular Disease, ed. by A. Yamamoto, Churchill Livingstone Japan, Tokyo, pp. 243–247 (1994)

CIGARETTE SMOKING AND VASOREACTIVITY TO ISCHEMIA: BENEFICIAL EFFECTS OF QUITTING SMOKING

Haruhisa Hashimoto

*Department of Internal Medicine, Yoshida General Hospital**

Key words: smoking, reactive hyperemia, vasoreactivity, vascular endothelium, microcirculation

Cigarette smoking is one of the three major risk factors for coronary heart disease, along with high blood pressure and hypercholesterolemia. Because both active and passive smoking affects people, cigarette smoking is a serious problem from the viewpoint of public health. Numerous epidemiological studies indicate that the degree of relative risk attributable to cigarette smoking increases approximately two-fold for coronary heart disease when taking all ages and both sexes together. Two-fold increase in relative risk has also been documented for peripheral arterial disease such as intermittent claudication in the Framingham study and in the Edinburgh artery study. It is important to note that cigarette smoking additively affects the cardiovascular system via a positive interaction with hypertension and hypercholesterolemia.

Cigarette smoking affects the cardiovascular system by means of a variety of different mechanisms. This includes the elevation of heart rate (10–20%), blood pressure (5–15%), myocardial oxygen consumption, and peripheral vasoconstriction through activation of the sympathetic nervous system mainly due to the effect of nicotine. Smoking affects the lipid profile adversely. Smokers, as a group, have lower high density lipoprotein (HDL)-cholesterol (10%) and higher free fatty acids than non-smokers. Another important contribution of smoking to atherosclerotic vascular disease is through its effects on hemostasis. Smoking increases fibrinogen, platelet adhesiveness and aggregability, as well as plasminogen activator inhibitor, all of which lead to an increased risk of thrombosis and atherosclerosis.

CIGARETTE SMOKING AND ENDOTHELIAL FUNCTION

The vascular endothelium has an important regulatory role in maintaining vascular tone and in the initiation and progression of atherosclerosis. Cigarette smoke can activate and injure the vascular endothelium and thereby affect the vasoreactivity and development of atherosclerosis. Actually, increased incidence of damage to the vascular endothelium has been reported in long-term cigarette smokers. In addition, morphological studies have confirmed a strong association between smoking and endothelial damage, as early as in newborn children of smoking mothers. As far as cigarette

* 217 Kou, Kitakohji, Yoshida, Kita-Uwa, Ehime 799-37, Japan.

smoking and endothelial function are concerned, two conflicting reports have been published. Rubinstein *et al* (1991) reported, using a hamster cheek pouch preparation, that cigarette smoke extract impaired the endothelium-dependent arteriolar relaxation to acetylcholine. While Rångemark and Wennmalm (1992), studying the human forearm, reported that endothelium-dependent vasodilation to acetylcholine was much greater in smokers than in non-smokers.

CIGARETTE SMOKING AND VASOREACTIVITY

Transient ischemia can cause a significant overshoot of blood flow, known as reactive hyperemia (Fig. 1). This phenomenon is considered as a compensatory mechanism for transient hypoxemia which occurs in the ischemic tissue due to the temporary cessation of blood flow. It has been shown that this compensatory mechanism is attenuated in long-term cigarette smokers (Richardson 1985; Carlsson & Wennmalm 1987; Hashimoto 1994).

To document the relationship between vasoreactivity to ischemia and smoking status, the present study investigated reactive hyperemia in 54 healthy subjects (18 never smokers aged 52 ± 5 years, 18 current smokers aged 50 ± 7 years, and 18 ex-smokers aged 51 ± 6 years) who were males with no family history of diabetes mellitus or hypertension. Ex-smokers had given up smoking for over a year and the mean duration of abstention was 4.4 years. Monitoring the microvascular blood flow with a laser Doppler flowmeter, arterial occlusion and release was performed at the base of the middle finger to elicit post-occlusive reactive hyperemia. The attenuated response of reactive hyperemia was observed in current smokers (Fig. 2). A attenuation of reactive hyperemia in current smokers was related to the intensity of the smoking habit. There was a significant negative correlation between the number of cigarettes smoked per day and the increase in flow ($r = -0.67$) and area under the response curve ($r = -0.77$). On the other hand, there was no correlation between the parameters of reactive hyperemia and the duration of the smoking habit. Ex-smokers showed a similar response to never smokers suggesting that reduced vasoreactivity to ischemia is potentially reversible on quitting smoking. This is interesting because the increased risk of coronary events

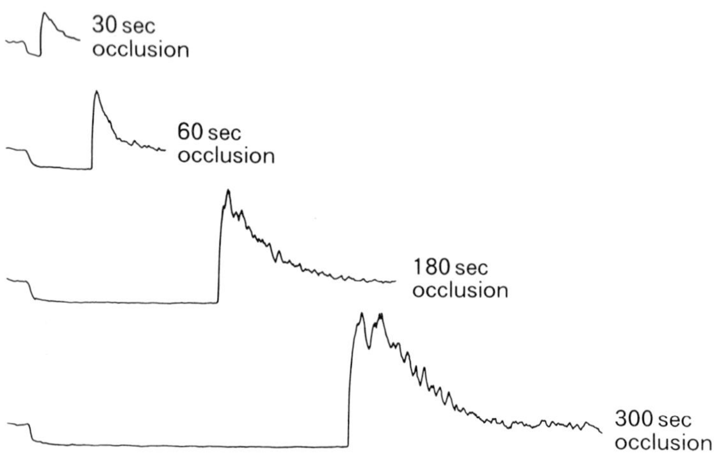

Fig. 1. Tracings of post-occlusive reactive hyperemia.
With increasing duration of arterial occlusion, the reactive hyperemic response is proportionally increased.

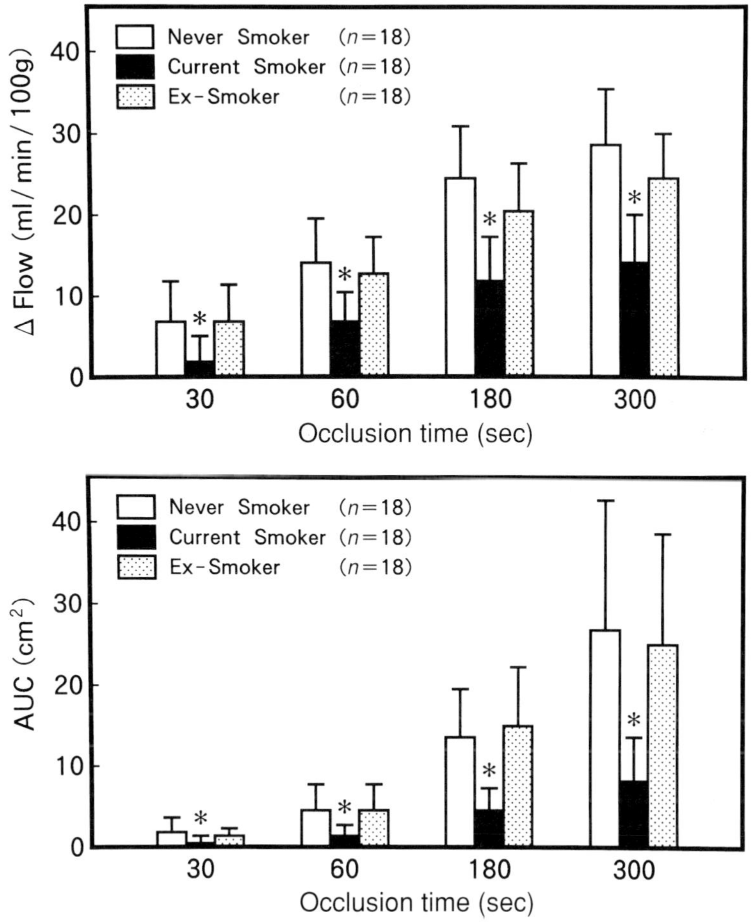

Fig. 2A. Delta flow following the release of arterial occlusion according to smoking status.
In current smokers, delta flow significantly decreased to 31–49% compared with never smokers.
Fig. 2B. Area under the response curve (AUC) following the release of arterial occlusion according to smoking status.
In current smokers, AUC significantly decreased to 16–34% compared with never smokers. Ex-smokers exhibited the same response as never smokers.

in smokers declines quite rapidly within several years to the same level as non-smokers, once the patient quits smoking.

POSSIBLE MECHANISM FOR ATTENUATED VASOREACTIVITY IN CIGARETTE SMOKERS

A precise mechanism has not yet been fully described for reactive hyperemia and it is likely that a number of vasodilating metabolites of endogenous compounds are responsible for reactive hyperemia. Possible candidates which might modulate reactive hyperemia are oxygen, adenosine, prostacyclin, endothelium-derived relaxing factor (EDRF, NO), ion channels (potassium, calcium, chloride), blood viscosity, and vascular rigidity.

Indomethacin, a cyclooxygenase inhibitor, causes the reduction of reactive hyperemia in non-smokers but not in smokers, suggesting the importance of prostaglandins in reactive hyperemia (Carlsson & Wennmalm 1987). Because nicotine has been shown to inhibit the synthesis/release of prostacyclin in isolated blood vessels, it appears that indomethacin was unable to attenuate further the reactive hyperemia in smokers. Dipyridamole, which inhibits the degradation of adenosine, potentiates reactive hyperemia in non-smokers. On the other hand, theophylline, an adenosine receptor antagonist, reduces the degree of reactive hyperemia, suggesting the involvement of adenosine in reactive hyperemia.

Accumulating evidence has shown that EDRF (NO) contributes significantly to the flow-induced vasodilation. Also, EDRF (NO) plays an important role in the leukocyte-vessel wall interaction. Although there is yet no direct evidence that EDRF (NO) is responsible for reactive hyperemia *in vivo*, dysfunction of EDRF (NO) synthesis/release due to injury of the vascular endothelium, is considered as possibly having an inhibitory effect on the reactive hyperemia seen in cigarette smokers. It has been shown that cigarette smoke increases leukocyte adhesiveness to the vascular endothelium possibly enhancing the expression of adhesion molecules. EDRF (NO), on the other hand, inhibits the expression of adhesion molecules such as intercellular adhesion molecule-1. Thus, it seems likely that EDRF (NO) is an important modulator not only of vascular tone but also of leukocyte adhesiveness to the vascular endothelium and plays a critical role in maintaining the microcirculation in cigarette smokers.

A consistent abnormality found in cigarette smokers is an elevated leukocyte count. In addition to their increased number, the functional alteration of leukocyte adhesiveness and deformability is important in the regulation of microvascular blood flow. Mechanical obstruction of the microvasculature by blood cells leads to disturbances in capillary flow, and this may possibly be related to the attenuated reactive hyperemia seen in cigarette smokers. The fact that in the present study there was a weak but significant negative correlation ($r = -0.37$, $n = 54$) between leukocyte count and the degree of reactive hyperemia suggests this was indeed a possibility. Leukocytes activated by cigarette smoke could release oxygen-derived free radicals during the early phase of reperfusion, which could then cause breakdown of NO. The vasodilatory capacity of EDRF (NO) may be limited by the counteraction of free radicals even if the EDRF (NO) synthesis/release process is normal in cigarette smokers. Oxygen-derived free radicals appear to be responsible for causing injury to the vascular endothelium because recent studies have indicated that cigarette smokers have impaired antioxidant defense mechanisms.

Another mechanism concerns the structural impairment of the arterial system. Pathological studies of human autopsy cases have shown a positive association between smoking and atherosclerosis in large arteries such as the coronary artery, abdominal aorta, and iliac and femoral arteries although the contribution from the cerebral and brachial arteries seems smaller. Accumulation of macrophages and fatty streaks is often observed in the arterial walls of long-term smokers. At the arteriolar site, thickening of the walls has been shown in smokers due to the proliferation of smooth muscle cells. Differences in mechanical properties such as the more rigid arterial or arteriolar walls in smokers may explain the reduced response of reactive hyperemia.

With regard to platelet function and smoking, there is an important interaction between prostacyclin and EDRF (NO) as far as preventing platelet aggregation is concerned. Each substance inhibits platelet aggregation with sufficient dose. The antiaggregatory effects of prostacyclin are potentiated by low dose EDRF (NO), which per se has no antiaggregatory effects and, conversely antiaggregatory effects of EDRF (NO) are potentiated by low dose prostacyclin, which per se has no antiaggregatory effects. Thus, dysfunction of EDRF (NO) and prostacyclin synthesis/release plays an important role in increased platelet aggregation in long-term cigarette smokers.

SUMMARY

Cigarette smoking is an established risk factor for atherosclerotic disease although the underlying pathophysiological mechanisms of its action are incompletely understood. To study the effects of quitting smoking on vasoreactivity to transient ischemia, I studied post-occlusive reactive hyperemia. Current smokers showed an attenuated response, while ex-smokers who had quit smoking for over a year showed the same response as never smokers, suggesting that impaired vasoreactivity can be reversed by quitting smoking. The present results support epidemiological data which indicate that the increased risk of ischemic cardiovascular disease attributable to smoking is reduced once the patient quits smoking.

Dysfunction of the vascular endothelium may be the most important factor causing attenuated vasoreactivity in cigarette smokers. However, more evidence is needed to confirm this hypothesis. In particular, the roles of EDRF (NO), prostacyclin, adhesion molecules, and oxygen-derived free radicals in smoking-related cardiovascular events need further investigation.

REFERENCES

Carlsson I, Sollevi A, Wennmalm Å 1987 The role of myogenic relaxation, adenosine and prostaglandins in human forearm reactive hyperemia. J Physiol 389: 147–161

Hashimoto H 1994 Impaired microvascular vasodilator reserve in chronic cigarette smokers — A study of post-occlusive reactive hyperemia in the human finger. Jpn Circ J 58: 29–33

Rångemark C, Wennmalm Å 1992 Endothelium-dependent and -independent vasodilation and reactive hyperemia in healthy smokers. J Cardiovasc Pharmacol 20 (suppl 12): S198–S201

Richardson DR 1985 Effects of habitual tobacco smoking on reactive hyperemia in the human hand. Arch Environ Health 40: 114–119

Rubinstein I, Yong T, Rennard SI, Mayhan WG 1991 Cigarette smoke extract attenuates endothelium-dependent arteriolar dilatation *in vivo*. Am J Physiol 261: H1913–H1918

Multiple Risk Factors in Cardiovascular Disease, ed. by A. Yamamoto, Churchill Livingstone Japan, Tokyo, pp. 249–253 (1994)

DETRIMENTAL EFFECTS OF SMOKING ON PROGNOSIS IN VARIANT ANGINA — ACCURATE ASSESSMENT OF SMOKING STATUS BY URINARY COTININE MEASUREMENT

Kunihisa MIWA

*The Second Department of Internal Medicine, Toyama Medical and Pharmaceutical University**

Key words: smoking, smoking cessation, variant angina, anginal attack

Smoking has been established as an important risk factor for coronary heart disease. Epidemiological evidence indicates that smoking cessation significantly improves the long-term prognosis in smokers with coronary heart disease. Long-term prognosis for patients with variant angina is reported to be relatively good when calcium antagonists are prescribed (Yasue *et al* 1988). However, Madias (1979) reported in his study that all 10 patients with variant angina who had acute myocardial infarction were smokers. A recent statistical analysis of clinical risk factors for coronary artery spasm (Nobuyoshi *et al* 1992) has identified smoking as the most significant risk factor in discriminating between patients with and without coronary artery spasm.

Although self-reporting is widely used to estimate the prevalence of cigarette smoking, it is known to underestimate the true prevalence in some populations. This underestimation may be higher when patients are unwilling participants in a forced education program for smoking cessation conducted by physicians. Misclassification of the smoking status may lead to the wrong evaluation as far as the effects of the smoking cessation on the prognosis in patients with coronary artery disease is concerned. Consequently, a reliable biologic marker is needed to validate that smoking has stopped. In the present study, urinary cotinine, a stable metabolite of nicotine, was used to examine the validity of self-reporting of smoking status and determine the effects of smoking cessation on the short-term prognosis for variant angina.

URINARY COTININE MEASUREMENT IN PATIENTS WITH VARIANT ANGINA

A total 48 consecutive patients (41 men and 7 women with a mean age of 55) with variant angina were recruited. ST-segment elevation during anginal attacks was confirmed in all the patients. All patients underwent coronary arteriography to determine the site of spasm and the extent of the organic coronary stenosis. At the time of hospitalization, 37 patients (77%) were current habitual smokers, 3 (6%) were former smokers, and 8 (17%) were non-smokers. The smokers were strongly advised to stop smoking. All 48 patients were discharged when anginal attacks

* 2630 Sugitani, Toyama 930-01, Japan.
This study was supported in part by grants from Japan Research Foundation for Clinical Pharmacology, Tokyo, Japan.

had been completely suppressed during their daily life by the use of medication, including calcium-entry blockers. The usual drug doses were 40–80 mg daily for nifedipine and 90–240 mg daily for diltiazem. When lower doses of each drug were in sufficient to prevent the occurrence of anginal attacks, higher doses were employed. Drug treatment was continued and subjects were followed-up at our out-patient clinic every month. Each patient's account of their current smoking status and anginal history during the previous 3 months was recorded at each visit. When they declared that at least 1 week had passed since their last cigarette, they were classified as current non-smokers or quitters by self-reporting. The urine samples from all patients were collected for cotinine measurement at 3 months and 1 year after their discharge. Urinary cotinine concentrations were determined by radioimmunoassay using ^{125}I-1-cotinine and cotinine antibody obtained from rabbits (Miwa *et al* 1993, 1994). Urinary cotinine concentration is expressed as nanograms per milliliter urine. The urinary cotinine level was 245 ± 178 (mean ± standard deviation) ng/ml in the 64 known smokers, smoking 3 or more cigarettes daily, and 2 ± 3 ng/ml in the 51 non-smokers who did not have significant involuntary exposure to tobacco smoke (Miwa *et al* 1993). The urinary cotinine concentration in the habitual smokers was always over 100 ng/ml. The urinary cotinine level was able to discriminate between smokers and non-smokers. In smokers, the urinary cotinine roughly correlated with the self-reported cigarette consumption. The urinary cotinine of non-smokers was always less than 50 ng/ml, regardless of the presence of their involuntary exposure to tobacco smoke. In the present study, regardless of their claims, they were classified as smokers by urinary cotinine if they had a urinary cotinine level above 50 ng/ml.

VALIDITY OF SELF-REPORTING

In the present study, the validity of self-reporting on the cigarette smoking status of patients with variant angina was examined against a biochemical marker of nicotine uptake, urinary cotinine. According to their self-reporting, smoking habits were main-

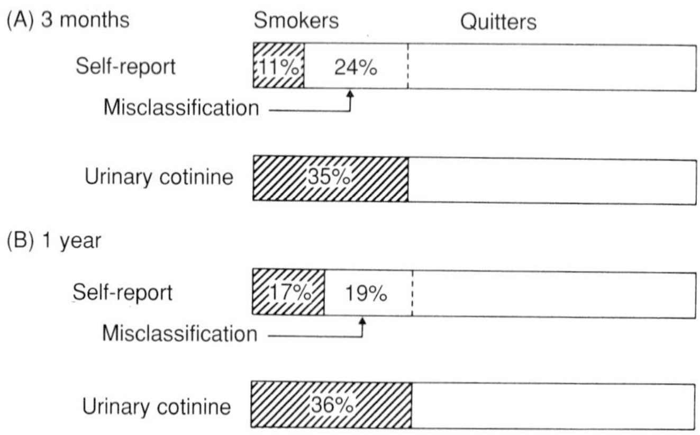

Fig. 1. Discrepancies in current smokers after the follow-up of 3 months (A) and 1 year (B) determined by self-reporting and urinary cotinine measurement.
Total number of the patients was 37 after 3 months and 36 after 1 year. Shaded area indicates current smokers, unshaded area, quitters.

tained at 3 months of follow-up in 4 (11%) of the smoking patients, at the time of hospitalization, educated for smoking cessation while they were seen in 13 (35%), as shown by the urinary cotinine assay (Fig. 1). Smoking habits after 1 year were still positive in 6 (17%) by self-reporting and 13 (36%) by urinary cotinine measurement. Our results clearly demonstrate the discrepancy in smoking prevalence rates between monitoring using self-reporting and urinary cotinine measurement. Urinary cotinine measurement revealed that all the "positive" patients in terms of smoking had urinary cotinine levels above 100 ng/ml and therefore, were voluntary smokers. A considerable number of patients lied about their smoking habits.

In the CARDIA study (Wagenknecht *et al* 1992) self-reporting underestimated the smoking prevalence by up to 4%. The misclassification rate was much higher in our patients; 9 (19%) of the total number of subjects were misclassified as non-smokers after 3 months and 7 (15%) after 1 year by self-reporting. This misclassification rate became higher in those smokers who, at the time of hospitalization, were receiving education for smoking cessation during follow-up periods (24% after 3 months and 19% after 1 year, Fig. 1). In the current smokers after follow-up, as many as 69% (9/13) after 3 months and 54% (7/13) after 1 year lied about their smoking status and were misclassified as current non-smokers by self-reporting. This high rate may be, at least in part, due to the pressure on these patients.

ANGINAL ATTACKS IN SMOKERS AND QUITTERS

Patients were divided into 3 groups according to their urinary cotinine levels; patients who continued smoking despite education for smoking cessation (smokers), patients who succeeded in stopping smoking (quitters), and patients, including non- and ex-smokers at the time of hospitalization, who never start smoking thereafter. When the current smoking status was determined by urinary cotinine assay, the prevalence rate of anginal attacks during the first 3 months was found to be significantly higher in the smokers (8/13, 62%) than in the quitters (5/24, 21%), although this rate was comparable when the classification of the patients was performed according to their self-reporting (Fig. 2).

BENEFICIAL EFFECTS OF SMOKING CESSATION ON THE PROGNOSIS FOR VARIANT ANGINA

Our data demonstrate, for the first time, that the beneficial effects of smoking cessation on

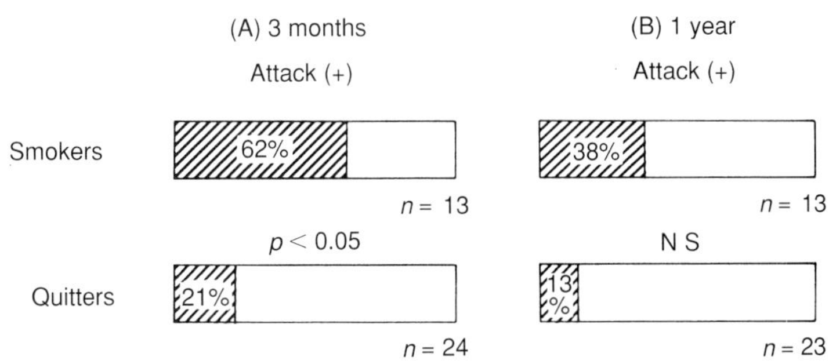

Fig. 2. A total of 37 patients were divided into smokers and quitters according to their urinary cotinine concentration.
Patients with anginal attacks after 3 months (A) and after 1 year (B) of follow-up are indicated by the shaded area. Anginal attacks were significantly ($p < 0.05$) more prevalent in current smokers (62%) than quitters (21%) after 3 months.

the prognosis of variant angina appears during the first 3 months. In earlier reports, favorable effects of smoking cessation became apparent in patients with coronary heart disease only after at least 2 years. The accurate evaluation of smoking status by urinary cotinine measurement probably helped in the disclosure of the beneficial effects of smoking cessation during a relatively short follow-up period. The prevalence rate of anginal attacks after 1 year was found to be also higher in smokers (5/13, 38%) than in quitters (3/23, 13%) (Fig. 2). However, this difference was not significant even after their smoking status was corrected using the urinary cotinine assay. The beneficial effects of smoking cessation appeared more marked during the first 3 months of follow-up. The high susceptibility to coronary spasm during the first 3 months, which is closely related to the occurrence of anginal attacks, appeared to be critically worsened by smoking.

The prevalence of patients with anginal attacks during the last 3 months was also compared between current smokers and current non-smokers, including non-smokers, ex-smokers and quitters. According to their self-reporting no significant differences were found in the ratio of the presence of anginal attacks between current smokers and current non-smokers after 3 months and after 1 year. However, the prevalence rate of anginal attacks was significantly higher in the current smokers than in the current non-smokers determined by the urinary cotinine assay after 3 months (8/13, 62% vs 10/35, 29%) and after 1 year (5/13, 38% vs 3/34, 9%). Anginal attacks were significantly more prevalent in the patients with a significant organic coronary artery stenosis after 3 months (13/21, 62% vs 5/27, 19%). However, this difference became insignificant after 1 year (5/21, 24% vs 3/26, 12%).

Non-fatal acute myocardial infarction developed at 14 months and within 1 month of the follow-up period in 2 male patients who failed to stop smoking, as shown by the urinary cotinine measurement. The data from a patient in whom acute myocardial infarction developed within 1 month were not included in the 1 year follow-up data. Although it has been reported that cardiac death and non-fatal myocardial infarction occur most often during the first 3 months of follow-up, in our patients, no cardiac death (only 1 acute non-fatal myocardial infarction) occurred during the first 3 months. The aggressive treatment with calcium entry blockers may have contributed to preventing the occurrence of cardiac events.

IMPORTANCE OF SMOKING CESSATION EDUCATION

Despite our intensive education aimed at smoking cessation, the prevalence rate of smokers after 1 year was 36%, essentially the same as that after 3 months (35%). Although the smokers were aware that their smoking status was being accurately monitored by a reliable objective method, the smoking cessation rate was not improved. Smoking cessation education during hospitalization appears to be important and should be increased.

CONCLUSIONS

In conclusion, smoking significantly worsens the prognosis of anginal attacks in patients with variant angina. The beneficial effects of smoking cessation on the attacks will be underestimated if the smoking status is evaluated exclusively by self-reporting.

SUMMARY

To examine whether smoking cessation would improve the short-term prognosis for patients with variant angina, 37 smokers with variant angina, who were discharged after the complete disappearance of angina following medical treatment with calcium blockers, were advised to stop smoking and followed-up for 1 year. Urinary cotinine radioimmunoassay was used to evaluate their current smoking status. Patients with a urinary cotinine concentration above 50 ng/

ml were classified as current smokers. The prevalence of smokers was underestimated by self-reporting (11% by self-reporting vs 35% by urinary cotinine measurements after 3 months; 17% by self-reporting vs 36% by urinary cotinine measurements after 1 year). The presence of angina during the first 3 months was significantly ($p < 0.05$) more prevalent in those who continued to smoke (8/13,62%) than in those who succeeded in smoking cessation (5/24, 21%) when the current smoking status was determined by urinary cotinine measurements. Smoking cessation definitely improved the prognosis for variant angina during a relatively short follow-up period.

Acknowledgment
Anticotinine sera from rabbits were kindly provided by Prof. Shigeru Matsukura of Miyazaki Medical University, Japan.

REFERENCES

Madias JE 1979 The syndrome of variant angina culminating in acute myocardial infarction. Circulation 59: 297–306

Miwa K, Miyagi Y, Asanoi H, Fujita M, Sasayama S 1993 Augmentation of education for smoking cessation by urinary cotinine measurement. Jpn Circ J 57: 775–780

Miwa K, Fujita M, Miyagi Y 1994 Beneficial effects of smoking cessation on the short-term prognosis for variant angina — validation of the smoking status by urinary cotinine measurements. Int J Cardiol 44: 151–156

Nobuyoshi M, Abe M, Nosaka M *et al* 1992 Statistical analysis of clinical risk factors for coronary artery spasm: identification of the most important determinant. Am Heart J 124: 32–38

Wagenknecht LE, Burke GL, Perkins LL, Haley NJ, Friedman GD 1992 Misclassification of smoking status in the CARDIA study: a comparison of self-report with serum cotinine levels. Am J Public Health 82: 33–36

Yasue H, Takizawa A, Nagao M *et al* 1988 Long-term prognosis for patients with variant angina and influential factors. Circulation 78: 1–9

Multiple Risk Factors in Cardiovascular Disease, ed. by A. Yamamoto, Churchill Livingstone Japan, Tokyo, pp. 255–258 (1994)

PLATELET SIZE (MEAN PLATELET VOLUME) AND CIGARETTE SMOKING

Kazuomi KARIO* and Takefumi MATSUO

Department of Internal Medicine, Hyogo Prefectural Awaji Hospital and Awaji-Hokutan Public Clinic

Key words: mean platelet volume, cigarette smoking, stopping smoking, cardiovascular risk factor, automated blood cell analyzer

Platelet behavior is as an important determinant of cardiovascular disease and recently, platelet size has been recognized as a cardiovascular risk factor (Martin *et al* 1991; Thompson *et al* 1990). Larger platelets have been shown to be more active than smaller ones, since they contain more granules and express greater enzymatic activity (Thompson *et al* 1990). Automated blood cell analyzers now enable us to easily measure mean platelet volume (MPV) and increases in MPV, which have been described in various arterial diseases, may play an important part in the progression of atherogenesis and thrombosis (Kristensen 1990). Cigarette smoking is widely recognized as a risk factor for cardiovascular disease, but it is still controversial whether smoking can alter platelet function. The effects of smoking on platelet aggregation have usually been studied *in vitro* and in healthy young subjects. Cigarette smoking may locally enhance the *in vivo* platelet-vessel interaction (Klein 1984), which is increased on the injured endothelium of elderly subjects, especially those with atherosclerotic diseases. The clinical significance of MPV and the effect of cigarette smoking and its cessation on MPV are discussed here.

* Correspondence to: Dr. Kario K, 480-2 Ikuha, Hokutan, Tsuna, Hyogo 656-16, Japan.

THE MEANING OF PLATELET VOLUME

Determination of MPV

MPV is a simple parameter providing information about the megakaryocyte-platelet-hemostasis axis. Platelets do not change their volume as they age, so a major determinant of MPV is now thought to be established before the time of megakaryocyte fragmentation into platelets and to express megakaryocyte activity (Thompson *et al* 1990).

Correlation of MPV with Platelet Activity

Larger platelets are more active than smaller ones, contain more granules and express greater enzymatic activity *in vitro* (Thompson *et al* 1990). Thus, MPV is correlated with platelet aggregation, platelet LDH, ATP, and β-thromboglobulin content as well as platelet serotonin and β-thromboglobulin release.

Clinical Significance of MPV

MPV may be an independent cardiovascular risk factor. MPV is found to increase at the onset of coronary artery diseases and acute cerebral infarction. The increase in MPV and megakaryocyte size are greater in patients dying suddenly from cardiac events than in those dying from road traffic accidents (Trowbridge *et al* 1984). In the recent prospective study of 1,716 men 6 months after myocardial infarction, MPV was found to be greater in the 126 who had a further recurrence during the 2 year-follow-up period compared with the 1,590 men who had no further events (Martin *et al* 1991). In the same study, MPV did not correlate with known cardiovascular diseases such as blood pressure, serum lipids, fibrinogen, white cell count, or plasma viscosity.

Measurement of MPV

To avoid the effect of artificial platelet swelling, the condition to measure MPV after blood collection should be considered. It has been reported that EDTA causes approximately a 15% increase in the measured MPV. However, the initial relative MPV is maintained, because all platelets increase proportionately. In our study (Kario *et al* 1992) the increase in MPV was 12% in blood samples collected in tubes containing EDTA measured 30 min after collection, compared with that measured immediately after collection. However, the change in MPV between 60 and 120 min in samples collected with EDTA was only 3.4%. Thus, we usually measure MPV in samples containing EDTA between 60 and 120 min after collection. Some authors have delayed measuring MPV until after 24 h, during which interval the MPV increases (Martin *et al* 1991).

EFFECT OF CIGARETTE SMOKING ON MPV

To study the effect of cigarette smoking on platelet size in arterial disease, we measured the MPV in 142 elderly smokers and non-smokers, with or without atherosclerotic risk factors (Kario *et al* 1992). MPV (mean ± SD) and plateletcrit (MPV × Platelet count) were significantly higher in the 20 atherosclerotic smokers than in the 42 non-smoking subjects without atherosclerotic disease (8.4 ± 0.7 vs 7.9 ± 0.9 fl, $p < 0.05$; 0.22 ± 0.005 vs 0.18 ± 0.004%, $p < 0.01$). An inverse relationship between MPV and platelet count was found in each group. The correlation coefficient was higher in the atherosclerotic smokers than in non-smoking group without atherosclerotic disease ($r = -0.54$, $p < 0.05$ vs $r = -0.32$, $p < 0.05$). When compared at the same platelet count, the MPV was higher in the atherosclerotic smokers than in the non-smoking group without atherosclerotic disease.

We also investigated the effect of smoking cessation on MPV in a longitudinal study. The changes in MPV in 8 smoking subjects in the atherosclerotic group who successfully gave up smoking are shown in Fig. 1. A significant decrease in MPV was found at 1–3 months after smoking cessation ($p < 0.05$). Two of the subjects who had stopped smoking resumed again after 4–6 months. Their MPV values increased after they started again. The plateletcrit also tended to decrease after smoking cessation, although the change was not significant (before smoking cessation: 0.18 ± 0.03%; 1–3 months after smoking cessation: 0.16 ± 0.04%). These changes were not found in the 8 control subjects who did not stop smoking.

A previous report has shown that smoking shortens, the platelet survival half-life, as determined by ^{51}Cr, and that smoking cessation or therapy with dipyridamole plus aspirin can reverse this (Fuster *et al* 1981). Others have reported that cigarette smoking enhances platelet-vessel interactions *in vivo* (Klein 1984), suggesting that platelet turnover is accelerated by smoking. This increased turnover seems to be greater in atherosclerotic vessels. Thus, increased platelet removal seems to activate megakaryocytes and subsequently is related to an increase in MPV (Fig. 2). Smoking cessation may weaken the platelet-vessel interaction, reduce platelet turnover and subsequently decrease MPV.

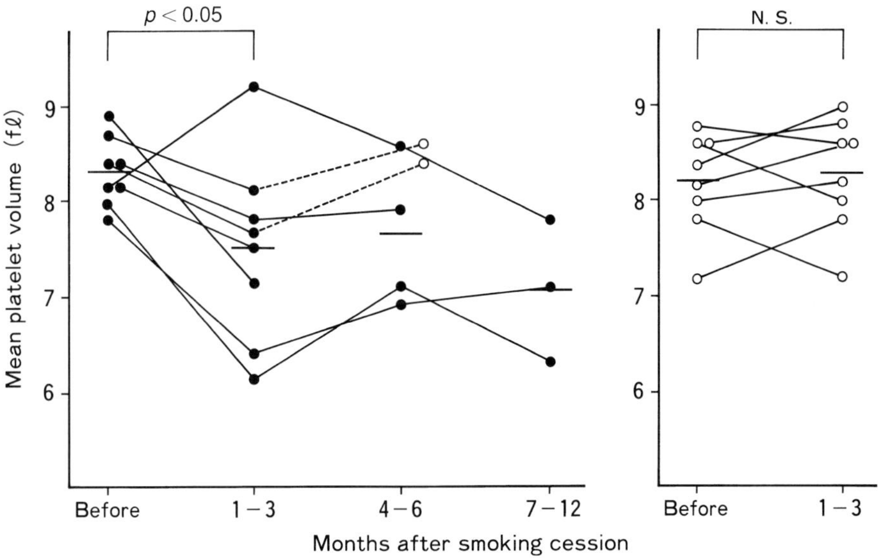

Fig. 1. The changes in mean platelet volume after smoking cessation.
Left: Subjects who stopped smoking. ●, time where stopping smoking was successful; ○, time where smoking was resumed.
Right: Control subjects who did not stop smoking.
The bars show the mean values. * $p < 0.05$, compared with before smoking cessation.

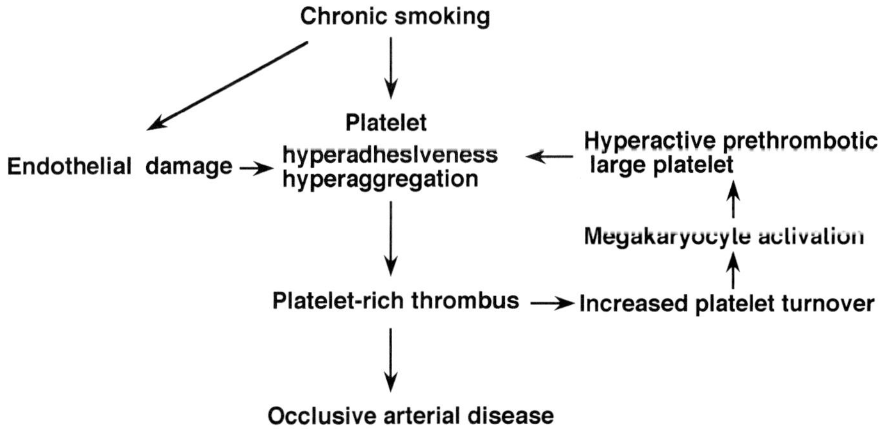

Fig. 2. Adverse platelet cycle produced by chronic smoking.
The appearance of large hyperactive platelets is expressed as an increase in MPV.

During steady-state thrombopoiesis, the platelet count and MPV of circulating platelets have been reported to be inversely correlated so as to maintain a constant plateletcrit (Thompson 1990). Our own research has shown that smoking increases both the platelet count and the MPV, as is also found after the stimulation of thrombopoiesis, and this occurs during periods of increased hemostatic demand. In our study, an inverse relationship between platelet count and MPV was found in each group, with the correlation being highest in the atherosclerotic smokers (Kario *et al* 1992). These results suggest that the simultaneous increase in platelet count and MPV produced by smoking may be related to compensation for increased platelet turnover.

A recent report demonstrated that the larger platelets, produced following platelet destruction by anti-platelet antibodies, are accompanied by an increase in megakaryocyte size and DNA content and that atherosclerosis is accelerated in rabbits fed a cholesterol-rich diet (Kristensen 1990). Thus. the increase in MPV due to smoking may also contribute to the acceleration of atherosclerosis.

SUMMARY

Smoking increases MPV, probably due to increased platelet turnover in atherosclerotic vessels and subsequent activation of megakaryocytes to produce more active larger platelets. Thus, an increase in MPV due to smoking may also contribute to the acceleration of atherosclerosis and should be considered as a risk factor for atherosclerotic disease. This harmful cycle is reversible by smoking cessation.

REFERENCES

Fuster V, Chesebro JH, Frye RL, Elveback LR 1981 Platelet survival and the development of coronary artery disease in the young adult: Effect of cigarette smoking, strong family history and medical therapy. Circulation 63: 546–551

Kario K, Matsuo T, Nakao K 1992 Cigarette smoking increases the mean platelet volume in elderly patients with risk factor for atherosclerosis. Clin Lab Haematol 14: 281–287

Klein LW 1984 Cigarette smoking, atherosclerosis and the coronary hemodynamic response: A unifying hypothesis. J Am Coll Cardiol 4: 972–974

Kristensen SD, Roberts KM, Kishk YT, Martin JF 1990 Accelerated atherogenesis occurs following platelet destruction and increases in megakaryocyte size and DNA content. Eur J Clin Invest 20: 239–247

Martin JF, Bath PMW, Burr ML 1991 Influence of platelet size in outcome after myocardial infarction. Lancet 338: 1409–1411

Thompson CB, Monroy RL, Skelly RR, Quinn PG, Jakubowski JA 1990 The biology of platelet volume heterogeneity. *In*: Martin JF, Trowbridge EA (Eds.) Platelet heterogeneity: Biology and pathology. Springer-Verlag, London, pp 25–35

Trowbridge EA, Slater DN, Kishk YT, Woodcock BW, Martin JF 1984 Platelet production in myocardial infarction and sudden cardiac death. Thromb Haemost 52: 167–171

Multiple Risk Factors in Cardiovascular Disease, ed. by A. Yamamoto, Churchill Livingstone Japan, Tokyo, pp. 259–265 (1994)

THEORY AND PRACTICE OF SMOKING-CESSATION EDUCATION

Edward K. Fujimoto

*Health Education Department, Tokyo Adventist Hospital**

Key words: smoking-cessation, disease intervention, smoking relapse, clinical intervention, behavior change

The risks of premature death and disability associated with smoking have been expressed in a variety of ways but the relative magnitude of risk can be described in stark terms as killing nearly 1 in every 10 persons alive today if current smoking patterns persist (Peto & Lopez 1991). Specifically, analysis of deaths in men in the U.S. show that 92% of all oral and pharyngeal cancers, 81% of laryngeal cancers, 90% of lung cancers, 45% of coronary heart disease and cerebrovascular disease for those under the age of 65, and 84% of chronic obstructive pulmonary disease are attributable to smoking (US DHHS 1989). The mortality costs, increased morbidity and associated costs from increased medical care and lost productivity provide a mandate for a concerted effort to decrease the prevalence of smoking in all populations.

DIRECT INTERVENTION BY SMOKING CONTROL

Smoking control activities — e.g. prevention, cessation, restriction, public and corporate smoking policies, community action, etc. — are direct interventions targeted at the most important source of preventable morbidity and premature mortality. In the 25 years that followed the publication of the landmark U.S. Surgeon General's report *Smoking and Health* in 1964 (US PHS 1964), interventive activities such as these have been credited with the avoidance or postponement of an estimated three-quarters of a million smoking-related deaths in the U.S., plus an additional 2.1 million projected in the 15 year period up to the year 2000 (US DHHS 1989).

UNDERSTANDING SMOKING BEHAVIOR

At the time of the 1964 Surgeon General's report, smoking behavior was understood using a simple 2-stage model — "taking up smoking" and "discontinuation of smoking". The current models involve several stages broadly categorized as development of smoking, habituation, cessation/relapse, with characteristic pharmacological/physiological processes and cognitive changes in each stage (US DHHS 1989). Exploration and initiation occurs during the development stage, usually during adolescence or early adulthood. The initial psychopharmacological effects then facilitate transition from

* 3-7-13 Amanuma, Suginami-ku, Tokyo 167, Japan

experimentation and trial to regular use, and smoking is viewed positively with poor awareness of health consequences and addictive potential. In the habituation stage, conditioned pharmacological effects of nicotine associated with the smoker's environment (e.g. work, stress, relaxation, recreation) become closely tied to smoking behavior, and addiction is developed. Health consequences are depersonalized or minimized, and smoking is viewed positively. During the cessation stage, withdrawal symptoms and conditioned effects of nicotine encourage relapse. There is greater awareness of the effect of smoking on personal health, and the benefits of cessation, and the smoker believes he can stop.

Processes involved in smoking cessation have been further categorized into substages, with one widely accepted model defining these as precontemplation, contemplation, action, maintenance, relapse, and recycling (Fig. 1). In precontemplation the smoker has no intention of stopping and has not yet initiated the processing of smoking-related health information. In the contemplation stage, the smoker has confronted smoking issues and is now thinking about stopping, and is actively processing information on health and how to stop smoking. During the action stage, the smoker is no longer smoking but for a period less than 6 months, while in the maintenance stage, smoking has been discontinued for a longer time. Inability to establish long-term abstinence results in relapse. From the relapse stage the smoker "recycles" to previous stages (US DHHS 1992).

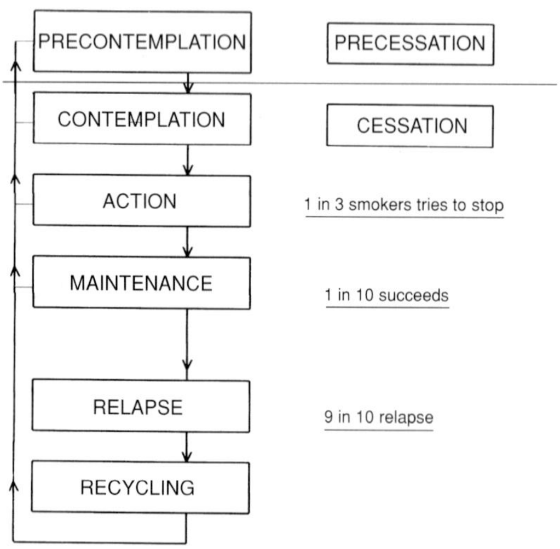

Fig. 1. A smoking cessation model. (Adapted from US DHHS 1989)

CESSATION METHODS

Significant evolution in the understanding of smoking behavior has been paralleled by an equally significant evolution in smoking cessation methodology. Conditioning processes, along with the pharmacological effects of smoking, e.g. addiction, are major factors influencing the act of cessation. Withdrawal symptoms, with both physical and psychological manifestations, e.g. strong urges to smoke, play a major role in early relapse. Attempts to counter these and other problems have generally been the objective of a large number of cessation methods that have been developed. Treatments based on pharmacological effects used for many years, such as herbs, spices (Schwartz 1969), and lobeline sulfate (Dorsey 1936), have been joined by silver acetate-containing chewing gums and sprays that cause a disagreeable taste when smoking (FDA 1982); citric acid sprays; the antihypertensive centrally-acting alpha-adrenergic agonist clonidine (Glassman *et al* 1988); nicotine-replacement methods using polacrilex gum (Lam *et al* 1987), dermal patches (Rose *et al* 1990), nasal drops and aerosols (Jarvis *et al* 1987); mecamylamine, a ganglionic-blocking agent that reduces the reinforcing effects of nicotine (Henningfield *et al* 1982). Some of these and others are still under study. Methods for reducing craving have also been introduced such as stimulus control, which alters situations that trigger smoking; acupuncture; hypnotism; aversion conditioning (e.g. electric shock and rapid smoking); and covert sensitization (unpleasant imagery). Behavior modification methods, professional counseling, avoidance training, and numerous others have been introduced, and some methods have become widely accepted (Hall *et al* 1984; Emmons *et al* 1988; Best & Hakstian 1978).

Relapse — a Universal Problem

A universal problem that has plagued all methods is that high end-of-treatment success rates are not necessarily preserved at one year or even six months post-treatment, with rates of 5 to 40% being typical (US DHHS 1989). Unlike strictly cognitive educational methods, smoking cessation goals are measurable changes in behavior — smoking cessation over a long period of time, typically 1 year — in response to the impact of the cessation methods on the multifactorial elements inherent in smoking — physiological, cognitive, psychological, and behavioral. The striking similarity between the relapse, over time, associated with smoking to that for alcohol and heroin, is due to the similarity or commonality in behavioral and cognitive components and not due to any common addictive agent (Hunt *et al* 1971).

THEORETICAL PROCESSES IN BEHAVIOR CHANGE

The educational process involved in behavior change can be described by a model involving three categories of factors that contribute to the process (Fig. 2): 1) predisposing factors such as knowledge, attitudes, beliefs, values, and perception, that provide the rationale or motivation for behavior; 2) enabling factors antecedent to behavior, such as personal skills and other resources that allow the realization of a motivation; 3) reinforcing factors such as family, significant others, social and work group, that provide continuing rewards, incentives, and disincentives, contributing to the maintenance or termination of a behavior. Initiation of the process starts with the motivation to act, followed by a deployment of supportive resources. Reaction to the behavior by others reinforces that behavior, and also affects the predisposing factors. Enabling factors act similarly in changing predisposing factors. The successful initiation of the behavior also affects the predisposing factors.

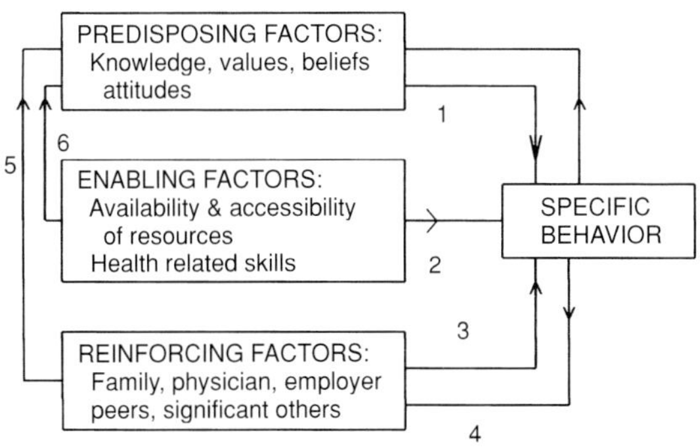

Fig. 2. Major factors which contribute to adoption of health behavior.
Numbers indicate the approximate order of the process. (Adapted from Green *et al* 1980)

Success rate differences in cessation methods appear to be largely due to differences in the program participants rather than the treatment methods themselves (Schwartz 1987). Therefore, while cessation techniques have mostly focused on enabling factors such as skills, more emphasis needs to be placed on methodology that has an impact on the smoker's values, beliefs, and attitudes — predisposing factors necessary for increasing the potential for a successful behavior change.

Locus of Control and Self-efficacy

The importance of this can be understood in terms of two concepts —"health locus of control" and "self-efficacy." The concept of locus of control, introduced by Rotter (1966) to describe how outcome expectations are under one's own control or the control of others, was applied to health by Wallston *et al* (1976). An individual who has an internal locus of control believes that he is responsible for, and has control of, influences on his health. One with an external locus of control, on the other hand, tends to believe that fate, chance, or powerful others determine one's destiny. In general, internally controlled persons are more likely to take control of their own health, seek health information, be informed about their illness, and maintain their well being, and consequently more likely to engage in health promoting activities. The health locus of control of a person appears to have an effect on their ability to adopt and maintain non-smoking behavior (Wallston & Wallston 1978). Persons who have a high level of internal locus of control appear to have greater probability of succeeding compared with persons with a "powerful others" or "fate" locus of control.

Self-efficacy, belief that one can successfully perform a behavior that is necessary to yield a particular outcome, is a concept from social learning theory by Bandura (1977). This concept explains how specific behaviors are adopted by an individual. Belief that one is able to adopt a particular behavior determines whether or not that person will attempt and maintain the behavior change. One's judgment of self-efficacy is a determinant of how much effort to expend and for what duration, and how long one will persist in the face of difficulty and aversive experience. How well a person copes with high-risk smoking situations and successfully survives, is related to his self-efficacy rating. Lack of confidence in one's ability to stop smoking not only deters the initial attempt to stop but, if attempted, the person will slacken efforts or give up altogether when the risk to smoke is encountered (O'Leary 1985).

MANAGEMENT OF RELAPSE

Approximately one-third of smokers attempt to quit each year, but 90% fail (US DHHS 1989). Relapse studies show that primary triggers of relapse include stress, interpersonal conflict, dysphoria, presence of other smokers, and alcohol consumption (Marlatt & Gordon 1980), with consistency in the role of the ability to cope with stress and negative affect (Baer & Lichtenstein 1988; Marlatt & Gordon 1980; Shiffman 1982). Lapses may diminish self-efficacy which may then lead to giving up altogether, the "abstinence violation effect," a cognitive and affective reaction that is a response to violation of an absolute state, that of abstinence (Marlatt & Gordon 1980). This failure, if interpreted as due to a personal shortcoming, diminishes self-efficacy. Changing a person's internality or locus of control, and increasing self-efficacy levels appear to be vital to success in smoking cessation. Changing a person's attitudes and self-perception by cognitive restructuring strategies, equipping the person with required skills for coping, and providing the opportunity to experience the expected change in behavior, directly or vicariously by model observation, strongly influence subsequent self-efficacy levels. Therefore, in any cessation method used, preserving or enhancing both internality and self-efficacy are vitally important. This is especially important in the case of the more than half of the participants in smoking cessation activities who relapse. Clearly these persons should be retained in the smoking cessation cycle. Each group that passes through the cycle yields successful non-smokers. With each recycling of a potential non-smoker, proper methods should increase his internality and self-efficacy to increase his potential for success.

CLINICAL INTERVENTION BY THE PHYSICIAN

It is estimated that 90% of those that succeed in stopping smoking do so on their own without recourse to formal programs (Fiore *et al* 1990). Therefore only 0.3% of all smokers attempt and succeed in smoking cessation as a result of a program. Triggering the smoking cessation process in a patient can be a highly significant function of personal physicians (Russell *et al* 1979; Kottke *et al* 1989; Wilson *et al* 1988). Ockene (1987) reports estimates that physicians have contact with at least 70% of all smokers each year. It is important that smokers hear very clearly and repeatedly from their physician that smoking is hazardous and that stopping is possible and of great benefit. Synergism of the clinical intervention with other smoking control activities, and the clear expression by the physician that non-smoking behavior is the social norm, can provide a highly effective source of support for patients entering the smoking cessation cycle. Contracting on a start date and on the target behavior, providing advice on stimulus control, urge management, stress management, and other techniques to avoid relapses, are valuable actions that the physician can take. Nicotine replacement aids, used judiciously, are helpful and will benefit if internality of locus of control and self-efficacy levels are enhanced. If the patient's efforts to stop smoking are diminished because of a perception of being a passive recipient of treatment, with the possibility of fall-back on pharmacological aids such as nicotine, long-term cessation or maintenance may be difficult. A program format having a periodic cycle of repeating may be more effective than a one-time campaign, since it provides support during the maintenance stage and manages recycling of recidivists.

CONCLUSION

While long-term maintenance of non-smoking behavior remains the greatest challenge, smoking cessation, as an interventive activity for cardiovascular disease, in synergism with current changes in society and individual norms regarding smoking, is unquestionably one of the most promising objectives.

SUMMARY

The acquisition of smoking behavior involves several stages of behavioral, pharmacological, physiological, and cognitive changes which develop into habituation with characteristic dependence and addiction to nicotine. The morbidity and mortality consequences of smoking are preventable by avoiding this behavior. Education in avoidance of this behavior is obviously of great benefit but, for those who are already smoking, the mandate is much more difficult to achieve due to high relapse rates in smoking cessation. Of those who attempt to stop only about 10% succeed. An estimated 90% of those who successfully stop do so outside of any formal programmed approach and few succeed after a single attempt. Various methods to counter the physical and psychological symptoms of withdrawal from nicotine, such as nicotine replacement, behavioral techniques, conditioning, etc., have been introduced to reduce early relapse and increase long-term cessation. These and approaches that impact factors that intervene in the process of behavior change, and that properly manage relapse, may increase the probability of success in stopping for an individual. A vital role which the personal physician can and should perform is to introduce smokers to the smoking cessation cycle. The smoker needs to consider stopping and the stimulus that triggers the process that develops into cessation may be the physician. Effective smoking cessation methods will improve the success of direct intervention in what is the most important cause of premature morbidity, mortality and disability.

REFERENCES

Baer JS, Lichtenstein E 1988 Classification and prediction of smoking relapse episodes: An exploration of differences. J Consult Clin Psychol 56: 104–110

Bandura A 1977 Self-efficacy: Toward a unifying theory of behavioral change. Psychol Rev 84: 191–215

Best JA, Hakstian AR 1978 A situation-specific model for smoking behavior. Addict Behav 3: 79–92

Dorsey JL 1936 Control of the tobacco habit. Ann Intern Med 10: 628–631

Emmons KM, Emont SL, Collins RL, Weidner G 1988 Relapse prevention versus broad spectrum treatment for smoking cessation: A comparison of efficacy. J Subst Abuse 1: 79–89

Fiore MC, Novotny T, Pierce J *et al* 1990 Methods used to quit smoking in the united states. Do cessation programs help? JAMA 263: 2760–2765

Food and Drug Administration 1982 Smoking deterrent drug products for over-the-counter human use: Fed Regist 47: 490–500

Glassman AH, Stetner F, Walsh T *et al 1988* Heavy smokers, smoking cessation, and clonidine: Results of a double-blind randomized trial. JAMA 259: 2863–2866

Green LW, Kreuter MW, Deeds SG, Partridge KB 1980 Health Education Planning — A Diagnostic Approach. Mayfield Publishing, Palo Alto, CA

Hall SM, Rugg D, Tunstall C, Jones R 1984 Preventing relapse to cigarette smoking by behavioral skill training. J Consult Clin Psychol 52: 372–382

Henningfield JE, Miyasato K, Johnson RE, Jasinski DR 1982 Rapid physiologic effects of nicotine in humans and selective blockade of behavioral effects by mecamylamine. *In*: Harris LS (Ed) Problems of drug dependance. National Institute on Drug Abuse Research Monograph Series 43. Government Printing Office. DHHS Publ No.(ADM) 83-1264: 259–265

Hunt WA, Barnett LW, Branch LG 1971 Relapse rates in addiction programs. J Clin Psychol 27: 455–456

Jarvis MJ, Hajek P, Russell MA, West RJ, Feyerabend C 1987 Nasal nicotine solution as an aid to cigarette withdrawal: a pilot clinical trial. Br J Addict 82: 983–988

Kottke TE, Brekke ML, Solberg LI, Hughes MR 1989 A Randomized Trial to Increase Smoking Intervention by Physicians: Doctors Helping Smokers Round I. JAMA 260: 2101–2106

Lam W, See PC, Sacks HS, Chalmers TC 1987 Metanalysis of randomized controlled trials of nicotine chewing gum. Lancet 2: 27–30

Marlatt GA, Gordon JR 1980 Determinants of relapse: Implications for the maintenance of behavior change. *In*: Davidson PO, Davidson SM (Eds) Behavioral medicine: Changing health lifestyles. Brunner / Mazel, New York, pp 410–452

Ockene JK 1987 Physician-delivered intervention for smoking cessation: Strategies for increasing effectiveness. Prevent Med 16: 723–737

O'Leary A 1985 Self-efficacy and Health. Behav Res Ther 23: 437–451

Peto R, Lopez AD 1991 Worldwide mortality from current smoking patterns *In*: Durston B, Jamrozik K (Eds) Tobacco and health 1990: The global war. Health Department of Western Australia, pp 66–68

Rose JE, Levin ED, Behm FM *et al* 1990 Transdermal nicotine facilitates smoking cessation. Clin Pharmacol Ther 47: 323–330

Rotter JB 1966 Generalized expectancies for internal versus external control of reinforcement. Psychology Monograph: General and Applied 80: p 1

Russell MAH, Wilson C, Taylor C, Baker CD 1979 Effect of general practitioners' advice against smoking. BMJ 6184: 231–235

Schwartz JL 1969 A critical review and evaluation of smoking cessation methods. Publ Health Rep 84: 483–506

Schwartz JL 1987 Review and evaluation of smoking cessation methods: United States and Canada, 1978–1985. US Department of Health and Human Services, Public Health Services, National Institutes of Health. NIH Publ No.87–2940

Shiffman S 1982 Relapse following smoking cessation: A situational analysis. J Consult Clin Psychol 50: 71–86

US Department of Health and Human Services 1989 Reducing the Health Consequences of Smoking: 25 Years of Progress. A Report of the Surgeon General U.S. Department of Health and Human Services, Public Health Services, Centers for Disease Control, Office on Smoking and Health. DHHS Publ No.(CDC) 89-8411

US Department of Health and Human Services 1992 Smoking and Tobacco Control Monograph No.1. US Department of Health and Human Services, National Institutes of Health, National Cancer Institute

US Public Health Service 1964 Smoking and Health. Report of the Advisory Committee to the Surgeon General of the Public Health Service. U.S. Department of Health Education and Welfare, Public Health Service, Center for Disease Control. PHS Publ No. 1103

Wallston BS, Wallston KA 1978 Locus of Control and Health: A Review of Literature. Health Educ Monogr 6: 107–117

Wallston BS, Wallston KA, Kaplan GD, Maides SA 1976 Development and validation of the Health Locus of Control (HLC) Scale. J Consulti Clin Psychol 44: 580–585

Wilson DM, Taylor DW, Gilbert JR *et al* 1988 A Randomized Trial of a Family Physician Intervention for Smoking Cessation. JAMA 260: 1570–1574

Multiple Risk Factors in Cardiovascular Disease, ed. by A. Yamamoto, Churchill Livingstone Japan, Tokyo, pp. 267–271 (1994)

TOBACCO CONTROL: EDUCATION IS NOT ENOUGH

Andrew PIPE

*Department of Family Medicine & University of Ottawa Heart Institute, Ottawa Civic Hospital**

Key words: tobacco control, tobacco addiction, nicotine, nicotine replacement therapy, tobacco advertising, smoking cessation

Tobacco addiction is a principal risk factor for the development of coronary heart disease and for atherosclerotic diseases in general. Tobacco's deadly role in the development of cardiovascular disease processes occurs as a consequence of its ability to damage vessel walls, promote smooth muscle cell proliferation, initiate the development of atherosclerosis, activate platelets, and increase the plasma viscosity and levels of fibrinogen and factor VII. Cigarette smoke serves to increase the heart rate, blood pressure, peripheral resistance, and myocardial oxygen demand at the same time as it lowers the threshold for ventricular fibrillation, impairs coronary artery autoregulation and potentiates arrhythmia development (McBride 1992). Not surprisingly, the United States Office of Technology Assessment calculates that one fifth of cardiovascular disease deaths in 1990 were attributable to smoking. Notwithstanding the abundant clinical and pathological evidence that identifies the important role that tobacco plays in the etiology of cardiovascular disease, attempts to deal with the public health hazard represented by tobacco consumption have traditionally relied solely on initiatives to 'educate' the public about the hazards represented by smoking. Such efforts while a *necessary* component of any attempt to deal intelligently with the leading cause of preventable disease, disability and death in the developed world, are not *sufficient*. They are, sadly, usually overshadowed by the lavishly financed advertising and sponsorship activities of the tobacco industry: an industry which is malevolent in its denial of the health consequences of tobacco consumption, obdurate in its attempts to evade all forms of regulation and control and almost unequaled in its power and wealth.

There is no greater challenge in the prevention of cardiovascular disease than to develop public health strategies designed to control the availability of tobacco, eliminate all forms of tobacco advertising and sponsorship, prevent children from becoming smokers, assist those already addicted to nicotine, and accelerate the development of an environment in which smoking is seen as socially unacceptable behavior. As smoking rates decline in the western world there is an added challenge: ensuring that the nations of Asia and those in the developing world, which have been targeted by the transnational tobacco companies as the customers

* 1053 Carling Ave., Ottawa, Ont K1Y 4E9, CANADA.

— and victims — of tomorrow, are appropriately protected from a burgeoning epidemic of tobacco-caused disease. The challenges will only be met by the implementation of strategies which are comprehensive, consistent and concerted. Central to their success is the development of appropriate 'healthy public policies.' To this end it is important that all health professionals recognize their particular responsibilities to act as advocates for the development of such policies. The German pathologist Rudolf Virchow once observed that 'there are two causes of disease; one is pathological, the other is political.' Political indifference to the necessity for appropriate tobacco control is a malady that merits our professional concern!

RESPONSIBILITIES OF HEALTH PROFESSIONALS

Physicians and other health professionals are uniquely placed to influence the smoking behavior of their patients. Surprisingly, many smokers have reported that they have never been advised by their physicians to stop smoking. The smoking status of all patients should be determined at the time of any clinical encounter and smokers can be advised in an unambiguous, non-judgmental way that it is in the best interests of their health for them to stop smoking. Given the highly addictive nature of nicotine such advice is appropriately accompanied by an offer to be of assistance in the process of smoking cessation. Many physicians feel a sense of frustration and helplessness in trying to help would-be non-smokers. Almost all practitioners understand the need for the identification and continued follow-up of those with hypertension or hyperlipidemia, but many fail to understand that exactly the same principles apply to helping those addicted to nicotine. Quitting smoking is a process, not a single-step phenomenon. The advent of nicotine replacement therapy (NRT) using chewing-gum, or more commonly, a nicotine-containing skin patch provides physicians with the opportunity to offer very effective assistance to those wishing to become non-smokers (Hurt *et al* 1994). All physicians, and particularly those involved in the treatment of cardiovascular disease, should become familiar with the use of such approaches.

In recent years the incidence of smoking among health professionals has declined significantly in many nations. However, in some countries, notably Japan and Spain, this has not been the case and rates of smoking by medical practitioners are unaccountably high (Audet 1994). Physicians can exercise implicit leadership in the battle against the tobacco-related diseases by becoming non-smokers and by ensuring that their offices and hospitals become smoke-free environments.

THE PROTECTION OF MINORS

Just as it is important to assist smokers in quitting it is equally important to ensure that, as far as possible, young people do not start smoking. There is considerable evidence that most smokers start tobacco use at an early age and quickly become addicted before any appreciation of the health consequences develop. Thus, any strategy to delay or prevent the onset of smoking behavior will have a significant effect on adult smoking rates and the predictable development of the health consequences of tobacco use. Health professionals may wish to use 'anticipatory guidance' in discussing the desirability of a non-smoking lifestyle in all their encounters with young non-smokers; it is equally important to advise all young smokers, with particular sensitivity, of the advantages of smoking cessation.

The most successful approaches to the prevention of smoking by the young will take the form of strategies applied at community level. Children are the particular targets of tobacco company advertising (Pierce *et al* 1994); the elimination of all forms of tobacco advertising and sponsorship should be viewed as a central component of any public health strategy designed to address the prevention of the tobacco-related diseases. School-based programs which emphasize the development of skills to resist the influences of peer pressure and 'lifestyle' advertising will equip youngsters with important lifeskills. The prevention of tobacco sales to minors via regulations which establish the age of majority as a criterion for tobacco purchase, mandate the licensing of all tobacco retailers, eliminate all tobacco vending machines and provide for realistic sanctions in the case of violations of such regulations will do much to limit the availability of tobacco to the young. Young people are particularly sensitive to changes in the price of tobacco and the most effective strategy in deterring smoking by the young is to ensure that tobacco products are appropriately taxed (see below). The challenge of preventing tobacco use among the young is the focus of the most recent report of the US Surgeon General (1994).

APPROPRIATE TOBACCO PRICING POLICIES

The relationship between price and the demand for consumer products exists for tobacco although it is blunted by the fact that smokers are addicted to nicotine. It is generally accepted that the price-elasticity for tobacco products is –0.4 (i.e. a 10% increase in price will result in a 4% decline in consumption); adolescents would appear to be more sensitive to tobacco price increases, presumably because they have less disposable income. Between 1980 and 1990 tobacco taxes increased eight-fold in Canada; such tax increases were felt to be instrumental in reducing adult tobacco consumption by 35% and teenage consumption by 62% (Sweanor 1992). It is unlikely that any other single strategy will be as effective in a) reducing the demand for tobacco and b) preventing the onset of smoking behavior among the young.

The development of such taxation policy is not easy given the formidable political influence wielded by the tobacco industry. But at a time when governments everywhere are concerned about rising health costs, a significant component of which are the costs associated with cardiovascular and other tobacco-caused diseases, the effectiveness of such policies will continue to attract more and more interest.

As an unfortunate measure of the influence of the tobacco industry's political influence it is sad to observe that the Canadian government has recently announced a reduction of tobacco taxes in response to what has officially been described as a concern about the problem of tobacco smuggling — a problem accentuated by the actions of the Canadian tobacco industry.

THE ELIMINATION OF TOBACCO ADVERTISING

Tobacco advertising might be considered the 'vector' by which the tobacco diseases are 'spread'. Despite strenuous denials by the tobacco industry advertising strategies have been specifically targeted at recruiting the young, women, and the citizens of Asia and the developing world as customers to replace those who are now dying as a consequence of the consumption of tobacco products. Advertising aimed at children seeks to portray smoking as a pleasurable, fashionable behavior common to successful, accomplished and sophisticated adults. Images of sporting and risk-taking behavior are particularly aimed at young males; young females see and hear messages relating to slimness, fashion and emancipated behavior. Advertising in Asia and the developing world suggests that smoking is the normal pursuit of affluent, educated and refined westerners or the typical behavior of that quintessential American icon — the cowboy. Given what is known today of the consequences of tobacco addiction such images represent a gross, cynical, and calculating distortion of the truth.

Advertising exists not only to sell tobacco products but also to establish a backdrop of social acceptability for smoking. Advertising also buys silence. Periodicals that carry tobacco advertisements are far less likely to jeopardize this advertising revenue by publishing articles on the health consequences of smoking (Warner *et al* 1992). Legislation banning such advertising was introduced in Canada in 1989; tobacco companies have, predictably, been cunning in the ways in which they have circumvented such regulations by creating "phantom corporations" and sponsoring all manner of sporting and cultural events in the name of such enterprises. In other jurisdictions the association of tobacco trademarks with a wide range of consumer goods, sporting and entertainment events has, regrettably, been commonplace. Any comprehensive strategy to deal with tobacco must include the elimination of tobacco advertising in all its forms.

SMOKE-FREE ENVIRONMENTS

The development of public policies designed to protect individuals from the risks of involuntary exposure to tobacco smoke has had a far broader impact. They have altered public perceptions regarding the social acceptability of smoking and made a non-smoking environment the norm in many communities. The public has come to accept, to appreciate and value, and to seek the clean air now to be found in many workplaces, health care and educational facilities, public transport, shopping centers, and other public spaces. Such initiatives are often best developed at the local level; impetus and support for their introduction can often be provided by the advocacy of health care professionals.

SUMMARY

To be successful modern approaches to the health problems posed by tobacco addiction must involve far more than *education* about the health consequences of smoking. Given the major role that tobacco addiction plays in the development of cardiovascular disease, physicians must be as committed to assisting their patients with smoking cessation as they are to the identification and management of hypertension and hyperlipidemic conditions. The creation of a social environment in which non-smoking is seen as the norm, in which the healthy choices are the easy choices, will require the development of comprehensive, consistent and community-based strategies. Health professionals must recognize the need for, and support the development of, public health policies which treat tobacco control realistically and in a manner consistent with tobacco's role as the leading cause of preventable disease, death and disability in developed societies. The influence, wealth and power of the tobacco industry must be recognized and countered.

'The public interest' observed the British parliamentarian, Edmund Burke, 'requires doing today those things that men of intelligence and goodwill would wish, five or ten years hence, had been done.' He might well have been thinking of tobacco control.

REFERENCES

Audet A 1994 When it comes to smoking, Japanese MD's do not set a good example for their patients. Can Med Assoc J 150: 1673–1674.

Hurt RD, Dale LC, Frederikson PA *et al* 1994 Nicotine patch therapy for smoking cessation combined with physician advice and nurse follow-up: One year outcome and percentage of nicotine replacement. JAMA 271: 595–600

McBride PE 1992 The health consequences of smoking: Cardiovascular diseases. *In*: Fiore MC (Ed) The Medical Clinics of North America. Cigarette smoking: A clinical guide to assessment and treatment. 76: 333–353

Pierce JP, Lee L, Gilpin EA 1994 Smoking initiation by adolescent girls, 1994 through 1988: An association with targeted advertising. JAMA 271: 608–611

Sweanor D 1992 Canada's tobacco tax policies: successes and challenges. Non-Smokers' Rights Association. Ontario (Canada)

US Dept of Health and Human Services 1994 Preventing tobacco use among young people: a report of the Surgeon General. US Dept of Health and Human Services, Public Health Service, Centers for Disease Control and Prevention, National Center for Chronic Disease Prevention and Health Promotion, Office on Smoking and Health. Atlanta

Warner KE, Goldenhar LM, Mclaughlin CG 1992. Cigarette advertising and magazine coverage of the hazards of smoking: a statistical analysis. N Engl J Med 32b: 305–309

SUBJECT INDEX